Clinics in Developmental Medicine No. 155
SLEEP DISTURBANCE IN CHILDREN
AND ADOLESCENTS WITH DISORDERS
OF DEVELOPMENT: ITS SIGNIFICANCE
AND MANAGEMENT

© 2001 Mac Keith Press

High Holborn House, 52–54 High Holborn, London WC1V 6RL

Senior Editor: Martin C.O. Bax
Editor: Hilary M. Hart
Managing Editor: Michael Pountney
Sub Editor: Pat Chappelle

First published in this edition 2001

British Library Cataloguing-in-Publication data:
A catalogue record for this book is available from the British Library

ISSN: 0069 4835
ISBN: 1 898683 24 7

Printed by The Lavenham Press Ltd, Water Street, Lavenham, Suffolk
Mac Keith Press is supported by Scope

Clinics in Developmental Medicine No. 155

Sleep Disturbance in Children and Adolescents with Disorders of Development: its Significance and Management

Edited by

GREGORY STORES
LUCI WIGGS

Department of Psychiatry
University of Oxford
Oxford, England

2001
Mac Keith Press

Distributed by 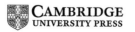 **CAMBRIDGE**
UNIVERSITY PRESS

CONTENTS

AUTHORS' APPOINTMENTS

Martin Bax, DM	Emeritus Reader in Paediatrics, Imperial College of Medicine, Department of Child Health, Chelsea and Westminster Hospital, London, England
Robert Beckerman, MD	Professor and Chief, Section of Pediatric Pulmonology, Department of Pediatrics, Tulane Hospital for Children, New Orleans, LA, USA
Georges Casimir, MD	Professor and Head of Paediatric Pneumology, University Hospital for Children, Free University of Brussels, Belgium
Gillian Colville, MPhil, CPsychol	Consultant Clinical Psychologist *and* Head of Paediatric Psychology Service, St George's Hospital, London, England
Penny Corkum, PhD	Assistant Professor, School Psychology Program, Department of Education, Mount Saint Vincent University, Halifax, Nova Scotia; *and* Co-director, Colchester East Hants Attention Deficit Hyperactivity Disorder Clinic, Truro, NS, Canada
Paolo Curatolo, MD	Professor and Head of Child Neurology and Psychiatry, University of Rome Tor Vergata, Rome, Italy
Ronald E. Dahl, MD	Associate Professor of Psychiatry and Pediatrics, University of Pittsburgh Medical Center, Pittsburgh, PA, USA

Bernard Dan, MD

Professor and Head of Paediatric Neurology, University Hospital for Children, Free University of Brussels, Belgium

Jean Duchâteau, MD

Professor and Head of Immunology Research Laboratory, University Hospital for Children, Free University of Brussels, Belgium

E. Jane Garland, MD, FRCPC

Clinical Associate Professor, University of British Columbia; and Director, Mood and Anxiety Disorders Clinic, Department of Psychiatry, British Columbia's Children's and Women's Health Center, Vancouver, BC, Canada

José Groswasser, MD

Head of Paediatric Sleep Laboratory, University Hospital for Children, Free University of Brussels, Belgium

André Kahn, MD, PhD

Professor and Chairman of Paediatrics, University Children's Hospital, Free University of Brussels, Belgium

Suresh Kotagal, MD

Senior Associate Consultant, Sleep Disorders Center, and Chair, Division of Child and Adolescent Neurology, Mayo Clinic, Rochester, MN, USA

Daniel S. Lewin, PhD

Post Doctoral Fellow in Child and Adolescent Psychiatry, University of Pittsburgh Medical School, The Western Psychiatric Institute and Clinic, Pittsburgh, PA, USA

Gerald M. Loughlin, MD

Professor of Pediatrics and Director of Eudowood Division of Pediatric Respiratory Sciences, The Johns Hopkins University School of Medicine, Baltimore, MD, USA

Marie José Mozin

Research Fellow, University Hospital for Children, Free University of Brussels, Belgium

Jesús Oliván-Palacios, MD

Staff Clinical Neurophysiologist, Clinical Neurophysiological Unit, Hospital Carlos III, Madrid, Spain

Cathleen C. Piazza, PhD

Director of Training, Marcus and Kennedy Krieger Institutes (Atlanta, GA, and Baltimore, MD); *and* Associate Professor, Department of Psychiatry, Johns Hopkins University School of Medicine, Baltimore, MD, USA

Amanda Richdale, PhD, MAPS

Senior Lecturer in Psychology, Department of Psychology and Disability Studies, RMIT University, Melbourne, Australia

Henry Roane, PhD

Instructor in Pediatrics, Division of Developmental Pediatrics, Emory University School of Medicine; *and* Case Manager, The Marcus Institute, Altanta, GA, USA

Avi Sadeh, PhD, ClinPsychol

Director, Laboratory for Children's Sleep Disorders, Department of Psychology, Tel Aviv University, Israel

Sonia Scaillet, MD

Research Fellow, University Hospital for Children, Free University of Brussels, Belgium

Stefano Seri, MD	Director, Neurosciences Programme, Birmingham Children's Hospital; *and* Honorary Senior Lecturer, University of Birmingham, Birmingham, England
Narong Simakajornboon, MD	Assistant Professor of Pediatrics, Pediatric Pulmonology and Sleep Medicine, Department of Pediatrics, Tulane University School of Medicine, New Orleans, LA, USA
Martine Sottiaux	Research Fellow, Paediatric Sleep Laboratory, University Hospital for Children, Free University of Brussels, Belgium
Gregory Stores, MA, MD, FRCP, FRCPsych	Professor of Developmental Neuropsychiatry, University of Oxford Department of Psychiatry (Child and Adolescent Section), Oxford, England
Rebecca Stores, PhD, CPsychol	Research Psychologist, University of Oxford Department of Psychiatry (Child and Adolescent Section), Oxford, England
Antonio Vela-Bueno, MD	Professor, Department of Psychiatry, Universidad Autónoma, Madrid, Spain
Alexandros N. Vgontzas, MD	Professor, A. Kales Endowed Chair in Sleep Medicine, and Director, Center for Sleep Disorders Medicine, Pennsylvania State University, Hershey, PA, USA
Luci Wiggs, DPhil, CPsychol	Research Psychologist, University of Oxford Department of Psychiatry (Child and Adolescent Section), Oxford, England

PREFACE:
HOW TO USE THIS BOOK

Section One of this book contains general information about sleep patterns in children and adolescents and an overview of the various sleep disorders from which they may suffer. It also discusses management issues, directing the reader to further reading where appropriate.

In the subsequent Sections Two to Five inclusive, sleep patterns associated with specific neurodevelopmental, neurological, paediatric and psychiatric disorders are described. To avoid repetition, general descriptions of sleep disorders and their treatment are not provided in each of these chapters as it is assumed that the reader has read the introductory section of the book. Aspects of sleep specific to the condition under consideration will, however, be highlighted.

It is therefore recommended that readers familiarize themselves with the contents of the first section of this book before reading any of the later chapters.

SECTION ONE

GENERAL ISSUES

1

SLEEP DISTURBANCE: A SERIOUS, WIDESPREAD, YET NEGLECTED PROBLEM IN DISORDERS OF DEVELOPMENT

Gregory Stores and Luci Wiggs

A neglected topic

The issue of sleep disturbance presents a curious paradox. There is ample evidence (Partinen and Hublin 2000) that, at all ages, sleep disturbance is very common in the general population. Also, the finding from both clinical observation and experimental work that such disturbance often has serious effects is compelling (Bonnet 2000). Not only is disturbed sleep distressing at the time that is occurs; if persistent it commonly causes much personal, educational, occupational and other social disadvantage and sometimes adverse physical effects with a huge overall cost to the national economy (National Commission on Sleep Disorders Research 1993, 1994).

And yet, the subject of sleep and its disorders usually features very little (if at all) in medical and other professional healthcare teaching and training, including that concerning children whose sleep problems are a cause of much concern to their families. UK medical students receive an average of only five minutes of formal teaching on the topic out of their typical five-year course (Stores and Crawford 1998), and there are no signs that this shortcoming is corrected at postgraduate level, even in specialties where sleep problems can be expected to be commonly encountered such as paediatrics (Royal College of Paediatrics and Child Health 1996). Nurses and psychologists generally fare no better (Cohen *et al.* 1992, Wiggs and Stores R 1996, Stores R and Wiggs 1998), despite the important role they can play in the assessment and treatment of many sleep disorders. Although some health visitors have taken the initiative and established sleep clinics for young children, there are very few centres providing clinical services across the whole range of children's sleep disorders. Where such a service is available, its effectiveness may well be restricted (at least for long-distance referrals) without the maintenance of a higher standard in the child's own locality of service provision and a commitment to the treatment recommendations made by the sleep disorders service (Stores G and Wiggs 1998).

Sleep disturbance in developmental disorders

These shortcomings are serious enough for the population at large, but much worse for children with disorders of development of a physical or psychiatric nature, in whom sleep problems

3

seem to be particularly common. Because of the neglect of the topic, accurate figures on the prevalence of sleep disturbance in childhood developmental disorders are not available. Whatever the precise proportions, however, it is very likely that the majority of such children and their families are affected because their condition or associated factors predispose them to sleep loss or disruption.

Predisposing factors in the child can be physical, psychological, or a combination of the two. A prime example of *physical predisposition* is the respiratory dysfunction seen in many neurodevelopmental disorders. As will be evident from later chapters, upper airway obstruction during sleep (Chapter 5) is widely distributed in such conditions as Down syndrome, the mucopolysaccharidoses, neuromuscular disorders and craniofacial syndromes. Similarly, epilepsy commonly accompanies many neurodevelopmental disorders and may contribute to sleep disruption, as discussed in Chapter 15. Other physical complications or accompaniments of certain disorders of this type that are likely to affect sleep include immobility or discomfort at night.

Developmental disorders of neurological or other physical origin are often complicated by *psychological disturbance* (Graham *et al*. 1999). The many reasons for this include direct influences of neurological dysfunction on learning and behaviour, the limitations and frustrations imposed on the child by his disability, and the effects of the disability on the family. The main types of psychological disturbance arising in these ways are difficult and antisocial behaviour, including conduct disorder and overactivity, and emotional problems such as anxiety and depression. As also discussed in the later chapters, sleep disturbance is a common feature of these forms of psychiatric disorder.

A potent way in which children with developmental problems are prone to sleep disturbance is the likely effects of the child's condition on his parents' attitudes, parenting ability and overall well-being. Once established, the child's sleep disturbance itself may add to the parents' difficulties in these respects. Depending on the nature and severity of the child's basic disorder (and their own temperament, personality and resilience), parents may be resourceful and effective or they may be overpermissive and inconsistent in their handling of the child, especially if they are themselves chronically anxious or depressed (Armstrong *et al*. 1998). This risk increases in the presence of family discord or disunity.

Developmental effects of sleep disturbance

The point has already been made that persistent sleep disturbance can have widespread and serious effects on the individual at any age. Conceivably, the adverse effects are most significant in young people, and possibly more so in children whose development is compromised in other ways.

Animal experiments have shown that total sleep loss for long periods is incompatible with survival. Fortunately there is no counterpart to this in normal human existence, but partial sleep deprivation seems to be very common in the population as a whole, especially in particular subgroups including those engaged in certain occupations, notably shiftworkers and junior doctors! Parents of sleepless children are another high-risk group. In the USA in particular, the term 'national sleep debt' is used to describe this supposedly endemic problem of inadequate sleep with its associated health risks.

Much of the experimental and clinical evidence that persistent sleep loss or disruption causes serious effects is based on adult studies and reports, but there is increasing evidence of adverse influences on various aspects of development in children.

COGNITIVE FUNCTION AND EDUCATIONAL PERFORMANCE

The potential seriousness of cognitive effects can be judged from adult studies showing the influence of sleep deprivation on memory, attention and visuospatial abilities, especially sustained attention, and possibly creative thinking. It has been calculated that the average level of functioning of sleep-deprived adults is equivalent to only the ninth percentile of non-sleep-deprived subjects (Pilcher and Huffcutt 1996). Impaired performance and accidents are described in the various occupational groups prone to sleep disturbance.

Comparable effects of experimental sleep deprivation in children (obviously limited by ethical considerations) on aspects of cognitive function have been reported, and there are consistent reports that sleep loss in children and adolescents is associated with daytime sleepiness and impaired performance at school (Wolfson and Carskadon 1998, Meijer *et al.* 2000). In keeping with adult studies, sleep-related breathing difficulties associated with impairment of sleep quality have been linked with impaired cognitive and academic performance (as well as other psychological deficits) in children with obstructive sleep apnoea (Gozal 1998) and asthma (Stores *et al.* 1998).

MOOD AND BEHAVIOUR

Pilcher and Huffcutt's (1996) meta-analysis indicated that mood may well be particularly affected by sleep deprivation. The main general effects reported in adults of irritability, aggression and depressed mood are paralleled by reports that attention deficit hyperactivity disorder (ADHD) symptoms and various other behavioural problems are commonly associated with sleep loss or disruption in children (Chapter 26).

Children may also show emotional and behavioural problems because they are distressed about their sleep, because of confrontation with their parents, or from fear or embarrassment about their sleep disorder. The emotional climate may well be affected within the family as a whole. This risk is increased if parents disagree about the nature or management of the problem, if the diagnosis is delayed, or if the advice given is inappropriate.

The consequences for *parenting* can be very serious. Quine (1992) has described mothers of children with an intellectual impairment and severe sleep problems as more irritable and concerned about their own health, and less affectionate towards their children (with greater use of physical punishment) than mothers of such children without sleep problems. It has also been suggested that marital discord and separation (and even physical abuse of children) can result from children's sleep problems (Chavin and Tinson 1980). Successful treatment of the sleep disorder can improve parental functioning and well-being (Wolfson *et al.* 1992, Minde *et al.* 1994).

PHYSICAL DEVELOPMENT

In certain circumstances, the adverse effects of chronic sleep disturbance can extend to physical processes. Impairment of growth and failure to thrive are known to be associated with early

onset obstructive sleep apnoea (Carroll and Loughlin 1995); and growth hormone deficiency, linked to abnormal sleep physiology, has been suggested as the cause of 'psychosocial dwarfism'. Also, there is increasing interest in the possible physical and psychological effects of immune system dysfunction associated with sleep disturbance (Moldofsky and Dickstein 1999).

Improving the care of children with sleep disorders
Given the harmful effects on development, early recognition of sleep problems is important, followed by effective treatment. Ideally, such problems would be prevented in the first place. At present, the help provided is generally inadequate even when sleep problems are particularly serious as in children with severe intellectual impairment (Wiggs and Stores G 1996).

To improve matters, the first requirement is for both the public and professionals to become more aware that sleep problems are common, their effects are potentially harmful in various ways, and for the most part (providing treatment is chosen on the basis of accurate diagnosis) they are treatable. Some parents show limited interest when offered help even when their child's sleep problems are severe. Reasons for this include the mistaken belief that the problems are an inevitable and untreatable accompaniment to intellectual impairment. Alternatively, parents may be disenchanted by previous treatments that have been inappropriately chosen or performed. Reassurance that appropriate and properly conducted treatment programmes are likely to be effective will be needed in these circumstances. Attitudes to the child may be improved in the process, as well as objective aspects of the child's sleep patterns (Wiggs and Stores 1998).

There is no point in raising expectations if no adequate service is available, although it can be argued that services will not improve until a demand for better provision is felt. Either way, there is every reason to raise professional knowledge and expertise concerning sleep disorders and their management by better teaching and training at undergraduate and postgraduate levels. The European Sleep Research Society is currently in the process of assessing how this might be done. Similar moves have been made in the USA.

Appropriate sources of information are, of course, essential for the success of these enterprises. Although much research is still needed on even fundamental aspects of children's sleep disorders, a considerable amount is already known that could improve the care of affected children if translated into clinical practice. This large body of knowledge about 'sleep disorders medicine' is contained in a number of recent publications such as the specialist textbook by Kryger *et al.* (2000) concerning sleep disorders in adults and its companion volume about children by Ferber and Kryger (1995); the comprehensive coverage of sleep-related breathing disorders in children by Loughlin *et al.* (2000); and the guidebook for clinicians by Stores (2001). *Especially in relation to Section One, the reader is referred to these sources for detailed referencing.* Practical guidelines for parents are also available (Ferber 1985, Quine 1997, Durand 1998).

Although the sleep problems and disorders of children with developmental disorders receive some coverage in these publications, they are not addressed in detail. As otherwise comprehensive books on other aspects of childhood developmental disorders contain very little about sleep disturbance, there is a need for an additional source that will help to fill

the gap. The present book is intended to serve that purpose, mainly for professionals involved in the care of children with developmental disorders who do not have a specialist interest in sleep and its disorders. The basic aim is to stimulate awareness of the nature, consequences and management of the sleep disorders that commonly add to the problems of children suffering from such disorders and that also increase the demands made on those who care for these children.

'Developmental disorders' is interpreted broadly to include neurodevelopmental disorders in the usual sense, other paediatric (including neurological) conditions, and additional disorders in which psychological aspects of development are primarily affected. This last group of disorders is important in its own right but also merits attention as a potential source of sleep disturbance because, as already discussed, psychological problems often accompany other abnormal developmental conditions. Both the European (World Health Organization 1992) and North American (American Psychiatric Association 1994) classification systems for psychiatric disorders are referred to in the text, depending upon the country of origin of the cited research.

The relative amount of space devoted to the different developmental disorders does not necessarily reflect how common they are compared with each other, or even the severity of the sleep problems encountered in each group. Rather, the sections are proportionate to what has been reported about sleep disturbance in each disorder. The topics of intellectual impairment and the epilepsies have needed relatively more extensive review because of their general nature. The balance between the different disorders is an indication of not only what is currently known but also what remains to be researched.

No attempt has been made to include discussion of sleep aspects of all the conditions contained in such accounts of developmental disorders as those by O'Brien and Yule (1995) or Goldstein and Reynolds (1999), for the good reason that there appears to be no published work on many of the disorders mentioned in these accounts. However, this should not be taken to mean that no sleep problems exist in children with the disorders that have not been systematically addressed. On the contrary, it is reasonable to assume that sleep will commonly be disturbed in all of these disorders because of the influence of the various physical and psychological factors considered earlier.

It is worth repeating that the present book is meant to complement the more general accounts of children's sleep disorders already cited, and to consider sleep disturbance in particular conditions and circumstances. Although they are very relevant to developmental disorders, certain sleep disorders (such as obstructive sleep apnoea or nocturnal enuresis) are not described in any detail because good accounts are already available in the sources mentioned.

Emphasis has been placed on clinical abnormalities of sleep; for the most part, reference is made to polysomnographic findings only if they are of likely clinical or theoretical importance. Some restriction has been placed on the number of references cited throughout the book to avoid overextensive referencing while at the same time acquainting the reader with the main sources of information.

The various terms used in the literature to mean that the child is intellectually impaired can be confusing. In particular, in the UK 'learning disability' or 'learning difficulty' are

the equivalent to USA descriptions of 'mental retardation' (and elsewhere the outmoded terms 'mental handicap' and 'mental subnormality') and not 'specific learning disability' such as a difficulty with reading or with numbers. For purposes of consistency the term 'intellectual impairment' is used throughout the text of this book. A further terminological matter of note is that, in places, the child is referred to as 'he' purely for the sake of convenience.

Chapters 2 to 6 are intended to provide a general background about sleep disorders in children and adolescents. The findings and recommendations in these chapters are generally applicable whether a child has a developmental disorder or not, and irrespective of the type of developmental disorder. With the publisher's permission, most of the tables in these chapters are taken from Stores (2001), sometimes with slight modification. In many of the later chapters it is assumed that these introductory chapters will have been read.

REFERENCES

American Psychiatric Association (1994) *Diagnostic and Statistical Manual of Mental Disorders, 4th Edn.* Washington, DC: APA.

Armstrong, K.L., O'Donnell, H., McCallum, R., Dadds, M. (1998) 'Childhood sleep problems: Association with prenatal factors and maternal distress/depression.' *Journal of Pediatrics and Child Health*, **34**, 263–266.

Bonnet, M.H. (2000) 'Sleep deprivation.' *In:* Kryger, M.H., Roth, T., Dement, W.C. (Eds.) *Principles and Practice of Sleep Medicine. 3rd Edn.* Philadelphia: W.B. Saunders, pp. 53–71.

Carroll, J.L., Loughlin, G.M. (1995) 'Obstructive sleep apnoea syndrome in infants and children: Clinical features and pathophysiology.' *In:* Ferber, R., Kryger, M. (Eds.) *Principles and Practice of Sleep Medicine in the Child.* Philadelphia: W.B. Saunders, pp. 163–191.

Chavin, W., Tinson, S. (1980) 'Children with sleep difficulties.' *Health Visitor*, **53**, 477–480.

Cohen, F.L., Merritt, S.L., Nehring, W.M., Mercer, P.W., Eshler, B.C. (1992) 'Curricular sleep content in graduate and undergraduate nursing programs.' *Sleep Research*, **21**, 187. *(Abstract.)*

Durand, V.M. (1998) *Sleep Better! A Guide to Improving Sleep for Children with Special Needs.* Baltimore: Paul H. Brookes.

Ferber, R. (1985) *Solve Your Child's Sleep Problems.* London: Dorling Kindersley.

—— Kryger, M. (Eds.) (1995) *Principles and Practice of Sleep Medicine in the Child.* Philadelphia: W.B. Saunders.

Goldstein, S., Reynolds, C.R. (1999) *Handbook of Neurodevelopmental and Genetic Disorders in Children.* New York: Guilford Press.

Gozal, D. (1998) 'Sleep disordered breathing and school performance in children.' *Pediatrics*, **102**, 616–620.

Graham, P., Turk, J, Verhulst, F. (1999) *Child Psychiatry. A Developmental Approach. 3rd Edn.* Oxford: Oxford University Press.

Kryger, M.H., Roth, T., Dement, W.C. (Eds.) (2000) *Principles and Practice of Sleep Medicine. 3rd Edn.* Philadelphia: W.B. Saunders.

Loughlin, G.M., Carroll, J.L., Marcus, C.L. (Eds.) (2000) *Sleep and Breathing in Children. A Developmental Approach.* New York: Marcel Dekker.

Meijer, A.M., Habekothé, H.T., Van Den Wittenboer, G.L.H. (2000) 'Time in bed, quality of sleep and school functioning of children.' *Journal of Sleep Research*, **9**, 145–153.

Minde, K., Faucon, A., Falkner, S. (1994) 'Sleep problems in toddlers: effects of treatment on their daytime behavior.' *Journal of the American Academy of Child and Adolescent Psychiatry*, **33**, 1114–1121.

Moldofsky, H., Dickstein, J.B. (1999) 'Sleep and cytokine-immune functions in medical, psychiatric and primary sleep disorders.' *Sleep Medicine Reviews*, **3**, 325–337.

National Commission on Sleep Disorders Research (1993) *Wake Up America: A National Sleep Alert. Vol. 1. Executive Summary and Report.* Bethesda, MD: Department of Health and Human Sciences.

—— (1994) *Wake Up America: A National Sleep Alert. Vol. 2. Working Group Reports.* Bethesda, MD: Department of Health and Human Sciences.

O'Brien, G., Yule, W. (Eds.) (1995) *Behavioural Phenotypes. Clinics in Developmental Medicine No. 138.* London: Mac Keith Press.

Partinen, M., Hublin, C. (2000) 'Epidemiology of sleep disorders.' *In:* Kryger, M.H., Roth, T., Dement, W.C. (Eds.) *Principles and Practice of Sleep Medicine. 3rd Edn.* Philadephia: W.B. Saunders, pp. 558–579.

Pilcher, J.J., Huffcutt, A.I. (1996) 'Effects of sleep deprivation on performance: a meta-analysis.' *Sleep*, **19**, 318–326.

Quine, L. (1992) 'Severity of sleep problems in children with severe learning difficulties: description and correlates.' *Journal of Community and Applied Social Psychology*, **2**, 247–268.

—— (1997) *Solving Children's Sleep Problems.* Huntingdon, Cambs: Beckett Karlson.

Royal College of Paediatrics and Child Health (1996) *Syllabus and Training Record for General Professional and Higher Specialist Training in Paediatrics and Child Health.* London: Royal College of Paediatrics and Child Health.

Stores, G. (2001) *A Clinical Guide to Sleep Disorder in Children and Adolescents.* Cambridge: Cambridge University Press.

—— Crawford, C. (1998) 'Medical student education in sleep and its disorders.' *Journal of the Royal College of Physicians of London*, **32**, 149–153.

—— Wiggs, L. (1998) 'Clinical services for sleep disorders.' *Archives of Disease in Childhood*, **79**, 495–497.

—— Ellis, A.J., Wiggs, L., Crawford, C., Thomson, A. (1998) 'Sleep and psychological disturbance in nocturnal asthma.' *Archives of Disease in Childhood*, **78**, 413–419.

Stores, R., Wiggs, L. (1998) 'Sleep education in clinical psychology courses in the UK.' *Clinical Psychology Forum*, **119**, 14–18.

Wiggs, L., Stores, G. (1996) ' Sleep problems in children with severe intellectual disabilities: What help is being provided?' *Journal of Applied Research in Intellectual Disabilities*, **9**, 160–165.

—— —— (1998) 'Behavioural treatment for sleep problems in children with severe learning disabilities and daytime challenging behaviour: Effect on sleep patterns of mother and child.' *Journal of Sleep Research*, **7**, 119–126.

—— Stores, R. (1996) 'Sleep education in undergraduate psychology degree courses in the UK.' *Psychology Teaching Review*, **5**, 40–46.

Wolfson, A., Lacks, P., Futterman, A. (1992) 'Effects of parent training on infant sleeping patterns, parents' stress and perceived parental control.' *Journal of Consulting and Clinical Psychology*, **60**, 41–48.

—— Carskadon, M.A. (1998) 'Sleep schedules and daytime functioning in adolescents.' *Child Development*, **69**, 875–887.

World Health Organization (1992) *The ICD-10 Classification of Mental and Behavioural Disorders.* Geneva: WHO.

2
NORMAL SLEEP INCLUDING DEVELOPMENTAL ASPECTS

Gregory Stores

The nature of sleep

Human existence is spent in three basic physiological states: wakefulness, non-rapid eye movement (NREM) sleep and rapid eye movement (REM) sleep. Each has its distinctive physiological characteristics. Sleep as a whole is a relatively inactive state that, however, is different from other states of reduced awareness and responsiveness (such as coma) partly because it is usually readily reversible but also because it is not simply a passive shut-down state as once supposed.

The onset of sleep and the occurrence of NREM and REM sleep involve activation of complex mechanisms, including different transmitter systems, in various parts of the brain.

The functions of sleep

Considering the need to sleep for so much of the time (a third of life in adults and much more in children, especially in the first few months of life), sleep must serve some fundamental purpose. The various theories advanced have emphasized physical and psychological restoration, energy conservation, consolidation of memories, discharge of emotions, brain growth, and other basic biological functions including the maintenance of immune systems. No one theory is adequate across all species and stages of development, and sleep is likely to serve multiple purposes (Rechtschaffen 1998).

What is clear is that persistent sleep loss has significant adverse effects as discussed in the previous chapter.

Sleep stages

By convention, different stages of sleep are distinguished from each other according to standardized physiological criteria, mainly concerning features of the electroencephalogram (EEG), the electro-oculogram (EOG) and the electromyogram (EMG). The main characteristic features in a healthy young adult of NREM sleep (including its four stages of increasing depth) and REM sleep are shown in Table 2.1, together with the proportions of overnight sleep usually contributed by these stages.

In *NREM sleep*, vertex sharp waves (Stage 1) and K-complexes (Stage 2) are transient arousal phenomena. Sleep spindles (brief spindle-shaped bursts of EEG activity) may accompany a K-complex. Stages 3 and 4 NREM sleep are referred to as slow wave sleep (SWS) or delta sleep. They are the deepest levels of sleep, from which awakening is most

TABLE 2.1
Sleep stages: main features

Stage	Features	% of main sleep period
Non-rapid eye movement (NREM) sleep		
Stage 1	Mixed EEG frequencies	4–5%
	Reduced alpha activity	
	Vertex sharp waves	
	Slow rolling eye movements	
Stage 2	More slow EEG activity	45–55%
	Sleep spindles	
	K-complexes	
Stage 3*	Yet more slow EEG activity	4–6%
Stage 4*	Predominantly slow activity	12–15%
Rapid eye movement (REM) sleep**		20–25%
	Low voltage, mixed frequency, non-alpha rhythm EEG	
	Spontaneous rapid eye movements	
	Skeletal muscle virtually paralysed	
	Variable heart rate, blood pressure and respiration	
	Body temperature regulation impaired	
	Penile and clitoral tumescence	

*Stages 3 and 4 are referred to as slow wave sleep (SWS), delta sleep or deep sleep.
**Most dreaming occurs in REM sleep.

difficult. SWS is particularly prominent in young children. The immature NREM sleep in infancy is referred to as 'quiet sleep'.

The high rate of brain metabolism in *REM sleep* is reflected in the EEG, which is similar to that seen in the alert awake state. Most dreaming occurs in this stage of sleep, during which the skeletal musculature is virtually paralysed. Because of the combination of the absence of muscle tone and high levels of brain activity, REM sleep has been called 'paradoxical sleep'.

REM sleep (or its equivalent in neonates, 'active sleep') accounts for 50 per cent or more of sleep in the term neonate, reducing to 20–25 per cent by 2 years of age and staying at that level thereafter. Infants often enter REM sleep at the start of their sleep period.

The high level of REM sleep early in development suggests a role in cerebral maturation but its true significance remains unclear.

'Indeterminate' or 'transitional' sleep in neonates is a mixture of active and quiet sleep.

Sleep architecture
Figure 2.1 shows in diagrammatic form the pattern of overnight sleep ('hypnogram') in a healthy child of school age. NREM and REM sleep alternate throughout the night several times. The amount of NREM sleep gradually lessens in successive sleep cycles, with SWS usually confined to the first two cycles. Conversely, the amount of REM sleep usually increases as the night progresses. Young children may have a final period of SWS before waking in the morning.

11

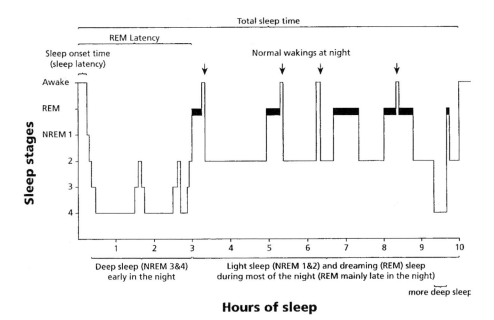

Fig. 2.1. Hypnogram showing characteristic progression of sleep stages overnight in healthy school-age child.

Sleep microstructure and sleep continuity

There is increasing interest in the finer details of sleep physiology than those considered in conventional sleep staging. Very brief physiological (mainly EEG) arousals, without waking, occur as an aspect of normal sleep, seemingly without ill effects. However, if they occur very frequently (either experimentally induced or in certain pathological conditions), the restorative nature of sleep is impaired and daytime psychological function is affected. Constant interruption of sleep continuity by repeated brief arousals of this type, or by others involving brief awakenings, is called 'sleep fragmentation' and is a main cause of *poor quality sleep*.

Sleep–wake rhythms

The timing of sleep (not its amount) is regulated by a *circadian clock* in the suprachiasmatic nucleus (SCN) of the hypothalamus. This clock also controls other biological rhythms including body temperature and cortisol production, with which the sleep–wake rhythm is normally synchronized. From an early age the sleep–wake rhythm has to be brought into line with the 24 hour day–night cycle ('entrainment'). In healthy children, sleep periods have largely shifted to night, and wakefulness to daytime, by 12 months of age, except for daytime napping. The main cue (or *'zeitgeber'*) by which this is achieved is light perception, but social cues, *e.g.* mealtimes and social activities, as well as ambient temperature and noise levels, and internal body signals such as hunger and temperature, are also important.

TABLE 2.2
Average daily sleep duration at different ages

Term birth	16–18 hours
1 year	15 hours
2 years	13–14 hours
4 years	12 hours
10 years	8–10 hours
Mid-adolescence	8.5 hours
Later adolescence	7–8 hours

The hormone *melatonin* is mainly produced in the pineal gland during darkness (the 'hormone of darkness'). It is suppressed by exposure to bright light. Melatonin influences circadian rhythms via the SCN pacemaker, which, in turn, regulates secretion of the hormone by relaying light information to the pineal gland. Complicated changes occur in melatonin production during the course of childhood, with night-time levels peaking between 1 and 3 years of age. After this the level declines, especially with the onset of puberty. At this stage of development there is also a change in the timing of melatonin secretion associated with a delay in the overnight sleep phase independent of social influences.

Within each 24 hour period the tendency to sleep is greater in the early hours of the morning, and again to a lesser extent in the early afternoon (the 'post-lunch dip'). Alertness is generally greatest in the evening before the onset of sleepiness as bedtime approaches (the so-called 'forbidden zone' when it is particularly difficult to sleep). However, individual differences are prominent, at least in the timing of peak alertness. 'Morning types' or 'larks' wake early and are very alert in the early part of the day before tiring in the evening and readily falling asleep. In contrast, 'evening types' or 'owls' are at their best in the evening and have particular difficulty getting up and functioning in the morning. Such differences may be apparent from an early age.

Most children between about 5 years and puberty sleep very soundly at night and are very alert during the day. In contrast, many adolescents are sleepy during the day. This is not wholly because of strong social influences to stay up late, pressures to get up early, or generally irregular sleep habits. Biological changes also play a part, namely proportionately less SWS than at an earlier age, physiological delay in the timing of the sleep phase, and a halt to the earlier steady decline in sleep requirements.

Duration of sleep
Table 2.2 shows the typical amounts of sleep reported to be taken at different ages in childhood and adolescence compared with the average seven to eight hours of overnight sleep for a young adult. However, individual differences are seen from an early age, with some children apparently needing less and others more than these average values. As discussed in the previous chapter, there is a belief that many people of all ages do not get enough sleep (or that the quality of their sleep is impaired), to the detriment of their general well-being. The figures quoted refer to total sleep per 24 hour period. Daytime *napping* is normal during the day up to the age of 3 to 5 years (occasionally later). The frequency of

13

daytime naps usually reduces from four to six in the newborn infant to only one per day by about 1 year.

REFERENCE

Rechtschaffen, A. (1998) 'Current perspectives on the function of sleep.' *Perspectives in Biology and Medicine*, **41**, 359–390.

3
SLEEP PROBLEMS AND SLEEP DISORDERS: GENERAL

Gregory Stores and Luci Wiggs

It is important to distinguish between a *sleep problem or complaint* and the underling cause of the problem, *i.e.* the *sleep disorder*. This distinction is often not made but it is essential for adequate diagnosis and choice of treatment.

Sleep problems

There are three basic types of sleep problem:
- difficulty getting to sleep or staying asleep
- sleeping too much
- disturbed episodes that interfere with sleep.

Each sleep problem can be caused by a variety of sleep disorders, of which over 80 are described in the International Classification of Sleep Disorders—Revised (ICSD-R) (American Sleep Disorders Association 1997). It is no more appropriate to refer to 'sleep-lessness' and its management, without considering the underlying sleep disorder, than to diagnose 'breathlessness' and try to treat it symptomatically without establishing the cause. For example, the common problem of children not going to sleep when their parents would like them to may be the result of poor sleep habits with no routine or discipline at bedtime, but other explanations (each requiring a different approach) should be considered. These include the child being put to bed too early (when he is physiologically not ready for sleep), a bedroom that is too stimulating or otherwise not conducive to sleep, or bedtime fears. The common practice of using hypnotic medication, irrespective of the reason why the child does not settle, is inappropriate, usually ineffective and possibly harmful.

Often the sleep problem is all too obvious such as bedtime struggles, demands for attention in the middle of the night, waking very early and causing a commotion, or having alarming experiences at night. However, some sleep problems do not come so readily to light. Families vary in the extent to which they cope with their child's disturbed sleep. Some may not seek help at all. At times, this is in the belief that the problems are inevitable and cannot be changed. This can occur in some intellectually impaired children with particularly severe sleep problems (Wiggs and Stores 1998). In other cases, the family's general way of life is so disorganized that no effort is made to improve matters. In these circumstances, there is a good argument in favour of tactful intervention in an attempt to treat the sleep disturbance because of its harmful effects on the child and possibly on the family as a whole.

TABLE 3.1
International Classification of Sleep Disorders—Revised*

Dyssomnias
Intrinsic sleep disorders
Extrinsic sleep disorders
Circadian rhythm sleep disorders
Parasomnias
Arousal disorders
Sleep–wake transition disorders
Parasomnias usually associated with REM sleep
Other parasomnias
Sleep disorders associated with mental, neurological or other medical disorders
Associated with mental disorders
Associated with neurological disorders
Associated with other medical disorders
Proposed sleep disorders

*American Sleep Disorders Association (1997).

In other instances, professionals themselves may need to be alerted to the likelihood of significant sleep disorder and the need to check routinely for this possibility as part of overall assessment. For example, in children with Down syndrome it is important to consider upper airway obstruction during sleep in view of the commonness of this problem in such children.

Sleep disorders
Sleep disorders are conditions or circumstances, of a physical or psychological nature (or both combined), that cause a sleep disturbance or problem of one type or another.

CLASSIFICATION
The many sleep disorders now recognized are described in the ICSD-R, which, however, is largely adult in its orientation and needs some modification in relation to children. The basic structure of the scheme is shown in Table 3.1.
- *Dyssomnias* are primary sleep disorders that cause either difficulty getting off to sleep or remaining asleep (sleeplessness or insomnia), or excessive sleepiness during the day. The dyssomnias are divided into *intrinsic sleep disorders* (originating from within the body), *extrinsic sleep disorders* (caused by external factors), and *circadian rhythm sleep–wake disorders* (related to the timing of sleep within the 24 hour period).
- *Parasomnias* (disturbances that intrude into the sleep process) are subdivided according to the phase of sleep with which they are associated: *arousal disorders* (arising from NREM sleep); *sleep–wake transition disorders*; and *parasomnias usually associated with REM sleep. Other parasomnias* are those that do not fall into these three categories.
- *Sleep disorders associated with mental, neurological or other medical disorders* are not primary sleep disorders but sleep-related manifestations of psychiatric or medical conditions.

16

- Conditions that need further assessment before each can be convincingly seen as a disorder in its own right are called *proposed sleep disorders*.

The ICSD-R provides summaries of each sleep disorder including its main characteristics, associated features and possible complications, course, predisposing factors, prevalence, age at onset, sex ratio, familial patterns, polysomnographic and other laboratory features, and differential diagnosis. Diagnostic, severity and duration criteria are also stated. By means of a three-axis system a patient's condition and treatment needs can be characterized in terms of the ICSD-R diagnosis of the sleep disorder, investigations performed and abnormalities demonstrated, and accompanying medical and psychiatric disorders. A glossary of basic terms and concepts is also provided.

Children compared to adults

The main ways in which children's sleep disorders differ from those in adults are as follows.
- Parenting factors or involvement feature prominently in the causation of many children's sleep disorders and in ways in which the disorders can be treated, as discussed previously.
- In general, the effects of persistent sleep disturbance are more wide-ranging in children, whose intellectual and behavioural development can be affected in various ways.
- Sleep disturbance may well result in overactivity and other forms of disturbed behaviour including so-called attention deficit hyperactivity disorder (ADHD), in contrast to adults who are more likely to be sleepy and underactive during the day (Chapter 1).
- For the most part, children's sleep disorders are very treatable (assuming accurate diagnosis of the disorder).

Assessment of sleep

The main requirement for the recognition and correct diagnosis of sleep disorders is careful history taking. This may seem an obvious point, but conventional history-taking schedules usually contain only superficial enquiries about sleep. To avoid sleep disturbance being overlooked, the following basic questions should be asked routinely about any child:
- Does he have difficulty getting off to sleep or staying asleep?
- Is he excessively sleepy/overactive during the day?
- Does he have any disturbed episodes at night?

If there is a positive answer to any of these questions, a detailed history (including a sleep history) should be taken followed by physical and mental examination of the child. Depending on the findings, special investigations may be needed.

SLEEP HISTORY

Parents are the usual main source of information, but children themselves, siblings and teachers may also need to be consulted for a full account. Important aspects to be covered are:
- the precise nature of the current sleep complaint and its development
- associated medical or other factors, including triggering factors or other patterns of occurrence
- effects on the child and others

TABLE 3.2
Review of child's 24 hour sleep–wake pattern*

Evening
What time is the child's last meal?
What activities typically take place between then and getting ready for bed?
Does he take any sleep medicine?

Going to bed
Who gets the child ready for bed and how? Is it always the same person and done in the same way?
Is there a bedtime routine? If so, what is the sequence of events? Does it include a wind-down period?
What time does he go to bed?
Is he put to bed awake or asleep?
Where and how does he fall asleep (own bed, parent's bed, downstairs, being rocked, nursed or fed, with or without a parent present)?
Does he need a bottle, dummy or special object to fall asleep or want someone else to sleep with?
Does he express fears about going to bed?
Does he have his own room?
Is the bedroom conducive to sleep or is it a place for entertainment or other arousing experiences?
Does he have any unusual experiences when going off to sleep?
Exactly what happens if he will not go to bed or does not go to sleep readily? Who deals with the problem and how consistently?

Night-time
Does the child wake during the night? If so, when and how often? Does he get up in the night to go to the toilet or to have a drink? Is he able to return to sleep easily or does he need his parents or join them in their bed? If so, what precisely happens, who is involved and what is the result?
Is the child's sleep disturbed in other ways, *e.g.* restlessness, sleep talking, sleep walking, head banging or rocking, teeth grinding, nightmares or terrified episodes, jerking or convulsive movements or other episodes of disturbed behaviour? How often do these things occur and at what time of night; how long do they last and does he seem awake at the time? What do his parents do?
Does he snore or have any difficulty breathing when asleep?
Does he wet the bed?
What is his usual period of continuous sleep?

Waking
What time does the child wake up? For how long has he slept?
Does he wake up spontaneously or have to be woken? Is he very difficult to awaken? Does he look tired? Is he irritable and in a bad mood?
Does he have any unusual experiences and how does he feel between waking up and getting out of bed?

Daytime
Is the child drowsy or does he sleep during the day? If he sleeps, can he resist doing so and does he fall asleep when engaged in activities?
What are the number, duration and timing of naps?
Do his muscles become weak when he laughs or is upset or surprised?
Does he find it difficult to concentrate?
Has his performance at school deteriorated?
Is he overactive, irritable or depressed?
Are there any unusual episodes during the day?
What is the total time spent asleep each 24 hours?

*Modified according to child's age.

TABLE 3.3
Basic principles of sleep hygiene in childhood and adolescence*

Sleeping environment should be conducive to sleep
Familiar setting
Comfortable bed
Correct temperature
Darkened, quiet room
Non-stimulating
No negative associations (*e.g.* punishment)

Encourage
Bedtime routines
Consistent bedtime and waking up times (weekdays, weekends, holidays)
Going to bed only when tired
Thinking about problems and plans before going to bed
Falling asleep without parents (young children)
Regular daily exercise, exposure to sunlight, and general fitness

Avoid
Excessive or late napping during the day
Overexcitement near bedtime
Late evening exercise
Caffeine-containing drinks late in the day
Smoking and alcohol
Large meals late at night
Too much time awake in bed (especially distressed)

*Relevance varies with age.

- past and present treatments and their effectiveness (the details are important as treatment may have been inappropriate or inadequately carried out).

The child's 24 hour *sleep–wake schedule* should be described (Table 3.2), including possible inconsistencies from night to night, or from weekday to weekend or during holiday periods (important in the sleep–wake cycle disorders described later). Features of particular diagnostic significance may come to light (*e.g.* chronic noisy breathing). The child's *sleep rhythm* (timing and duration of overnight sleep and daytime naps) and *overall amount of sleep* each 24 hours should be established. Other important aspects are:
- the child's *sleep associations* (important in determining his ability to go to sleep readily, preferably without his parents' attention as discussed in the next chapter)
- *sleep hygiene, i.e.* whether the sleeping environment and the child's general activities are conducive to sleep (Table 3.3).

These clinical enquiries can be supplemented by means of a general screening *sleep–wake questionnaire* (*e.g.* Bruni *et al.* 1996) or by one directed at sleep-disordered breathing (Chervin *et al.* 2000). The Epworth Sleepiness Scale (ESS) (Johns 1998) is a well-established brief measure of the tendency to fall asleep in various everyday situations. The adult form can be adapted for use with children, for whom, however, it has not been standardized. A *sleep diary* kept over about a two-week period is often very revealing compared with retrospective general impressions by parents. Typical information that might be gathered is shown in Figure 3.1.

Date	*Monday June 12th*
Time woke/woken	*7.30am (woken by alarm)*
Time got up	*7.50am (dragged out of bed by Mum)*
What did he do in between waking and getting up?	*Dozed in bed listening to radio. He seemed really tired and did not want to get up.*
Time and length of all daytime naps	*Fell asleep watching TV when he got home from school (4.30pm until 5.15pm). Woken at 5.15pm by Mum.*
What did he do in the hour before bedtime?	*Watched TV, played a computer game with his sister, had a bath then came downstairs again for a story which Dad read to him. When asked to go to bed he said he wasn't tired and moaned a bit about going to bed but went after about 10 minutes of arguments!*
Time to bed	*8.45pm*
Time to sleep	*11.30pm*
What happened in between going to bed and falling asleep?	*Mum took him upstairs, said goodnight and left the room. At 9pm he came downstairs asking for a drink. Dad gave him some water and took him back to bed. He read in bed until 10pm. Mum called up that it was time to put the light out and he did. Heard him tossing and turning but he stayed in bed after this time. Sid said, the next morning, that he couldn't sleep because he was worrying about his maths test at school tomorrow.*
Time and length of all wakes during the night. Please describe what happened.	*1.30pm he woke and went to the toilet. Returned to bed straight away and was asleep within 5 minutes.*
Anything else of importance?	*Sid seemed a bit unwell today. I think he may be coming down with a cold.*

Fig. 3.1. Example of sleep diary entry.

OVERALL REVIEW

Factors contributing to the sleep problems may well be revealed by a review of:
• the child's developmental, medical and psychiatric history
• family history (often positive in arousal disorders, enuresis and narcolepsy)
• physical symptoms of possible significance (*e.g.* breathing difficulties or nocturia).

PHYSICAL AND MENTAL STATE EXAMINATION

This should include special attention to:
• neurological, cardiorespiratory or other diseases that might affect sleep
• obesity, or facial or pharyngeal abnormalities predisposing to upper airway obstruction in particular
• overactivity, depression or other psychiatric disorders likely to affect sleep
• evidence of intellectual impairment (including signs of specific syndromes) relevant to possible sleep disturbance.

SLEEP STUDIES INCLUDING POLYSOMNOGRAPHY (PSG)

Audiovisual recordings, including those obtained with the family's own video equipment, can be very instructive about night-time events, sometimes providing a very different account than descriptions given in the clinic. The mode of onset of any nocturnal episodes may be particularly useful diagnostically, and this should be emphasized to parents if they are making recordings at home.

Actigraphy (or *actometry*)involves monitoring body movements by use of small, wrist-watch-like movement sensors and applying validated algorithms to the data, which permits the scoring of sleep and wake states (American Sleep Disorders Association 1995). Although conventional sleep staging is not possible, actigraphy may be a particularly useful method of obtaining objective data on children who are unable to tolerate PSG, or where basic sleep–wake patterns (*i.e.* timing, continuity, duration) are the main interest. A further advantage is that it can be used as an outpatient procedure.

Polysomnography (Broughton 1999) provides detailed physiological information about the occurrence of conventional sleep stages. This is needed in only a minority of cases. Main indications are:
• the investigation of excessive daytime sleepiness (Chapter 5), including assessment of the objective degree of sleepiness by means of the Multiple Sleep Latency Test (MSLT) (American Sleep Disorders Association 1992). The MSLT measures the time the child takes to fall asleep during five opportunities (at two-hourly intervals) to do so in standardized conditions during the day
• the diagnosis of complicated parasomnias, the nature of which remains unclear despite careful clinical evaluation
• as an objective check on the accuracy of the sleep complaint or response to treatment.

Standard PSG involves recording EEGs, EOGs and EMGs, from which basic measures of NREM sleep, REM sleep and sleep continuity can be made. Where necessary, PSG can be extended to include a range of respiratory measures (for sleep-related breathing problems), additional EEG channels (if epilepsy is suspected), or anterior tibialis EMG recording for

TABLE 3.4
Examples of treatment approaches for sleep disorders

General principles
Explain the problem, reassure where appropriate and provide support
Encourage good sleep hygiene
Where possible treat any underlying cause of sleep disturbance
    Medical
    Psychiatric
Safety or protective measures (hazardous parasomnias)

Specific measures
Psychological (mainly for sleeplessness)
    Bedtime routine
    Appropriate associations with bedtime
    Promotion of self-soothing
    Setting limits
    Reinforcement of good behaviour
    Systematic desensitization
    Self-control training (*e.g.* approaches using relaxation, imagery etc.)
Chronobiological (circadian sleep–wake rhythm disorders)
    Sleep phase retiming
    Light therapy
Medication
    Hypnotics (selectively and short term)
    Stimulants (excessive sleepiness)
    Melatonin (some circadian rhythm disorders)
Physical measures
    Continuous positive airway pressure (obstructive sleep apnoea)
Surgery
    Adenotonsillectomy (obstructive sleep apnoea)

the detection of periodic limb movements in sleep. Home PSG (Stores 1994), using small portable recording systems, is generally more acceptable to children than admission to a sleep laboratory, of which there are very few that are designed specially for children. Normative data for children's home PSG are now available for conventional sleep variables (Stores *et al.* 1998) and also for brief arousals (Stores and Crawford 2000).

OTHER SPECIAL INVESTIGATIONS
Depending on the outcome of other enquiries, further investigations may be appropriate. These include haematological, biochemical or endocrinological tests, urinalysis, drug toxicity screening, ENT evaluation, and more detailed EEG studies for further consideration of epilepsy.

Treatment approaches
There is a wide variety of treatments from which to choose, depending on the nature of the child's sleep disorder (Table 3.4). In general, there is still undue reliance on hypnotic medication for sleeplessness despite the evidence that it is rarely helpful and can be harmful. The effectiveness of behavioural treatments, on the other hand, is well established, but they

are often not employed. Melatonin has yet to be shown to deserve the sometimes enthusiastic claims made for it as a treatment for various sleep disorders and needs to be much better researched (Zhdanova 2000). Sleep hygiene principles are an important adjunct to the specific treatments mentioned in the coming chapters and are sometimes effective by themselves. Further, preventive measures to encourage the development of appropriate sleep habits in young children deserve greater emphasis.

REFERENCES

American Sleep Disorders Association (1992) 'The clinical use of the Multiple Sleep Latency Test.' *Sleep*, **15**, 268–276.

—— (1995) 'The role of actigraphy in the evaluation of sleep disorders.' *Sleep*, **18**, 288–302.

—— (1997) *ICSD—International Classification of Sleep Disorders, Revised: Diagnostic and Coding Manual.* Rochester, MN: American Sleep Disorders Association.

Broughton, R.J. (1999) 'Polysomnography: Principles and applications in sleep and arousal disorders.' *In:* Niedermeyer, E., Lopes da Silva, F. (Eds.) *Electroencephalography: Basic Principles, Clinical Applications and Related Fields. 4th Edn.* Baltimore: Williams & Wilkins, pp. 858–895.

Bruni, O., Ottaviano, S., Guidetti, V., Romoli, M., Innocenzi, M., Cortesi, F., Giannotti, F. (1996) 'The Sleep Disturbance Scale for Children (SDSC). Construction and validation of an instrument to evaluate sleep disturbances in childhood and adolescence.' *Journal of Sleep Research*, **5**, 251–261.

Chervin, R.D., Hedger, K., Dillon, J.E., Pituch, K.J. (2000) 'Pediatric Sleep Questionnaire (PSQ): Validity and reliability of scales for sleep-disordered breathing, snoring, sleepiness, and behavioral problems.' *Sleep Medicine*, **1**, 21–32.

Johns, M. (1998) 'Rethinking the assessment of sleepiness.' *Sleep Medicine Reviews*, **2**, 3–15.

Stores, G. (1994) 'Investigation of sleep disorders including home monitoring.' *Archives of Disease in Childhood*, **71**, 184–185.

—— Crawford, C. (2000) 'Arousal norms for children age 5–16 years based on home polysomnography.' *Technology and Health Care*, **8**, 285–290.

—— Selman, J., Wiggs, L. (1998) 'Home polysomnography norms for children.' *Technology and Health Care*, **6**, 231–236.

Wiggs, L., Stores, G. (1998) 'Behavioural treatment for sleep problems in children with severe learning disabilities and daytime challenging behaviour: Effect on sleep patterns of mother and child.' *Journal of Sleep Research*, **7**, 119–126.

Zhdanova, I.V. (2000) 'The role of melatonin in sleep and sleep disorders.' *In:* Culebras, A. (Ed.) *Sleep Disorders and Neurological Disease.* New York: Marcel Dekker, pp. 137–157.

4
SLEEPLESSNESS

Luci Wiggs and Gregory Stores

Sleeplessness is an overall term for delay in getting to sleep or difficulty staying asleep. 'Insomnia' tends to be used for people who are old enough to complain about these problems. In one form or another, sleeplessness is the most common sleep problem at any age. Unfortunately, it is all too often treated symptomatically (and ineffectively) by means of hypnotic medication with little attempt to identify the underlying cause, of which there are many possibilities. Perhaps 20 to 30 per cent of children in the general population have a significant degree of difficulty sleeping. Rates are very much higher in children with a developmental disorder, and, at least in those with an intellectual impairment, the problem tends to be very long-lasting (Stores 1992).

It is necessary to describe the problem in detail, making the distinction between:
- bedtime difficulties (either reluctance to go to bed or difficulty getting to sleep)
- waking at night and not being able to go back to sleep
- waking very early
- other aspects of the child's sleep called (misleadingly) sleeplessness or poor sleep, *e.g.* frequent nightmares or restlessness without actual waking.

Combinations of these types of sleeplessness are not uncommon.

As the sleep disorders underlying these different types of sleeplessness tend to be different, treatment will vary from one type to another. A detailed description of the child's sleep problem as perceived by the parents sometimes reveals that sleep is, in fact, within normal limits and that the parents' mistaken views or expectations need to be corrected. In the simplest case, information on what is normal will be sufficient. If the misperception is part of a generally distorted view of the child (*e.g.* because the parent is seriously depressed), more substantial help will be required.

Aetiology: general factors
There are a number of possible influences on the adequacy or otherwise of a child's sleep.
- Parenting practices and other *parental factors* (*e.g.* personality, state of health) are often relevant, even when physical causes of the sleep problems predominate.
- *The sleeping environment* is important and may reflect the family's general circumstances including financial resources and housing conditions.
- *Medical disorders*, affecting any system and present in their own right or complicating some other childhood disorder, can disturb sleep.
- *Genetic factors* are being increasingly recognized in certain sleep disorders (Zai *et al.* 2000), although behavioural factors are also likely to be involved.

TABLE 4.1
**Factors to consider in sleepless children at
different ages**

Infancy
'Colic'
Cow's milk intolerance
Middle ear disease
Frequent night-time feeds
Inappropriate sleep associations

Early childhood (1–3 years)
Inappropriate napping
Poor bedtime routine
Stressful or otherwise undesirable sleep onset
  associations
Poor limit setting
Too early bedtime

Middle childhood (4–12 years)
Difficulty getting to sleep
Persistence of earlier problems
Night-time fears
Overarousal
Worry and anxiety
Conditioned insomnia
'Owl' sleep–wake pattern
Idiopathic insomnia
Night waking
Parasomnias
Early morning waking
Environmental disturbance
Advanced sleep phase syndrome
'Lark' sleep–wake pattern
Reduced sleep requirements
Conditioned early waking

Adolescence
Erratic sleep–wake schedules
Delayed sleep phase syndrome
Sleep-disrupting substances (recreational, illicit)
Worry and anxiety
Major psychiatric disorder
Idiopathic insomnia

The types of factors underlying sleep disturbance vary somewhat with the child's age, although there is some overlap. A strict developmental sequence is less likely to be seen in children with a neurodevelopmental abnormality. This is partly because of developmental delay, but also because of other possibly strong influences (such as parental handling of the child) or individual differences in the severity and effects of the disorder.

The following account of the causes of sleeplessness in children of different ages is necessarily much abbreviated to provide only general guidelines to the factors to be considered (summarized in Table 4.1) and the treatments that are appropriate.

Infancy

Particularly at this early age, certain medical possibilities should be considered as a primary explanation of the child's sleeplessness, although convincing evidence of their relevance is required. Main examples are:

- *infantile colic:* traditionally considered to be a cause of settling difficulty, although its validity as an intestinal condition distinct from other patterns of intense crying in children has been doubted
- *allergies*, including cow's milk intolerance (Chapter 20)
- *gastro-oesophageal reflux*
- from 6 months onwards, *teething* is sometimes thought by parents to disturb sleep.

Other aspects of early development to consider include too frequent night-time feeds. This impedes the acquisition of a pattern of predominantly daytime feeding, may make the infant uncomfortable from wet nappies, and encourages a need for his parents to be there.

Early childhood (1–3 years)

Medical causes should also be excluded at this age and, indeed, later. For example, chronic *middle ear disease* can cause night-time waking and distress because of an increase in middle ear pressure and discomfort. Settling to sleep at night may be difficult if the child's *daytime naps* are too frequent, too long, too close to bedtime, or if they are inadequate causing 'overtiredness' at night. The pattern of napping can be improved by gradual changes. However, the main and very common cause of problems is that the child has not learnt appropriate sleep behaviour. Difficulty getting the child to sleep and/or night waking where the child demands his parents' attention are the most prevalent types of these 'behavioural' sleep difficulties.

The following general principles should be encouraged in order ideally to prevent these problems, or at least to minimize them (the same principles underlie many of the programmes of behavioural treatment, discussed later, for use when the sleep problem has become well established):

- a consistent *bedtime routine* including a *wind-down period* before the child is expected to go to sleep
- *sleep-onset associations* that are conducive to sleep. Bed should be associated with going to sleep rather than stimulating activities or upsetting experiences such as punishment. When the child wakes in the night (which is normal at any age), he should be able to go back to sleep without needing his parents' attention (*i.e.* to be 'self-soothing'). As this is much easier if he has not needed to be with his parents when going to sleep at bedtime, it is generally best to teach the child to go to sleep alone
- consistent rules for going to bed and settling to sleep (*limit setting*). If parents give in to the child's attempts to delay bedtime, the settling problem will be reinforced
- the child should not be put to bed too early in the pre-sleep period when he is very alert (the *'forbidden zone'*). Instead, bedtime should be when he is 'sleepy tired'. This allows bed to become associated with falling asleep quickly rather than lying awake or struggling with his parents.

Cognitive and behavioural treatments for established settling and waking problems have been reviewed by Owens *et al.* (1999), and also by Wiggs and France (2000) who considered them specifically in children and adolescents with physical illness, psychological problems and intellectual impairment.

For these treatments to be properly implemented, parents need to be convinced that they are usually very effective even in long-standing and difficult cases of sleeping difficulty. As mentioned previously, sometimes they lack this conviction because inadequate or inappropriate treatment programmes have been attempted in the past. It is also important that parents are emotionally capable of seeing the programme through, especially if the child's sleep problems worsen before they improve, and that they are capable of organizing themselves to use the treatment consistently. For these reasons, it is usually important for a health visitor or psychologist to design the treatment programme in conjunction with the parents and to support and advise them during its use.

The various types of behavioural treatments are as follows.

- *Ignoring the child* once he is put to bed, or if he wakes during the night, despite his protests or demands for his parents' attention. Although apparently effective quite quickly, this method is rarely appropriate. Parents cannot usually bear their child's distress and, indeed, it is ill-advised if the child has a medical condition that might worsen in the night.
- *Variations on complete ignoring* involve different ways in which parents gradually reduce their reinforcing contact with the child when he protests or cries. This may be achieved by parents *gradually reducing their proximity* to the child in his bed, the *time* they spend with him there, or repeated brief *checking* with minimal contact with the child. Other methods of this general type involve parents *remaining in the child's room but ignoring him.* There is some evidence that a combination of a short-term hypnotic drug and an ignoring procedure helps in otherwise resistant cases. The particular method chosen depends upon parents' preference. It may be necessary to try different methods, although each should be fully attempted before moving on to another.
- For children able to understand them, the use of *reward systems* (such as a star chart) can be effective in addition to the above methods and sometimes on their own.

Early morning waking can also be a problem in early childhood. One cause may be *going to sleep unusually early* for the child's age so that his sleep requirements have been met well before other family members are ready to wake up (*advanced sleep phase syndrome*). Re-establishing appropriate sleep times is best done gradually, by delaying when the child is put to bed over a period of time, with the intention that final wake-up time will be delayed spontaneously. Daily delays of 15 minutes or longer can be used. Often, other important daily time cues, such as meal times and nap times, are also somewhat too early, and shifting the child's whole daily pattern, in line with bedtime, is usually required. Ferber (1995) provides a clear discussion of these behavioural and chronobiological aspects of management.

Middle childhood (4–12 years)

Some of the problems just considered may persist, but at this age children in the general population mainly have difficulty getting off to sleep. This may be the result of:

27

- being *overaroused* at bedtime because of boisterous or exciting activities (*e.g.* computer games) or frightening stories or television
- night-time fears, which are common and often more complicated as the child grows up, and possibly accompanied by nightmares. A variety of treatments may be useful, including self-control strategies (such as relaxation training, guided imagery and positive self-statements), reward programmes and systematic desensitization (Owens *et al.* 1999). In severe cases psychiatric treatment may be necessary
- *stress, worry or upset* about family or school issues or other daytime experiences
- *conditioned or learned insomnia, i.e.* when the habit of lying awake for long periods persists even when the original source of anxiety no longer exists. Altering sleep schedules, along with attention to sleep hygiene, is required in such cases
- *idiopathic insomnia* (which is unusual).

Waking at night is unusual at this age but sleep may be interrupted by *parasomnias* (Chapter 6). For many parasomnias, treatments employing cognitive restructuring may be particularly appropriate for this age of child (Owens *et al.* 1999). 'Growing pains' are an ill-understood condition that should not be confused with definite physical causes of night-time discomfort or pain.

Early morning waking becomes a problem if the child is noisy, demands attention, is liable to injure himself (or others), or is destructive if left unattended. Causes to consider include:
- *environmental* (early morning light or noise)
- *advanced sleep phase syndrome* (less common in middle childhood than in early childhood);
- a *'lark'* sleep–wake pattern (Chapter 2)
- the child *needing much less sleep* than others
- *conditioned* early waking (rare).

Adolescence

High rates of sleeplessness are reported at this age. Possible causes are:
- *erratic sleep–wake schedules* caused by inconsistent sleep habits, possibly made worse by excessive consumption of caffeine-containing drinks, alcohol or nicotine, or by the use of illegal substances
- difficulty getting off to sleep as part of the *delayed sleep phase syndrome* (Chapter 5), in which a previous habit of going to sleep late becomes a physiological inability to do otherwise because the circadian sleep–wake clock has become reset
- *worries and anxieties* causing difficulty getting to sleep and disrupted sleep
- major *psychiatric disorder* such as severe depression
- *idiopathic insomnia*, which may present at this time.

A variety of social, psychological and physical factors combine to make adolescence a time when sleeplessness may be especially likely. However, there is surprisingly little research to evaluate interventions in this particular age-group. Given that there can be large differences between the adolescent's and parents' perception of the 'problem', and also in their motivation to correct the problem, treatment decisions should be based upon discussions with the adolescent and his parents in order to be realistic and (hopefully) effective.

REFERENCES

Ferber, R. (1995) 'Circadian rhythm sleep disorders in childhood.' *In:* Ferber, R., Kryger, M. (Eds.) *Principles and Practice of Sleep Medicine in the Child*. Philadelphia: W.B. Saunders, pp. 91–98.

Owens, J.L., France, K.G., Wiggs, L. (1999) 'Behavioural and cognitive–behavioural interventions for sleep disorders in infants and children: a review.' *Sleep Medicine Reviews*, 3, 281–302.

Stores, G. (1992) 'Sleep studies in children with a mental handicap.' *Journal of Child Psychology and Psychiatry*, **33**, 1303–1317. *(Annotation.)*

Wiggs, L., France, K. (2000) 'Behavioural treatments for sleep problems in children and adolescents with physical illness, psychological problems or intellectual disabilities.' *Sleep Medicine Reviews*, **4**, 299–314.

Zai, C., Wigg, K.G., Barr, C.L. (2000) 'Genetics and sleep disorders.' *Seminars in Clinical Neuropsychiatry*, **5**, 33–43.

5
EXCESSIVE SLEEPINESS

Gregory Stores

Daytime sleepiness sufficient to interfere significantly with daytime functioning has been reported in 5 per cent or more of young adults. The comparable figure for children is not known, but, as it is associated with many conditions, it cannot be uncommon. However, because it is less obviously troublesome than other types of sleep problem it may not be recognized as a serious matter perhaps until the child has difficulties at school or with other aspects of living. Even then, sleepiness may be misinterpreted as laziness or disinterest. The consequences of not recognizing and correcting excessive sleepiness can be very serious in view of the many adverse consequences in adults, including poor work performance and accidents (Mitler 1996), for which there must be counterparts in children.

Suggestive signs that a child is excessively sleepy are:
• sleeping several hours longer than most children of his age
• napping beyond the age at which it would normally cease (*e.g.* after starting school)
• being sleepy when other children of the same age are active and alert
• sleeping much more than previously.

It is important to note, however, that young children may manifest their sleepiness as over-activity or other features of attention deficit hyperactivity disorder (ADHD).

Ideally, 'sleepy tiredness' should be distinguished from 'physical tiredness' (*i.e.* lethargy, fatigue, exhaustion or lack of energy), which tends to have a physical cause, although depression and, of course, the chronic fatigue syndrome (Chapter 28) may be responsible. Sleepy tiredness is most evident if the child falls asleep when doing something active; lesser degrees involve sleeping when in a comfortable setting or being drowsy with yawning, stretching and the other signs of sleepiness.

As shown in Table 5.1, causes of excessive sleepiness can be grouped as:
• insufficient sleep (including circadian sleep–wake cycle disorders)
• disturbed overnight sleep (*i.e.* poor quality sleep)
• conditions in which sleep requirements are increased.

Insufficient sleep including circadian sleep–wake cycle disorders

This is probably the main cause of excessive sleepiness. People of all ages are thought to suffer from chronic sleep deprivation partly because modern lifestyles reduce the hours of sleep below that required for optimal functioning during the day. Clinically, therefore, the various causes of sleeplessness discussed in the previous chapter should be considered in explaining the individual case. In addition, abnormalities of the circadian sleep–wake cycle, which are said to be particularly common in adolescents and young people and which are

TABLE 5.1
Differential diagnosis of excessive sleepiness in older children and adolescents

Insufficient sleep (including circadian sleep–wake cycle disorders)
Sleeplessness (Chapter 4)
Irregular sleep–wake schedule
Delayed sleep phase syndrome
Non-24-hour sleep–wake schedule

Disturbed sleep
Recreational drugs (caffeine, alcohol, nicotine)
Illicit drugs, including withdrawal
Medical and psychiatric disorders
Medication effects
Upper airway obstruction
Other sleep disorders (frequent parasomnias, periodic limb movements)

Increased need for sleep
Narcolepsy
Idiopathic CNS hypersomnia
Depression
Neurological disease or other physical illness
Congenital long sleeper
Kleine–Levin syndrome (intermittent sleepiness)
Menstruation-related hypersomnia (intermittent sleepiness)

described in some of the neurodevelopmental disorders considered in later chapters, are likely to cause excessive daytime sleepiness.

An *irregular sleep–wake schedule*, with disorganized and ever-changing sleep and behaviour patterns, can be the result of lack of consistency and routine in family functioning. However, irregular mealtimes, inconsistent late-night activities, variable bedtimes and waking up times, stress, and (in adolescence) the use of recreational and even illicit drugs can combine to disrupt circadian rhythms to a serious extent. Learning and behaviour are likely to be affected. In theory, the young person's lifestyle, or the way the family functions as a whole, needs to be altered and consistent regular routines established. This may be difficult to achieve.

Reference was made in Chapter 4 to the *delayed sleep phase syndrome* (DSPS). This condition is characterized by a physiological difficulty getting to sleep until very late and by great difficulty getting up in time for school or work, as well as sleepiness during the day because of insufficient sleep. Adolescents are again especially prone to this sleep disorder, largely because of psychosocial influences on their sleep pattern, but sleep phase delay may develop at younger ages if bedtime has been delayed persistently for any reason.

Treatment of DSPS consists of moving the sleep phase forward to a more appropriate time. This might be achieved by gradually advancing the bedtime if the shift in the child's sleep phase is not too severe. In more serious cases, it is necessary to successively delay the sleep phase around the clock by about three-hour periods each night (Sheldon *et al.* 1992). Advancing the sleep phase may be aided by the use of bright natural or artificial light after waking in the morning. To prevent relapse, the corrected sleep schedules must be rigidly

maintained after the course of treatment has been completed. Patients must be strongly motivated, and their families well organized, for this 'chronotherapy' to be successful. Sometimes the young person has a vested interest in maintaining the abnormal sleep pattern (*e.g.* as part of school refusal), in which case psychological help will be needed.

A *non-24-hour sleep–wake schedule* is the result of failure to entrain to the 24 hour light–dark cycle. As discussed in Chapter 18, it is seen in blind children and also in neurological conditions in which there is damage or maldevelopment of the cerebral mechanisms that control the sleep–wake cycle. Characteristically, the ability to fall asleep slips later and later each night causing great difficulty getting up in the morning and also daytime sleepiness. As the sleep period gradually works around the clock, there is a phase when normal sleep–wake timing is completely reversed, but, later, another when the timing is normal before the cycle repeats itself. The psychological consequences of this highly abnormal sleep–wake pattern are likely to disrupt the child's sleep pattern further. Treatment consists of maximizing the effects of environmental cues to whether it is day or night, and firmly fixing bedtime and wake-up time as well as other daily activities.

Disturbed overnight sleep
As described in Chapter 2, continuity of sleep is important for its restorative function. Sleep can be disrupted and its quality impaired in many ways.

GENERAL FACTORS
These include:
- caffeine-containing drinks (notably coffee and cola drinks)
- tobacco and alcohol
- hypnotic drugs (including rebound effects during the night)
- illicit drugs (including their withdrawal effects)
- frequent parasomnias
- medical conditions (such as asthma, nocturia or epilepsy) or psychiatric disorder.

PERIODIC LIMB MOVEMENTS IN SLEEP (PLMS)
These are brief, stereotyped contractions, mainly affecting the legs, usually occurring in NREM sleep and possibly associated with physiological evidence of arousal with each movement. If frequent (*'periodic limb movement disorder'*) PLMS can disrupt sleep enough to cause daytime sleepiness. They may occur in association with other sleep disorders such as obstructive sleep apnoea or narcolepsy. Sometimes PLMS are accompanied by the *restless legs syndrome* in which distressing leg sensations and an irresistible urge to move the legs make it difficult to get to sleep.

Previously considered rare in children, PLMS have recently been described in some children and adolescents with ADHD whose daytime symptoms are thought to be the result of sleep disturbance caused by the movements. Treatment with dopaminergic medication is said to improve both sleep and behaviour (Chapter 26). PLMS have also been reported in children with Williams syndrome, whose sleep improved with the use of clonazepam (Chapter 14).

UPPER AIRWAY OBSTRUCTION (UAO)

The increasing awareness of *obstructive sleep apnoea* (OSA), a severe form of UAO, in adults and its potentially serious psychological and physical effects, has not been paralleled by acknowledgement that this is also a common and harmful condition in children. Estimates of its prevalence in children in the general population are around 1 per cent, the main cause being enlarged tonsils and adenoids. UAO is particularly important because in many groups of children with a developmental disorder this figure is greatly exceeded. The main examples are:

• Down syndrome
• craniofacial syndromes
• mucopolysaccharidoses
• fragile X syndrome
• some cases of Prader–Willi syndrome
• some forms of cerebral palsy
• neuromuscular disease
• spina bifida/myelomeningocele
• hydrocephalus
• Arnold–Chiari malformation
• achondroplasia.

A predisposition to UAO is also seen in other conditions such as sickle cell disease and disorders in which upper airway tissues become infiltrated or impinged upon.

Detailed accounts of the clinical manifestations, pathophysiology, diagnosis and treatment are provided elsewhere (Loughlin *et al.* 2000). UAO in some of the above conditions is considered in later chapters of this book. The following account mainly outlines some basic aspects of UAO in children.

Increasingly, the obstructive sleep apnoea syndrome (OSAS) is being viewed as the most severe end of a continuum of UAO. Lesser (but significant) degrees of obstruction are referred to as the *'upper airways resistance syndrome'* (UARS). Although UARS does not involve apnoeic episodes, its disruptive effects on sleep and daytime function are said to be indistinguishable from OSAS. In children, apnoeas are not in themselves necessary for a serious sleep-related breathing disorder to be present.

Children with UAO are different from adults with the condition in a number of ways:

• the usual cause is different (mainly enlarged tonsils and adenoids)
• only a minority are obese, and some will fail to thrive if the onset is very early
• partial obstruction with hypoventilation and hypercapnia is more usual than discrete cyclical obstructive apnoeas
• as with other causes of excessive sleepiness, it may present as school failure or behavioural disturbance rather than obvious sleepiness.

A main guideline to its recognition is chronic loud snoring or other sounds of breathing difficulty, but there are a number of other features occurring during sleep, on waking and during the day about which enquiries should be made (Table 5.2). History alone is thought not to distinguish clearly between different degrees of UAO, *i.e.* between UARS and OSA or, indeed, *'primary snoring'* (*i.e.* snoring without any obvious evidence of sleep disruption

TABLE 5.2

Night-time and daytime features of upper airway obstruction

During sleep

Chronic loud snoring

Other sounds of breathing difficulty (gasping, snorting)

Other evidence of increased respiratory effect (retractions of
   chest wall muscles, paradoxical inward movement of the chest
   during inspiration with outward movement of the abdomen)

Rapid breathing

Apnoeic episodes

Nasal flaring

Mouth breathing

Cyanosis

Unusual sleeping positions including kneeling or neck extension

Very restless sleep

Profuse sweating

Enuresis

Awakenings and associated parasomnias (night terrors,
nightmares)

On waking

Difficulty waking up, disorientation, grogginess

Bad mood

Headache

Dry mouth

Daytime

Sleepiness

Concentration and memory problems, poor school progress

Irritability and other emotional or behavioural problems

---

or daytime symptoms and exhibited by many children). Screening methods are much debated. Home audiovisual recordings may clarify descriptions obtained in the clinic. Abnormal findings on overnight oximetry indicate UAO severe enough to require treatment, but normal results do not exclude lesser although possibly significant degrees of obstruction. To diagnose and assess the severity of UAO, polysomnography (PSG) including respiratory measures is ideally required, but, as such investigations for all children with noisy breathing during sleep are not feasible, selection criteria for PSG have to be based on the presence of such additional features as:

- parental observations that their child stops breathing (other than the normal periodic breathing of infancy)
- daytime sleepy tiredness or overactivity
- failing performance at school or otherwise inexplicable behavioural problems
- enlarged tonsils and adenoids
- repeated upper airway infection
- poor growth rate or failure to thrive.

Table 5.3 lists factors to consider in the physical examination of a child with evidence of UAO. If PSG is performed, special requirements for children (including paediatric norms) must be considered.

TABLE 5.3

**Main factors to consider on physical examination of
the child with upper airway obstruction**

Nasal obstruction
Congenital stenosis
Deviated septum
Nasal polyps
Foreign body
Rhinitis (seasonal or perennial)

Nasal and oropharynx
Enlarged tonsils and adenoids
Large tongue
Abnormal hard palate including cleft palate repair
Abnormal soft palate including abnormal uvula
Micrognathia

Craniofacial structures
Midface hypoplasia
Mandibular hypoplasia

General
Obesity
Adenoidal facies
Growth
Muscle tone
Evidence of neurodevelopmental syndromes (*e.g.* Down
  syndrome)
Chest, cardiac or neurological abnormalities

For many children in the general population, removal of tonsils and adenoids is the appropriate treatment and this may also be beneficial in some children where the cause of the obstruction is more complicated (*e.g.* in Down syndrome). Continuous positive airway pressure (CPAP) or bilevel positive airway pressure (BiPAP) has been used for some children where removal of tonsils and adenoids is not appropriate or has been ineffective. Other measures include weight reduction in obese children and reconstructive upper airway surgery in some children with neurodevelopmental disorders.

Conditions in which sleep tendency is increased
Narcolepsy is the best-known example of a disorder that intrinsically involves an increased need to sleep. It is mainly an abnormality of REM sleep and has a strong genetic component. Occasionally it is thought to be symptomatic of some other neurological disorder such as Niemann–Pick disease type C. Narcolepsy is not a rare condition (the prevalence is usually quoted as about 4–6 per 10,000). Onset of symptoms occurs during childhood and adolescence in at least a third of patients.

The classic combination of sleep attacks (episodes of irresistible sleep), cataplexy (sudden loss of tone in response to intense emotion experience), hypnagogic hallucinations and sleep paralysis eventually occur together in less than 50 per cent of cases. The excessive sleepiness is the basic feature; some consider cataplexy to be an essential accompaniment

for the diagnosis to be made but this is not justified when the condition first declares itself in childhood. Childhood narcolepsy is often different from the adult form in other respects (Stores 1999). These include difficulties in detecting the main features (especially in modified form, such as partial forms of cataplexy, or when they are concealed or denied), or when secondary complications (such as fear or other psychological reactions) dominate the clinical picture. Narcolepsy is often missed or misdiagnosed with delays of several years in its proper recognition.

The correct diagnosis can usually be made clinically, but convincing evidence may not be apparent in the early stages and repeated assessment is then required. PSG should be performed in suspected cases, partly to exclude other sleep disorders but also to see if the characteristic findings of a short interval between sleep onset and the first period of REM sleep ('short REM latency') and also disruption of overnight sleep are present. In children above the age of about 8 years the Multiple Sleep Latency Test (MSLT) is a useful check on abnormal sleepiness and the tendency to rapidly enter REM sleep. A negative result on human leucocyte antigen (HLA) typing (especially for type DQBI*0602) makes the diagnosis of narcolepsy unlikely.

Management, which needs to be lifelong, consists of stimulant medication to combat the child's sleepiness and (if necessary) antidepressant-type drugs such as clomipramine for cataplexy and the other components of the narcolepsy syndrome. Further medication possibilities have been discussed by Guilleminault and Pelayo (2000). Other important measures include planned daytime naps and explanation of the condition to all concerned (to prevent misinterpretation of the symptoms), as well as long-term support and advice.

Other causes of an increase in sleep tendency are:
- the rare condition of *idiopathic CNS hypersomnia* (sometimes of early onset and consisting of considerable difficulty waking or staying awake during the day in spite of sound sleep but without the characteristic features of narcolepsy)
- the *Kleine–Levin syndrome* (classically a condition of males, starting in adolescence, in which periods of excessively long sleep accompanied by overeating, hypersexuality and other abnormal behaviours alternate with periods of normality)
- *seasonal affective disorder* or *SAD* (excessive sleepiness combined with depression and other abnormal behaviour confined to the winter months)
- *menstruation-related hypersomnia*
- *chronic medical conditions* (often with 'physical tiredness')
- *toxic states*
- *sedative medication* or the effects of *illicit drugs*
- (rarely) *nonconvulsive status epilepticus.*

Persistent sleepiness may also follow various *infections* such as infectious mononucleosis and Lyme disease.

A constitutional tendency to sleep for long periods (*congenital long sleeper*) should not be diagnosed without the various other explanations being considered. The rare condition (especially in children) of *idiopathic recurring stupor* (caused by an endogenous benzodiazepine-like substance and reversible with flumazenil) can be mistaken for a sleep disorder.

REFERENCES

Guilleminault, C., Pelayo, R. (2000) 'Narcolepsy in children. A practical guide to its diagnosis, treatment and follow up.' *Paediatric Drugs*, **2**, 1–9.

Loughlin, G.M., Carroll, J.L., Marcus, C.L. (Eds.) (2000) *Sleep and Breathing in Children.* New York: Marcel Dekker.

Mitler, M.M. (1996) 'Sleepiness and human behaviour.' *Current Opinion in Pulmonary Medicine*, **2**, 488–491.

Sheldon, S.H., Spire, J-P., Levy, H.B. (1992) 'Sleep wake schedule disorders.' *In:* Sheldon, S.H., Spire, J-P., Levy, H.B. (Eds.) *Pediatric Sleep Medicine.* Philadelphia: W.B. Saunders, pp. 106–118.

Stores, G. (1999) 'Recognition and management of narcolepsy.' *Archives of Disease in Childhood*, **81**, 519–524.

6
EPISODIC DISTURBANCES OF SLEEP (PARASOMNIAS)

Gregory Stores

The parasomnias are recurrent episodes of behaviour, experiences and/or physiological changes that occur exclusively or predominantly in relation to sleep. Some are *primary* sleep phenomena, others are *secondary* in the sense that they are manifestations of a physical or psychiatric disorder. There are many types of parasomnias that, it seems, are often confused with each other. This problem often occurs in children with nocturnal epilepsy, as discussed shortly. Children may have more than one variety of parasomnia.

The essential requirement for correct diagnosis is careful clinical description of the episodes in question, combined with an awareness of the characteristic features of each type of parasomnia. In any episodic disturbance it is important to obtain, as far as possible, details of the sequence of objective and subjective events from the very first change until the episode is concluded. The timing and circumstances in which the episodes occur are also very important. Audiovisual recordings (including home recordings) can be a valuable means of obtaining an accurate description.

Polysomnography (PSG) is only required if the diagnosis remains unclear despite a careful description, if there might be more than one type of parasomnia, if there might be coexisting different types of sleep disorder, or (rarely) if the physiological findings are required for a precise diagnosis (as in REM sleep behaviour disorder, discussed later). Sometimes it is useful to know from PSG if the child is actually asleep during the episodes as there are some reports of disturbed behaviour being enacted during apparent sleep.

Most primary parasomnias, however dramatic they might appear, do not mean that the child is physically ill or psychologically disturbed, and most cease spontaneously in time. Possible exceptions requiring further investigation (especially into psychological aspects) are those that are very frequent, start at a later age than usual, persist well beyond the age at which they normally cease, or recur after previously having stopped. If they follow some form of traumatic experience they may be one aspect of a serious emotional disturbance.

Table 6.1 shows the main types of primary parasomnia grouped according to the stage or phase of sleep in which they usually occur. This basis for classifying the parasomnias may not wholly apply in children with brain dysfunction severe enough to seriously affect sleep architecture. Parasomnias have been little studied in such children.

Presleep and sleep onset
Many people experience sudden single bodily jerks when drifting off to sleep. This is one

TABLE 6.1
The primary parasomnias

Sleep onset	REM sleep
Sleep starts	Nightmares
Hypnagogic hallucinations	REM sleep behaviour disorder
Sleep paralysis	
Rhythmic movement disorder	**Waking**
Restless legs syndrome	Hypnopompic hallucinations
	Sleep paralysis
Light NREM sleep	
Bruxism	**Inconsistently related to stage of sleep**
Periodic limb movements in sleep	Sleep talking
Deep NREM sleep	Nocturnal enuresis
Arousal disorders (confusional arousals,	Other primary parasomnias
sleepwalking, sleep terrors)	Overlap parasomnia disorder
	Sleep-related eating disorder

form of *sleep start*, which can also take the form of a loud bang, snap, or other sudden, very brief and often alarming sensory experience. Almost always these experiences are benign. Repetitive sleep starts have sometimes been mistaken for myoclonic seizures in neurologically impaired children. *Hypnagogic hallucinations* in various sensory modalities may accompany sleep starts and can also form part of the narcolepsy syndrome, but far more often they occur sporadically as an isolated phenomenon. Again, although potentially alarming, they do not signify serious disorder. *Hypnopompic hallucinations* is the term used to describe their equivalent on waking. *Sleep paralysis*, on going to sleep or waking up, can also be part of the narcolepsy syndrome but is also quite common as an isolated phenomenon, again capable of being very frightening but in itself benign. Tricyclic drugs are effective for these hallucinatory phenomena and for sleep paralysis if treatment is required.

The term *rhythmic movement disorder* covers head banging, head rolling, body rolling and other repetitive stereotypic movements, usually before going to sleep. Possibly the movements facilitate sleep onset, or return to sleep if they occur during the night. Such movements occur in perhaps the majority of very young children, usually stopping spontaneously by 3–4 years of age at the latest. They can be alarming for parents to witness (especially if the child bangs his head against the cot sides or other hard surface) and generally disruptive if the impact of the movements is noisy, or if the child makes loud rhythmic noises as well. In fact, the child is usually otherwise normal and is unlikely to seriously injure himself, although padding or some other protective measure may be needed. Where necessary, various behavioural treatments can be effective (Thorpy 1990). These sleep-related rhythmic movements should be distinguished from similar movements occurring during the day as part of a widespread behavioural disturbance in children with severe neurodevelopmental or psychiatric disorders.

Restless legs syndrome was mentioned in the last chapter.

Light sleep (NREM stages 1 and 2)
Bruxism or teeth grinding is common. Its main significance is that, if severe, it can cause facial pain or headache and damage to the teeth. Its relation to stress is uncertain.

Periodic limb movements in sleep (Chapter 5) can also be considered as a form of parasomnia.

Deep sleep (NREM stages 3 and 4 or slow wave sleep): arousal disorders
Parasomnias arising in this level of sleep usually occur early in the night when slow wave sleep (SWS) is mainly seen (Chapter 2). This group of parasomnias are called arousal disorders because they involve a sudden partial arousal from SWS to a lighter stage of sleep. The child does not wake up at the time but the arousal is accompanied by various behaviours that can be complicated and even dramatic.

A genetic predisposition to arousal disorders is usual, but sleep loss or disruption, irregular sleep–wake patterns, stress or acute illness influence the frequency of the episodes. Although spontaneous remission eventually occurs in most cases, embarrassment and accidental injury can be problems in the meantime.

There are three basic types of arousal disorder: confusional arousals, sleepwalking and sleep terrors. In all types there is a curious combination of seeming to be awake in some respects yet actually remaining asleep. The patient is unaware that the episode has occurred unless (as happens more in adolescence or adulthood) awakening occurs at the end of the episode, often with a report of threatening experience (but not the unfolding narrative typical of a nightmare).

Confusional arousals occur mainly in small children who may appear very agitated and distressed but unresponsive to their parents' attempts to console them. *Sleepwalking* can consist of relatively calm wandering in a semi-purposeful way (again, only partly responsive at most) or moving about frenetically in an agitated fashion. Habitual behaviour during sleep-walking can involve a complicated sequence of actions. As accidental injury (for example, from falling downstairs or through a bedroom window) is a serious risk, the environment should be made as safe as possible. There is a similar risk with *sleep terrors* (or *night terrors*), in which the degree of agitation and apparent fear is particularly striking, with the child possibly rushing about in a seeming attempt to escape danger.

In all these dramatic episodes, parents understandably feel the need to comfort the child and may make vigorous attempts to bring them round in order to do so. This should be discouraged. It is difficult to rouse someone from deep sleep, but, if achieved, this is likely to cause real confusion and distress. Instead, the episode should be allowed to subside of its own accord until the child resumes restful sleep, often quite rapidly in the case of sleep terrors. There may be little point telling the child about the night's events if he has not woken up and does not know about them.

Arousal disorders should be distinguished from other dramatic disturbances at night such as epileptic attacks and nightmares. The main distinguishing features are shown in Table 6.2. Other conditions to consider include gastro-oesophageal reflux in young children, awakenings associated with obstructive sleep apnoea (OSA) and panic attacks in older children.

Management, in addition to the advice already mentioned, involves explanation and (in most cases) reassurance. Good sleep hygiene is also important. If the episodes are frequent and the timing of the episodes consistent, 'scheduled awakening' (in which, over

TABLE 6.2
Comparison of main features of partial arousals, nightmares and nocturnal seizures

	Partial arousals	*Nightmares*	*Nocturnal seizures**
Time of night	Usually first third of night	Middle to last third of night	Variable
Usual stage of sleep	Deep NREM	REM	Variable
Behaviour	Variable but usually dramatic apart from calm sleepwalking; often inaccessible and cannot be comforted; may resist intervention	Distressed by frightening dream, accessible and welcomes comforting	Variable, may be undirected violence or distress during or after attack
Level of consciousness	Unaware during episode, confused if awakened or following episode	Asleep during episode, fully awake afterwards	Variable
Likelihood of injury	Moderate	Low	Low
Memory for events	None	Vivid recall	Variable
Family history	Common	None	Variable
Prevalence	Common	Common	Much less common

*In view of the wide range of types of epileptic seizure associated with sleep, the descriptions given are generalizations, but certain clear exceptions to the general rule should be noted (see text).

a period of about two weeks, the child is regularly woken for a short period of time before the arousal is due) might reduce the frequency of the episodes. Short-term medication (*e.g.* a benzodiazepine) is sometimes justified. Increasing feelings of self-control over the episodes has also been suggested as being useful.

REM sleep parasomnias

Being frightening dreams, *nightmares* are obviously related to REM (or dreaming) sleep. Typically they occur late in the night when REM sleep is most prominent (Chapter 2). The term should be reserved for genuine nightmares, avoiding the tendency to refer to any dramatic nocturnal episode as a nightmare. Nightmares are common and not usually particularly significant, although they can be precipitated by illness or by stress in which case there may be accompanying night-time fears. Abrupt withdrawal from REM-suppressing medication can also trigger nightmares because of the rebound effect of increased REM sleep later in the night. The extent of treatment depends on cause and severity. Behavioural and cognitive–behavioural approaches are said to be effective (Owens *et al.* 1999).

In *REM sleep behaviour disorder* the usual paralysis of the skeletal musculature seen in REM sleep is absent with the result that dreams can be enacted. Depending on dream content, this can result in dramatic, even violent, behaviour in which injury can occur. The condition is described mainly in adults, often in association with neurodegenerative disorders or medication, but childhood cases are reported. Diagnosis depends on a combination of clinical description and PSG demonstration of the atypical REM sleep features. In adult series, treatment with clonazepam has almost always been effective.

Waking

Hypnopompic hallucinations and *sleep paralysis* were described earlier.

Primary parasomnias inconsistently related to stage of sleep

These include *sleep talking*, which can occur in various sleep disorders or independently.

Nocturnal enuresis (recurrent involuntary bedwetting above the age of 5 years) is very common, persisting into the teenage years in perhaps 1 per cent of the general population. It is said to be 'primary' if bladder control has never been achieved (the majority of cases) and 'secondary' if there is a loss of control after being dry at night for at least six months. In most cases enuresis seems to be a problem of delayed maturation, but unsatisfactory toileting practices, overall developmental delay and psychological stress (especially in secondary enuresis) are sometimes implicated. It is important to exclude organic causes of bedwetting such as urinary tract abnormalities, epilepsy and diabetes insipidus. The most effective forms of treatment are conditioning by means of an alarm system and reward programmes. Desmopressin and also tricyclic drugs (less favoured because of potential cardiotoxic effects) are effective second-line treatments but with a high relapse rate when withdrawn. Other aspects of management include bladder training, improvement of possible negative attitudes to the child and, where necessary, psychiatric help.

Other primary parasomnias

Complex parasomnias have been described, sometimes in children, in which features of different primary parasomnias are combined. *Overlap parasomnia disorder* refers to a combination of arousal disorder and REM sleep behaviour disorder. *Sleep-related eating disorders* are described in people (including adolescents) with daytime eating disorders, but perhaps their association is more with other sleep disorders such as sleepwalking, OSA, narcolepsy or other causes of disrupted sleep.

Secondary parasomnias (Table 6.3)

The clinical manifestations of many physical and psychiatric disorders include disturbances during sleep.

Nocturnal epilepsy is a prime example. In the following epilepsies encountered in children, seizures are closely linked to sleep:

- *mesial frontal epilepsy* characterized by complicated motor automatisms and vocalizations to the extent that the seizures are often not recognized as epileptic at all. The brief type of paroxysmal nocturnal dystonia is a form of this type of epilepsy
- *benign partial epilepsy with centro-temporal (rolandic) spikes*, a common form of childhood epilepsy in which seizures usually have characteristic orofacial features
- some *seizures of temporal lobe origin* including those with prominent affective symptoms, which can be mistaken for night terrors
- the same mistake can be made in *benign epilepsy with affective symptoms*
- *benign occipital epilepsy* can also involve behaviour reminiscent of dramatic primary parasomnias.

Recognition of these forms of epilepsy depends on accurate clinical descriptions and

TABLE 6.3
Secondary parasomnias

Nocturnal epilepsies

Other physical disorders
Headaches
Respiratory disorders
Gastrointestinal conditions
Nocturnal muscle cramps
Cardiac arrhythmias
Sustained sleep starts
Some cases of restless legs syndrome or
  periodic limb movements in sleep

Psychiatric disorders
Post-traumatic stress disorder
Nocturnal panic attacks
Other (including psychogenic dissociative
  states and 'pseudoparasomnias')

appropriate EEG studies, preferably including recordings taken during the attacks. The possibility of a combination of epilepsy and other sleep disorders, such as OSA, should be considered.

Other parasomnias of physical origin include headaches of a migrainous type, respiratory events (*e.g.* in asthma or OSA), gastro-oesophageal reflux and cardiac arrhythmias.

Parasomnias secondary to psychiatric disorders and sometimes seen in children include:
• acute disturbances during sleep as part of *post-traumatic stress disorder*. Although often referred to as 'nightmares', they may take the form of different types of parasomnia
• nocturnal *panic attacks*, the key features of which are intense sympathetic arousal and a fear of sudden death or other serious illness. Sometimes there are no associated panic attacks during the day
• *'psychogenic dissociative states'* in which dramatic behaviour is enacted at night but while actually awake as demonstrated by PSG. The degree of conscious awareness in such episodes may vary from one case to another. The term 'pseudoparasomnia' has been used when consciousness is preserved.

REFERENCES

Owens, L.J., France, K.G., Wiggs, L. (1999) 'Behavioural and cognitive–behavioural interventions for sleep disorders in infants and children: a review.' *Sleep Medicine Reviews*, **3**, 281–302.
Thorpy, M.J. (1990) 'Rhythmic movement disorder.' *In:* Thorpy, M.J. (Ed.) *Handbook of Sleep Disorders.* New York: Marcel Dekker, pp. 609–629.

SECTION TWO

NEURODEVELOPMENTAL
DISORDERS

7
GENERAL ASPECTS OF SLEEP AND INTELLECTUAL IMPAIRMENT

Luci Wiggs and Gregory Stores

The connection between intellectual impairment and sleep disorders deserves particular attention because many of the developmental disorders discussed in the later chapters are often associated with such impairment, and also because intellectual impairment may give rise to sleep disturbance in a variety of ways.

Severe and often persistent sleep problems are reported by parents of intellectually impaired children, mostly taking the form of sleeplessness of one type or another (Chapter 4). Predictably, such problems can seriously affect parental health and family cohesion. These findings are important, but an understanding of the ways in which the sleep problems have arisen is often hampered by the mixed nature of the groups studied with regard to such factors as the cause of the child's condition and its severity, associated problems and family circumstances. As there is likely to be considerable advantage in studying sleep disorders in much more homogenous groups, the present book is concerned with separate types of disorder in the belief that this aids understanding of the origins of the sleep problems associated with each condition and what needs to be done to help.

That apart, there are certain general points that can be made about the psychosocial (including family) factors that might contribute to the development or maintenance of sleep problems in children with an intellectual impairment. Further, as a reflection of the currently available literature, reference has been made to studies of heterogeneous groups of children insofar as they illustrate general management issues.

Sleep disturbance
Reports of sleep and sleep disturbance in young people with intellectual impairment have generally taken one of two forms—accounts of sleep physiology (with or without reference to any clinical manifestations accompanying the detected abnormalities), or descriptions of sleep problems or presenting symptoms—unfortunately often without consideration of the basic underlying sleep disorders.

PHYSIOLOGY OF SLEEP IN CHILDREN WITH AN INTELLECTUAL IMPAIRMENT
The sleep physiology of children with intellectual impairments has been the subject of research although the findings need to be treated with some caution due to a number of factors. First, investigations have often been concerned with describing groups of children with intellectual impairment of mixed aetiology and different degrees of severity. Second,

epilepsy is, of course, more common in people with intellectual impairments, but the disrupting effect of this condition or its treatment upon sleep (see Chapter 15) is often not considered. This is of particular concern as Quine (1991) found epilepsy to be one of the factors associated with a severe sleep problem in the intellectually impaired children that she studied. However, certain points arising from the literature are of interest.

Not surprisingly, the extent to which sleep physiology is disrupted depends on the extent of brain damage or dysfunction.

Okawa and Sasaki (1987) have described how extensive and severe brain damage, usually occurring in the perinatal period, produces an 'acerebrate' state with little response to external stimuli and usually a highly irregular sleep–wake pattern. This is attributable to damage to the many integrated systems, notably the brainstem ascending reticular formation on which wakefulness depends, pontine and forebrain structures that regulate REM and NREM sleep, and the suprachiasmatic nuclei and connections that control sleep–wake rhythms. In these circumstances, usual sleep phenomena described in Chapter 2 (such as sleep spindles and vertex sharp waves) are absent. As a result, it is difficult to physiologically distinguish awake and asleep states ('monostage sleep'). Even in cases where this distinction could be made clinically to some extent, non-ambulant, profoundly intellectually impaired children and adults were described by Landesman-Dwyer and Sackett (1978) as spending almost 21 hours per day in sleep or low-level activity and only three hours in moderate to high levels of wakefulness. The timing of sleep and wakefulness was highly irregular.

Children with less severely damaged brains, but still lacking normal sensory appreciation of their environment, and with limited development of social relationships, may have abnormal sleep–wake patterns, perhaps because of a combination of damage to basic brain structures and failure to register the other cues to day and night also described in Chapter 2.

The relationship between REM sleep and intellectual level has been an issue since early studies of sleep physiology in intellectually impaired children. Partly because the proportion of REM sleep is high in neonates and decreases as the infant matures, it has been considered that this stage of sleep is particularly involved in information processing and other aspects of the learning process. Interestingly, a relative deficiency or other abnormalities in REM sleep have been described as a nonspecific finding in intellectual impairment of various aetiologies. There have been reports of fewer and/or shorter REM sleep periods and fewer eye movements ('low REM density') (Feinberg et al. 1969), generally more obvious the lower the child's level of intelligence (Grubar 1983).

Attention has also been given to sleep spindle activity (normally a feature of Stage 2 NREM sleep) as another possible indication of intellectual impairment at a given age. In intellectually impaired children in general, abnormalities are often seen. They may be absent, unusually diffusely distributed, high-voltage and continuous ('extreme spindles'), or their amount in infancy and their subsequent pattern of development may be abnormal (Shibagaki et al. 1982). As in the REM sleep abnormalities just described, the interest in these various unusual features is the evidence that they indicate abnormal brain development. The other polysomnographic features inconsistently described in children with an intellectual

impairment, such as an increase in Stage 4 NREM sleep (Petre-Quadens and Jouvet 1967) and prolonged time to the first REM sleep period, are not specific to intellectual impairment.

Despite the various abnormalities described in these reports, it seems that the overall pattern of developmental changes seen in children in general (*e.g.* decrease in total sleep time and in the proportion of REM sleep) are the same in even severely intellectually impaired children (Shibagaki *et al.* 1985, Piazza *et al.* 1996).

SLEEP PROBLEMS

Although there have been only a limited number of studies looking at sleep problems in intellectually impaired children and adolescents, the available evidence suggests that the prevalence of these problems is alarmingly high in this population. Pahl and Quine (1984) studied 200 children, aged up to 18 years, and found that 51 per cent were described by mothers as having settling difficulties and 67 per cent as having night waking at least a few times a week. Bartlett *et al.* (1985) reported that of 214 intellectually impaired children up to 16 years old, 86 per cent of those under 6 years, 81 per cent of those aged 6 to 11 years, and 77 per cent of the 12- to 16-year-olds were reported by parents to have 'sleep problems'. Settling difficulties and night waking were the most common problems, with 56 per cent waking on average once a night and 56 per cent being difficult to settle once in bed (53 per cent were reluctant to go to bed in the first place). Similarly high prevalences of settling and night-waking difficulties were reported by Pahl and Quine (1984). Somewhat lower rates were described by Clements *et al.* (1986) in their questionnaire study of 155 children under 15 years old. Sleep problems were present in 34 per cent, with about 13 per cent having night waking, 13 per cent limited sleep duration, and 8 per cent both night waking and limited sleep duration. The fact that settling difficulties were not considered, as well as the somewhat eclectic nature of the sample (*i.e.* the sample included children with intellectual impairment *and* those receiving special education who also displayed some behaviour found in early childhood psychoses), may explain the reduced occurrence of sleep problems compared with other studies. Piazza *et al.* (1996) used a momentary time-sampling observational method to investigate the sleep of 51 young people (aged 3–21 years) with sleep problems and severe behaviour disorder on an inpatient unit. They reported reduced total sleep time and night-time sleep, compared to peers, mainly due to delayed sleep onset, night wakings and early wakings.

The above publications have focused on sleeplessness but Wiggs and Stores (1996a) gathered questionnaire data on 209 children (aged 5–16 years) with severe intellectual impairment, asking parents to report on the whole range of sleep problems (*i.e.* types of sleeplessness, excessive sleepiness and parasomnias). Although all forms of sleep disturbance were represented, it was sleeplessness problems that predominated, with severe (*i.e.* occurring most nights or every night) settling, night-waking and/or early-waking problems in 44 per cent of the sample.

These types of sleeplessness frequently coexist (Quine 1992, Wiggs and Stores 1996a) and appear to be very persistent. Quine (1991) performed a three-year follow-up of the subjects in an earlier study (Pahl and Quine 1984) and found that 48 per cent of children with settling problems still had such problems, as did 66 per cent of the children with night-waking

problems. In addition, 21 per cent of children had developed sleep problems that were not present three years previously.

Aetiological factors

Various physical and psychosocial factors might combine to predispose children with intellectual impairments to the development of disturbed sleep.

- The physiological abnormalities associated with severe and extensive brain maldevelopment or damage have already been described.
- Teaching an intellectually impaired child good sleep habits may be more than usually difficult. Possible reasons for this include problems of communication with the child, which featured prominently in Quine's (1991) analysis of factors associated with sleep problems in children with severe intellectual impairments.
- Out of compassion for their child and because of guilt feelings, parents may feel unable to impose discipline in the way that is usually needed to avoid bedtime problems and to avoid the child's overdependence on them when settling to sleep or on waking during the night.
- The task of establishing good sleep habits is made more difficult if the child is emotionally or behaviourally disturbed, and such problems are encountered in intellectually impaired children more than in other children (Borthwick-Duffy 1994). As mentioned earlier, the same is true if the child's parents are demoralized or psychologically disturbed, or there is disharmony between them including in relation to their approach to the child's problems. Unfortunately, these also are not uncommon difficulties in families with intellectually impaired children.
- Even in the absence of such additional complications, parents of intellectually impaired children may view sleep difficulties as an inevitable part of the child's basic condition. Unless told otherwise, they may well not realize that with appropriate early advice it may be possible to prevent or minimize such problems, or to treat them effectively even when the sleep problem is severe or of long standing and also despite the child's behaviour being severely disturbed (or 'challenging') (Wiggs and Stores 1998).

Management considerations

As with all childhood sleep problems, management decisions need to be based on careful assessment of the individual child. While an individualized approach may be particularly appropriate for children with intellectual impairments, all of whom have different abilities and needs, the same types of treatments for sleep disorders that are used with children from the general population are increasingly being found to be of use for children with intellectual impairments. For example, as reviewed by Lancioni et al. (1999) and Wiggs and France (2000), behavioural treatments have been used successfully to treat problems of sleeplessness, excessive sleepiness and certain forms of parasomnias; chronotherapy has been reported as useful for sleep–wake cycle disorders; and melatonin has also been employed, although results have been mixed (perhaps unsurprisingly given the inconsistencies and uncertainties surrounding its use). The overwhelming message seems to be that intellectual impairment (and any coexisting problems including physical conditions and severe behaviour problems)

should not be viewed as inevitable obstacles to successful resolution of childhood sleep problems.

However, certain aspects of management need special consideration in the case of children with intellectual impairments.

- Behavioural approaches that employ 'ignoring' the child (so-called 'extinction' procedures, discussed in Chapter 4), whilst they have been used effectively, may well be less appropriate than modifications of such methods (*i.e.* 'graduated' procedures) for a variety of reasons. This is particularly the case if a child has a coexisting physical condition (such as epilepsy, breathing disorder or difficulty changing his position in bed) that may require his parents' attention during the night. Understandably, parents find extinction techniques unacceptable in these circumstances.
- Reports and clinical experience suggest that, while the majority of parents of children with intellectual impairments will have had past experience of severe sleep problems in their child, they may have had little positive experience of successful treatment for these sleep problems (Wiggs and Stores 1996b). Therefore, the therapist needs to be sensitive to their possible scepticism about the likely success of a further course of treatment. It is appropriate to strike an optimistic note that treatment is likely to be effective if carried out consistently and with conviction.
- On a more positive note, it may be that, for children attending school, the parents and the therapist may be particularly likely to find practical support for any treatment from the child's teachers. The exchange of information (*e.g.* about the child's behaviour, sleepiness or nap schedules) between parents and teachers of children with intellectual impairments is often more frequent and more complete than for other children (*e.g.* daily diary notebooks are often standard). Further, teachers at special schools are often particularly familiar with behavioural approaches and willing to reinforce any home-based interventions in any way they can.

The associations between sleep disturbance and daytime functioning, including learning and behaviour (and also parenting) were outlined in Chapter 1. Because children with intellectual impairments are already psychologically compromised, it is especially important to address any potentially modifiable factors, such as sleep disturbance, that might be compounding their problems (or affecting the health and welfare of other family members, notably parents). Indeed, the treatment of the sleep disorder may offer one of the few opportunities to significantly help the intellectually impaired child and his family when the basic condition cannot be influenced.

REFERENCES

Bartlett, L.B., Rooney, V., Spedding, S. (1985) 'Nocturnal difficulties in a population of mentally handicapped children.' *British Journal of Mental Subnormality*, **31**, 54–59.
Borthwick-Duffy, S.A. (1994) 'Epidemiology and prevalence of psychopathology in people with mental retardation.' *Journal of Consulting and Clinical Psychology*, **62**, 17–27.
Clements, J., Wing, L., Dunn, G. (1986) 'Sleep problems in handicapped children: a preliminary study.' *Journal of Child Psychology and Psychiatry*, **27**, 399–407.
Feinberg, I., Braun, M., Shulman, E. (1969) 'EEG sleep patterns in mental retardation.' *Electroencephalography and Clinical Neurophysiology*, **27**, 128–141.

Grubar, J.C. (1983) 'Sleep and mental deficiency.' *Review of Electroencephalography and Neurophysiology*, **13**, 107–114.

Lancioni, G.E., O'Reilly, M.F., Basili, G. (1999) 'Review of strategies for treating sleep problems in persons with severe or profound mental retardation or multiple handicaps.' *American Journal on Mental Retardation*, **104**, 170–186.

Landesman-Dwyer, S., Sackett, G.P. (1978) 'Behavioral change in nonambulatory, profoundly mentally retarded individuals.' *Monographs of the American Association of Mental Deficiency*, **3**, 55–144.

Okawa, M., Sasaki, H. (1987) 'Sleep disorders in mentally retarded and brain-impaired children.' *In:* Guilleminault, C. (Ed.) *Sleep and its Disorders in Children*. New York: Raven Press, pp. 269–290.

Pahl, J., Quine, L. (1984) *Families with Mentally Handicapped Children: A Study of Stress and of Service Response*. Canterbury: University of Kent, Health Services Research Unit.

Petre-Quadens, O., Jouvet, M. (1967) 'Sleep in the mentally retarded.' *Journal of Neurological Science*, **4**, 354–357.

Piazza, C.C., Fisher, W.W., Kahng, S.W. (1996) 'Sleep patterns in children and young adults with mental retardation and severe behaviour disorders.' *Developmental Medicine and Child Neurology*, **38**, 335–344.

Quine, L. (1991) 'Sleep problems in children with severe mental handicap.' *Journal of Mental Deficiency Research*, **35**, 269–290.

—— (1992) 'Severity of sleep problems in children with severe learning difficulties: description and correlates.' *Journal of Community and Applied Social Psychology*, **2**, 247–268.

Shibagaki, M., Kiyono, S., Watanabe, K. (1982) 'Spindle evolution in normal and mentally retarded children: a review.' *Sleep*, **5**, 47–57.

—— —— Yutaka, M. (1985) 'Nocturnal sleep of severely mentally retarded children and adolescents: Ontogeny of sleep patterns.' *American Journal of Mental Deficiency*, **90**, 212–216.

Wiggs, L., France, K (2000) 'Behavioural treatments for sleep problems in children and adolescents with physical illness, psychological problems or intellectual disabilities.' *Sleep Medicine Reviews*, **4**, 299–314.

—— Stores, G. (1996a) 'Severe sleep disturbance and daytime challenging behaviour in children with severe learning disabilities.' *Journal of Intellectual Disability Research*, **40**, 518–528.

—— —— (1996b) 'Sleep problems in children with severe learning disabilities: What help is being provided?' *Journal of Applied Research in Intellectual Disabilities*, **9**, 160–165.

—— —— (1998) 'Behavioural treatment for sleep problems in children with severe learning disabilities and daytime challenging behaviour: Effect on sleep patterns of mother and child.' *Journal of Sleep Research*, **7**, 119–126.

8
SLEEP AND DOWN SYNDROME

Rebecca Stores

Down syndrome is the most common genetic cause of intellectual impairment. It occurs in approximately 1 in 600 live births, the incidence increasing with maternal age. First described by Dr James Langdon Down in 1866, its underlying chromosomal abnormality (trisomy 21) was identified by Lejeune and colleagues in 1959. Three main genotypes are now recognized: trisomy 21 (accounting for about 95% of cases), translocation (4%) and mosaicism (1%). Roizen (1997) provides a comprehensive account of the condition.

The most common physical features associated with the condition are upward and outward slanting eyes, epicanthic folds at the inner corners, flattened appearance of the face, small ears, mouth, hands and feet, incurving little finger and often a single transverse crease on the palm. The head is small and stature short and there is generalized hypotonia. Children with Down syndrome have an increased risk of abnormality in many bodily systems, especially congenital heart defects, visual and hearing impairment, endocrine abnormalities, dental problems and skin disorders. Perhaps as many as 15 to 20 per cent develop Alzheimer's disease from the age of 40 years.

Virtually all children with Down syndrome have some degree of developmental delay, with cognitive, language, social and motor development being the most affected. The range of intellectual impairment is wide with some children falling within the normal range for the general population and capable of coping within mainstream education. The conventional stereotype of the child with Down syndrome as always good tempered, affectionate and cheerful is not supported by research in which a wide range of behaviours have been reported including different types of behavioural problems such as conduct disorders, aggressive behaviour and attention deficit hyperactivity disorder (ADHD) (Cuskelly and Dadds 1992).

Recent research has led to a much better understanding of the ways in which Down syndrome can affect physical and psychological development, and assessment and intervention programmes are now being implemented to minimize or prevent the various problems to which such children are prone. The impression gained, however, is that sleep problems and their psychological consequences are often not sufficiently considered.

Types of sleep disturbance
Studies of sleep abnormalities in children with Down syndrome can be grouped into the following three main types.

SLEEP DISTURBANCES REPORTED BY PARENTS
High rates of sleep disturbance, compared with other non-intellectually-impaired children, have been described consistently.

Cunningham *et al.* (1986) studied the sleep problems, as reported by parents, of children with Down syndrome aged 5 to 10 years. Compared with a general population sample, a significantly higher proportion were said to have settling and night-waking problems at all ages. The authors considered that these sleep difficulties were mainly related to difficulties within the family such as maternal stress, poor mother–child relationships and lack of family cohesion. This interpretation was different to that of Quine (1992), who, in her investigations of sleep problems in children with severe intellectual impairment of various aetiologies, emphasized the role of child development factors such as poor communication and self-help skills. In the same series of studies, Quine (1991) reported that 44 per cent of children with Down syndrome showed sleep problems, compared to 56 per cent of those children within her sample who had nonspecific forms of intellectual impairment.

Parental questionnaires were used by Epstein *et al.* (1992) in their study in which 69 per cent of children with Down syndrome were said to have difficulty settling to sleep and 46 per cent had troublesome night-waking. In addition, snoring or otherwise noisy breathing at night was reported in over a third to nearly a half of the children, and 12 per cent of parents described obvious apnoeas during sleep. About a third of the children were said to habitually sit up in bed during sleep for reasons that were unclear. Settling and night-waking problems, as well as sitting up in bed and restless sleep, were also found by Fields *et al.* (1995) to be significantly more common in a group of children with Down syndrome, aged 6 months to 19 years, than in the general population.

Using a parental questionnaire that covered a wide range of possible symptoms of childhood sleep disturbance, Stores *et al.* (1996) compared children with Down syndrome, their siblings, children with intellectual disability other than Down syndrome, and children from the general population. The four groups were broadly comparable for age, sex ratio and socioeconomic background. The children with Down syndrome and the mixed intellectually disabled group were similar regarding type of school attended, and were population-based rather than drawn from children referred to specialized centres. In keeping with other reports, the main findings were that although children with intellectual disability (irrespective of its cause) had significantly more sleep problems in general than their non-intellectually-impaired counterparts, the pattern of the reported sleep problems was distinctive in the children with Down syndrome. Settling and night-waking problems were equally prominent in the two groups, but, characteristically, the children with Down syndrome also displayed features suggestive of sleep-related breathing problems. Sleep patterns in the siblings of the children with Down syndrome were no different to those of children in the general population. Overall, the findings support the need to make a distinction in children with intellectual impairment between 'behavioural' sleep problems (*i.e.* settling and night-waking problems mainly resulting from failure to learn satisfactory sleep habits) and 'physical' sleep disorders reflecting organic influences, which, in the case of Down syndrome, concern disordered respiratory function during sleep.

THE ANATOMICAL AND PHYSIOLOGICAL BASIS OF SLEEP-RELATED BREATHING PROBLEMS
There is now ample objective evidence that children with Down syndrome are especially

prone to sleep-related breathing problems, although the exact prevalence is unclear because of possible referral bias in the series of children studied. As discussed in Chapter 5, it is acknowledged that there are different types of upper airway obstruction (including the upper airway resistance syndrome) and that clinically significant types will be overlooked if only the full-blown, classical obstructive sleep apnoea (OSA) syndrome is considered. Also, it is likely that many other cases do not come to medical attention because of a general unfamiliarity with upper airway obstruction to which children with Down syndrome are predisposed. This predisposition is caused by such anatomical abnormalities as midfacial and mandibular hypoplasia, large posteriorly placed tongue, enlarged tonsils and adenoids from upper respiratory tract infections, congenital narrowing of the trachea, obesity, and hypotonia of the pharyngeal musculature.

In a number of reported series of children with Down syndrome who have undergone polysomnography, the occurrence of OSA or hypoventilation has been between 50 and 80 per cent (Loughlin *et al.* 1981, Southall *et al.* 1987, Marcus *et al.* 1991, Stebbens *et al.* 1991). More recently, Ferri *et al.* (1997) have emphasized the importance of central apnoea (associated with significant desaturation), which they found to be much more common than obstructive apnoea in a series of 10 children with Down syndrome. They suggested that this might be the result of brainstem dysfunction, reflected by abnormalities in brainstem auditory evoked potentials in such children (Ferri *et al.* 1996). Conceivably, the atlantoaxial subluxation or instability described in a proportion of children with Down syndrome can compromise brainstem control of respiratory function. Other respiratory abnormalities contributing to hypoventilation include pulmonary hypoplasia (Cooney and Thurlbeck 1982). It is thought that nocturnal hypoxia might contribute to the high incidence of pulmonary hypertension in children with Down syndrome (Loughlin *et al.* 1981).

OTHER ASPECTS OF PHYSICAL SLEEP DISTURBANCE
Early physiological sleep studies of children with Down syndrome compared with non-disabled children demonstrated various abnormalities of sleep architecture including disrupted sleep and the nonspecific sleep spindle and REM sleep abnormalities seen in intellectually impaired children in general (Fukuma *et al.* 1974, Clausen *et al.* 1977, Hamaguchi *et al.* 1989). The administration of 5-hydroxytryptophan (on the grounds that people with Down syndrome are deficient in 5-hydroxytrytamine or 5HT) (Petre-Quadens and De Lee 1975) or butoctamide hydrogen succinate (involved in 5HT metabolism) (Gigli *et al.* 1987) was shown to improve REM sleep, but the clinical significance of the changes was unclear.

Another finding in some of these studies was apparently more restless sleep (*i.e.* increased body movements). This was also reported by Levanon *et al.* (1999) in their study of children with Down syndrome aged 1.7 to 8 years, compared with children with primary snoring and healthy control groups. Other features of the children with Down syndrome in that study were more arousals or awakenings and a greater number of shifts from deeper to light levels of NREM sleep. These aspects of 'sleep fragmentation' (Chapter 2) were only partly related to OSA. The authors point to various origins of sleep fragmentation including the less obvious forms of sleep-related breathing disorder. This serves as a reminder of possible comorbid conditions capable of disturbing sleep in children with

Down syndrome. These include the common psychological disorders to which reference has already been made, and associated physical disorders such as sensory deficits (Chapters 18 and 19) and, in a small proportion of cases, epilepsy (Chapter 15) or hypothyroidism.

Significance of sleep disturbance in children with Down syndrome
The above sleep abnormalities are likely to affect the lives of children with Down syndrome in various ways, both psychological and physical.

The adverse effects on cognitive, emotional and behavioural development (and on other members of the family) of persistently disturbed sleep were discussed in Chapter 1. OSA, whatever the cause, has been associated with a wide range of learning and daytime behavioural problems, and psychological improvements have been reported following successful treatment. Although there is much more to be learnt about the relationships between children's sleep-related breathing problems and daytime psychological function (Guilleminault and Pelayo 2000), it is reasonable to assume that improvement of the sleep of children with OSA and related conditions is likely to benefit the child and others involved in his care. Indeed, in intellectually impaired children, where prospects of altering the basic condition are limited, the promotion of better sleep may be a significant way of improving learning and behaviour.

As in other groups of children, those with Down syndrome who have sleep problems are more likely to show cognitive and behavioural disturbance compared with those who sleep well (Brooks *et al.* 1995). In a study of children with Down syndrome by Stores *et al.* (1998), behaviour problems (including irritability and overactivity) and mothers' complaints of their own well-being were most evident where the children's sleep was disrupted at night by repeated waking and extreme restlessness compared with other forms of sleep disturbance, although all reported sleep abnormalities were associated with behavioural problems and maternal stress.

Recognized physical complications of severe OSA (Arens 2000) include cardiovascular abnormalities (especially pulmonary hypertension, which may progress to cor pulmonale and heart failure if untreated) and growth failure, including failure to thrive with very early onset of the sleep-related breathing problem. The cause of the growth impairment remains unclear, but adenotonsillectomy may result in catch-up growth.

Assessment
It follows from the discussion so far that children with Down syndrome merit close attention to their sleep. The assessments described in Chapter 3 for the detection and characterization of sleep disorders are required as a matter of routine in the expectation that behavioural and/or physical disturbances of sleep will be present. Ideally, assessment of respiratory function and also careful sleep studies, as described, for example, by Lefaivre *et al.* (1997), would be performed to identify appropriate forms of treatment. Unfortunately, this degree of detailed assessment appears to be unusual.

Treatment possibilities
Treatment of behavioural sleep disorders by behavioural means (Chapter 4) in children with

Down syndrome should, in principle, be as successful as in other children including those with severe intellectual disability and long-standing sleep problems, even in the presence of severe behavioural disturbance (Wiggs and Stores 1998). However, there seems to have been no systematic study of the effects of behavioural treatment specifically in this group of children. Research on this topic needs to acknowledge the multifactorial origin of sleep disturbance in children with Down syndrome.

Treatment of sleep-disordered breathing in children with Down syndrome appears to be difficult, especially in those with the most impaired neuropsychological function (Brooks *et al.* 1997). Various treatments have been described. The results of adenotonsillectomy have been mixed (Bower and Richmond 1995). More complicated surgical procedures (for the correction of soft tissue and/or skeletal causes of obstruction) might be justified in individual cases (Jacobs *et al.* 1996, Lefaivre *et al.* 1997). Prompt antibiotic treatment of respiratory infections may reduce the likelihood of obstruction (Strome and Strome 1992). Nasal continuous positive airway pressure may be an appropriate and tolerable form of treatment for some children (Marcus *et al.* 1995).

Research

The need for further research on sleep disturbances and their consequences in children with Down syndrome is obvious from this review. The extent of behavioural and physical sleep disorders, including the different types and severity of sleep-related breathing problems, is not known; likewise, the details of different effects on learning and behaviour. Clearly, treatment approaches (based on accurate diagnosis of the sleep disorder) require careful evaluation, and preventive possibilities for the behavioural sleep disturbances need to be explored.

Conclusions

Children with Down syndrome are at risk of various types of sleep disturbance, including sleep-related breathing disorders, the psychological and physical consequences of which can be serious. As part of overall assessment, these possibilities should be considered routinely by means of detailed clinical enquiries and special investigations, as appropriate. Treatment of the sleep disorder is likely to benefit the child and the family as a whole.

REFERENCES

Arens, R. (2000) 'Obstructive sleep apnea in childhood: Clinical features.' *In:* Loughlin, G.M., Carroll, J.L., Marcus, C.L. (Eds.) *Sleep and Breathing in Children.* New York: Marcel Dekker, pp. 575–600.
Bower, C.M., Richmond, D. (1995) 'Tonsillectomy and adenoidectomy in patients with Down syndrome.' *International Journal of Pediatric Otorhinolaryngology*, **33**, 141–148.
Brooks, L.J., Bacevice, A.M., Beebe, A., Taylor, H.G. (1995) 'Relationship between sleep disorders and cognitive function in children with Down syndrome.' *Sleep Research*, **24**, 383. *(Abstract.)*
—— —— —— —— (1997) 'Relationship between neuropsychological function and success of treatment for OSA in children with Down syndrome.' *American Journal of Respiratory and Critical Care Medicine*, **155**, A710. *(Abstract.)*
Clausen, J., Sersen, E. A. Lidsky, A. (1977) 'Sleep patterns in mental retardation: Down's syndrome.' *Electroencephalography and Clinical Neurophysiology*, **43**, 183–191.
Cooney, T.P., Thurlbeck, W.M. (1982) 'Pulmonary hypoplasia in Down's syndrome.' *New England Journal of Medicine*, **307**, 1170–1173.

Cunningham, C., Sloper, T., Rangecroft, A., Knussen, C., Lennings, C., Dixon, I., Reeves, D. (1986) *The Effects of Early Intervention on the Occurrence and Nature of Behaviour Problems in Children with Down's Syndrome.* University of Manchester, Hester Adrian Research Centre.

Cuskelly, M., Dadds, M. (1992). 'Behavioural problems in children with Down's syndrome and their siblings.' *Journal of Child Psychology and Psychiatry*, **33**, 749–761.

Epstein, R., Pillar, D., Tzichinsky, O., Herer, P., Lavie, P. (1992) 'Sleep disturbances in children with Down's syndrome.' *Journal of Sleep Research*, **1**, Suppl. 1, 68. *(Abstract.)*

Ferri, R., Del Gracco, S., Elia, M., Musumeci, S.A., Stefanini, M.C. (1996) 'Age- and height-dependent changes of amplitude and latency of somatosensory evoked potentials in children and young adults with Down's syndrome.' *Neurophysiologie Clinique*, **26**, 321–327.

—— Curzi-Dascalova, L., Del Gracco, S., Elia, M., Musumeci, S.A., Stefanini, M.C. (1997) 'Respiratory patterns during sleep in Down's syndrome: importance of central apnoeas.' *Journal of Sleep Research*, **6**, 134–141.

Fields, D., Egers, J., Griffin, I. (1995) 'Patterns of sleep behavior in children with Down syndrome.' *Sleep Research*, **24**, 95. *(Abstract.)*

Fukuma, E., Umezawa, Y., Kobayashi, K., Motoike, M. (1974) 'Polygraphic study of the nocturnal sleep of children with Down's syndrome and endogenous mental retardation.' *Psychiatrica Neurologia Japonica*, **28**, 333–345.

Gigli, G.L., Grubar, J.C., Colognola, R.M., Amata, M.T., Pollicina, C., Ferri, R., Musumeci, S.A., Bergonzi, P. (1987) 'Butoctamide hydrogen succinate and intensive learning sessions: effect on night sleep of Down's syndrome patients.' *Sleep*, **10**, 563–569.

Guilleminault, C., Pelayo, R. (2000) 'Neuropsychological consequences of disordered breathing during sleep.' *In:* Loughlin, G.M., Carroll, J.L., Marcus, C.L. (Eds.) *Sleep and Breathing in Children.* New York: Marcel Dekker, pp. 575–600.

Hamaguchi, H., Hashimoto, T., Mori, K., Tayama, M. (1989) 'Sleep in the Down syndrome.' *Brain Development*, **11**, 399–406.

Jacobs, I.N., Gray, R.F. Todd, N.W. (1996) 'Upper airway obstruction in children with Down syndrome.' *Archives of Otolaryngology – Head and Neck Surgery*, **122**, 945–950.

Lefaivre, J.F., Cohen, S.R., Burstein, F.D., Simms, C., Scott, P.H., Montgomery, G.L., Graham, L., Kattos, A.V. (1997) 'Down syndrome: Identification and surgical management of obstructive sleep apnea.' *Plastic and Reconstructive Surgery*, **99**, 629–637.

Levanon, A., Tarasiuk, A. Tal, A. (1999) 'Sleep characteristics in children with Down syndrome.' *Journal of Pediatrics*, **134**, 755–760.

Loughlin, G.M., Wynne, J.W., Victoria B.E. (1981) 'Sleep apnea as a possible cause of pulmonary hypertension in Down syndrome.' *Journal of Pediatrics*, **17**, 281–297.

Marcus, C.L., Keens, T.G., Bautista, D.B., von Pechman, W.S., Davidson Ward, S.L. (1991) 'Obstructive sleep apnea in children with Down syndrome.' *Pediatrics*, **88**, 132–139.

—— Ward, S.L.D., Mallery, G.B., Rosen, C.L., Beckerman, R.C., Weese-Mayer, D.E., Brouilette, R.T., Trang, H.T., Brooks, L.J. (1995) 'Use of nasal continuous airway pressure as treatment of childhood obstructive sleep apnea.' *Journal of Pediatrics*, **127**, 88–94.

Petre-Quadens, O., De Lee, C. (1975) '5-hydroxytryptophan and sleep in Down's syndrome.' *Journal of the Neurological Sciences*, **26**, 443–453.

Quine, L. (1991) 'Sleep problems in children with severe mental handicap.' *Journal of Mental Deficiency Research*, **35**, 269–290.

—— (1992) 'Severity of sleep problems in children with severe learning difficulties: description and correlates.' *Journal of Community and Applied Social Psychology*, **2**, 247–268.

Roizen, N.J. (1997) 'Down syndrome.' *In:* Batshaw, M.L. (Ed.) *Children with Disabilities.* Baltimore: Brookes, pp. 361–376.

Southall, D.P., Stebbens, V.A., Mirza, R., Lang, M.H., Croft, C.B. Shinebourne, E.A. (1987) 'Upper airway obstruction with hypoxaemia and sleep disruption in Down's syndrome.' *Developmental Medicine and Child Neurology*, **29**, 734–742.

Stebbens, V.A., Dennis, J., Samuels, M.P., Croft, C.B. Southall, D.P. (1991) 'Sleep-related upper airway obstruction in a cohort with Down's syndrome.' *Archives of Disease in Childhood*, **66**, 1333–1338.

Stores, R., Stores, G., Buckley, S.J. (1996) 'The pattern of sleep problems in children with Down's syndrome and other learning disabilities.' *Journal of Applied Research in Intellectual Disabilities*, **9**, 145–159.

—— —— Fellows, B., Buckley, S. (1998) 'A factor analysis of sleep problems and their psychological

associations in children with Down's syndrome.' *Journal of Applied Research in Intellectual Disabilities*, **11**, 345–354.

Strome, M., Strome, S. (1992) 'Recurrent otitis and sleep obstruction in Down syndrome'. *In:* Lott, I.T., McCoy, E.E. (Eds.) *Down Syndrome Advances in Medical Care.* New York: Wiley-Liss, pp. 127–133.

Wiggs, L., Stores, G. (1998) 'Behavioural treatment of sleep problems in children with severe learning disabilities and challenging daytime behaviour: effect on sleep patterns of mother and child.' *Journal of Sleep Research*, **7**, 119–126.

9
SLEEP DISORDERS AND PRADER–WILLI SYNDROME

Antonio Vela-Bueno, Jesús Oliván-Palacios and Alexandros N. Vgontzas

The Prader–Willi syndrome (PWS) is a congenital condition characterized initially by a decrease in fetal activity, then by muscular hypotonia, obesity, short stature, small hands and feet, hypogonadotropic hypogonadism and mental retardation. Other features include almond-shaped eyes and triangular mouth, as well as insatiable appetite and various behavioural abnormalities. Complications include diabetes, scoliosis and cor pulmonale (Prader *et al.* 1956, Laurance *et al.* 1981, Cassidy 1984, Clarke *et al.* 1989, Butler 1990, Holm *et al.* 1993).

PWS is an autosomal dominant disorder that develops from a failure to express paternally derived genes in the q11–q13 region of chromosome 15 (Nicholls 1993). Deletions in the paternally derived chromosome 15 occur in 70 per cent of PWS patients. The majority of the remaining cases present maternal uniparental disomy 15 (Mascari *et al.* 1992). A failure in normal hypothalamic development has been suggested as a probable mechanism by which the phenotype is expressed.

Characteristic sleep disorders
Early reports on PWS did not include sleep disorders among its clinical features. However, more recent clinical descriptions have identified excessive daytime sleepiness (EDS) as a common finding and a disabling symptom for the patients and a problem for the caretakers (Laurance *et al.* 1981, Vela-Bueno *et al.* 1984, Clarke *et al.* 1989, Kaplan *et al.* 1991, Helbing-Zwanenburg *et al.* 1993, Hertz *et al.* 1993, Clift *et al.* 1994). In keeping with studies of other groups with an intellectual disability, Richdale *et al.* (1999) reported an association between EDS and daytime behavioural disturbance in young people with PWS.

The presence of EDS in a high proportion of PWS patients has been objectively demonstrated by polygraphic sleep studies, such as those using the multiple sleep latency test (Hertz *et al.* 1993, Clift *et al.* 1994), the recording of two one-hour naps (Vgontzas *et al.* 1996a) or the ambulatory monitoring of the sleep–wake continuum (Helbing-Zwanenburg *et al.* 1993). Polygraphic studies have shown a great variability in the nocturnal sleep patterns of PWS patients. This variability is consistent with the heterogeneity of the families' reports about nocturnal sleep, with some patients having normal sleep, others having long sleep duration and others having difficulties falling and staying asleep (Vela-Bueno *et al.* 1984). However, two recent studies showed an association between EDS and depth of nocturnal sleep (Hertz *et al.* 1993, Vgontzas *et al.* 1996a).

The most striking observation in PWS patients since the first polygraphic study (Vela-Bueno *et al.* 1984) has been that of REM sleep abnormalities, the most typical being sleep onset in REM sleep (SOREM). This finding has been confirmed in several night-time studies (Vela-Bueno *et al.* 1984, Sforza *et al.* 1991, Hertz *et al.* 1993). While some other authors did not report REM stage at sleep onset, some of their patients had short REM latencies (Clift *et al.* 1994, Vgontzas *et al.* 1996a). During daytime sleep testing, several studies found SOREM (Sforza *et al.* 1991, Hertz *et al.* 1993, Vgontzas *et al.* 1996a). One study reported SOREM but did not clearly state whether it was at night or during the day (Helbing-Zwanenburg *et al.* 1993). Finally, two studies did not report SOREM at night (Kaplan *et al.* 1991) or during the day (Clift *et al.* 1994). A great variability of REM latencies both between and within subjects has been pointed out (Vela-Bueno *et al.* 1984, Hertz *et al.* 1993, Clift *et al.* 1994, Vgontzas *et al.* 1996a). An increase in the number of REM periods in adult patients has also been reported (Hertz *et al.* 1993), especially in those with shortened REM latencies (Vgontzas *et al.* 1996a). Several studies described the mixture of signs of REM sleep with those of stage 2 (Vela-Bueno *et al.* 1984, Hertz *et al.* 1993, Clift *et al.* 1994), as well as REM fragmentation (Helbing-Zwanenburg *et al.* 1993, Hertz *et al.* 1993).

Only one study (Helbing-Zwanenburg *et al.* 1993) reported symptoms resembling the auxiliary ones of the narcoleptic tetrad. These authors described cataplexy-like episodes in six of their 21 patients.

Although families and caretakers quite often report snoring, noisy respiration, choking (Vela-Bueno *et al.* 1984) and even apnoea (Hertz *et al.* 1993, Clift *et al.* 1994), most studies on samples of PWS patients have not demonstrated that sleep apnoea is common. Some have not found it at all (Vela-Bueno *et al.* 1984, Helbing-Zwanenburg *et al.* 1993, Vgontzas *et al.* 1996b). One study showed only mild sleep apnoea in some patients (Kaplan *et al.* 1991). Another study found significant sleep apnoea in only two children, with most adults showing mild degrees of it (Hertz *et al.* 1993). Finally, one study reported clinically relevant sleep apnoea in most patients (Clift *et al.* 1994). A common finding of several studies was the presence of episodes of spontaneous oxygen desaturation during REM sleep (Vela-Bueno *et al.* 1984, Kaplan *et al.* 1991, Hertz *et al.* 1993, Clift *et al.* 1994).

Aetiological factors

In the first published sleep laboratory study (Vela-Bueno *et al.* 1984) it was speculated that the hypothalamic dysfunction characteristic of PWS could be involved in the mechanisms leading to EDS and REM abnormalities. More recently, other authors have proposed the same hypothesis (Hertz *et al.* 1993). We also postulated a role for such a dysfunction in the origin of nocturnal oxygen desaturation. Obesity has been shown to have a role in the development of sleep-related breathing abnormalities and oxygen desaturation in PWS patients (Hertz *et al.* 1995). Obesity and sleep apnoea, when present, can be compounding factors; when they are corrected (Sforza *et al.* 1991, Vgontzas *et al.* 1995) the sleep abnormalities persist, demonstrating their independence from those factors.

Only one study (Helbing-Zwanenburg *et al.* 1993) has suggested that the sleep disturbances of PWS could be the expression of a narcoleptic syndrome. However, this possibility seems

very unlikely since cataplexy was not well documented and there was no support from the HLA findings. In fact, a recent study suggested that the daytime and night-time sleep profiles of PWS patients with EDS and narcoleptics are quite dissimilar (Vgontzas *et al.* 1996a). Specifically, the intensity of sleepiness in PWS is less than that of narcolepsy, whereas narcolepsy is associated with higher amounts of nocturnal wakefulness than in PWS.

Therefore, EDS and REM abnormalities in PWS are not the consequence of obesity and sleep apnoea (although both may aggravate them) or of a narcoleptic syndrome. Most likely they are expressions of a hypothalamic dysfunction. In fact, morphological changes in the suprachiasmatic nuclei of some PWS patients have been reported (Swaab *et al.* 1987).

It has been suggested that the primary mechanism underlying those sleep abnormalities is a generalized 24 hour hypoarousal (Vgontzas *et al.* 1996a). EDS and REM abnormalities in PWS cannot be explained based on a single genetic model. However, both phenotypes seem to be more common in patients with paternal deletions than in those with maternal uniparental disomy (Vgontzas *et al.* 1996b).

Special considerations of management

The difficult management of the sleep disturbances in patients with PWS has to take into consideration several factors. First of all, complicating conditions such as obesity and sleep apnoea should be treated. However, the use of continuous positive airway pressure may be limited by the low tolerance of some subjects (Clift *et al.* 1994). In some severe cases, tracheostomy may be indicated (Gozal *et al.* 1996).

Stimulant drugs in PWS patients with EDS must be used with caution because of the danger of provoking or exacerbating mood and psychotic disorders, in addition to the risk of dependence. The use of antidepressants such as serotonin reuptake inhibitors, venlafaxine or reboxetine may have a positive impact on alertness, weight, mood and, in some cases, breathing.

REFERENCES

Butler, M.G. (1990) 'Prader–Willi: Current understanding of cause and diagnosis.' *American Journal of Medical Genetics*, **35**, 319–332.

Cassidy, S.B. (1984) 'Prader–Willi syndrome.' *Current Problems in Pediatrics*, **14**, 1–55.

Clarke, D.J., Waters, J., Corbett, J.A. (1989) 'Adults with Prader–Willi syndrome: abnormalities of sleep and behaviour.' *Journal of the Royal Society of Medicine*, **82**, 21–24.

Clift, S., Dahlitz, M., Parkes, J.D. (1994) 'Sleep apnoea in the Prader–Willi syndrome.' *Journal of Sleep Research*, **3**, 121–126.

Gozal D., Torres, J.E., Menendez, A.A. (1996) 'Longitudinal assessment of hypercapnic ventilatory drive after tracheotomy in a patient with the Prader–Willi syndrome.' *European Respiratory Journal*, **9**, 1565–1568.

Helbing-Zwanenburg, B., Kamphuisen, H.A.C., Mourtazaev, M.S. (1993) 'The origin of excessive daytime sleepiness in the Prader–Willi syndrome.' *Journal of Intellectual Disability Research*, **37**, 533–541.

Hertz, G., Cataletto, M., Feinsilver, S.H., Angulo, M. (1993) 'Sleep and breathing patterns in patients with Prader–Willi syndrome (PWS): effects of age and gender.' *Sleep*, **16**, 366–371.

—— —— —— (1995) 'Developmental trends of sleep-disordered breathing in Prader–Willi syndrome: The role of obesity.' *American Journal of Medical Genetics*, **56**, 188–190.

Holm, V.A., Cassidy, S.B., Butler, M.G., Hanchett, J.M., Greenswag, L.R., Whitman, B.Y., Greenberg, F. (1993) 'Prader–Willi syndrome: Consensus diagnostic criteria.' *Pediatrics*, **91**, 398–402.

Kaplan, J., Fredrickson, P.A., Richardson, J.W. (1991) 'Sleep and breathing in patients with the Prader–Willi syndrome.' *Mayo Clinic Proceedings*, **66**, 1124–1126.

Laurance, B.M., Brito, A., Wilkinson, J. (1981) 'Prader–Willi syndrome after age 15 years.' *Archives of Disease in Childhood*, **56**, 181–186.

Mascari, M.J., Gottlieb, W., Rogan, P.K., Butler, M.G., Waller, D.A., Armour, J.A.C., Jeffreys, A.J., Ladda, R.L., Nicholls, R.D. (1992) 'The frequency of uniparental disomy in Prader–Willi syndrome: Implications for molecular diagnosis.' *New England Journal of Medicine*, **326**, 1599–1607.

Nicholls, R.D. (1993) 'Genomic imprinting and candidate genes in the Prader–Willi and Angelman syndromes.' *Current Opinion in Genetics and Development*, **3**, 445–456.

Prader, A., Labhart, A., Willi, H. (1956) 'Ein Syndrom von Adipositas, Kleinwuchs, Kryptorchismus und Oligophrenie nach myatonieartigem Zustand im Neugeborenenalter.' *Schweizerische Medizinische Wochenschrift*, **86**, 1260–1261.

Richdale, A.L., Cotton, S., Hibbit, K. (1999) 'Sleep and behaviour disturbance in Prader–Willi syndrome: a questionnaire study.' *Journal of Intellectual Disability Research*, **43**, 380–392.

Sforza, E., Krieger, J., Geisert, J., Kurtz, D. (1991) 'Sleep and breathing abnormalities in a case of Prader–Willi syndrome: the effects of acute continuous positive airway pressure treatment.' *Acta Paediatrica Scandinavica*, **80**, 80–85.

Swaab, D.F., Roozendaal, B., Ravid, R., Velis, D.N., Gooren, L., Williams, R.S. (1987) 'Suprachiasmatic nucleus in aging, Alzheimer's disease, transsexuality and Prader–Willi syndrome.' *Progress in Brain Research*, **72**, 301–310.

Vela-Bueno, A., Kales, A., Soldatos, C.R., Dobladez-Blanco, B., Campos-Castello, J., Espino-Hurtado, P., Olivan-Palacios, J. (1984) 'Sleep in the Prader–Willi syndrome: clinical and polygraphic findings.' *Archives of Neurology*, **41**, 294–296.

Vgontzas, A.N., Bixler, E.O., Kales, A., Vela-Bueno, A. (1995) 'Prader–Willi syndrome: effects of weight loss on sleep-disordered breathing, daytime sleepiness and REM sleep disturbance.' *Acta Paediatrica*, **84**, 813–814.

—— —— —— Centurione, A., Rogan, P.K., Mascari, M., Vela-Bueno, A. (1996a) 'Daytime sleepiness and REM abnormalities in Prader–Willi syndrome: Evidence of generalized hypoarousal.' *International Journal of Neuroscience*, **87**, 127–139.

—— Kales, A., Seip, J., Mascari, M.J., Bixler, E.O., Myers, D.C., Vela-Bueno, A., Rogan, P.K. (1996b) 'Relationship of sleep abnormalities to patient genotypes in Prader–Willi syndrome.' *American Journal of Medical Genetics (Neuropsychiatric Genetics)*, **67**, 478–482.

63

10
SLEEP DISORDERS AND CRANIOFACIAL SYNDROMES

Narong Simakajornboon and Robert Beckerman

Structural and functional airway narrowing in children who have a variety of craniofacial anomalies (CFAs) may lead to sleep-disordered breathing (SDB) and are major predisposing factors to their morbidity and mortality. Maintenance of upper-airway patency during sleep is the result of complex interactions between abnormal airway anatomy and alteration of the normal physiology of neuromuscular control of breathing (see Chapter 17). Close follow-up with anticipatory guidance, selective performance of physiological studies and early intervention can reduce both the short- and long-term complications of SDB in children with CFAs. The emphasis in this chapter is placed on sleep disorders of physical origin. It is likely that many children with CFAs will also have behaviourally determined sleep problems as described in earlier chapters due to the impact of the condition on the family as a whole.

Aetiological factors
Several unique features in infants and children predispose them to upper airway obstruction and respiratory failure. The airway diameter of the infant is proportionately smaller than that of the adult, thereby imposing significantly increased resistance to breathing in both awake and sleep states. Because the relationship between decreasing radius and increasing resistance is exponential (resistance $\propto 1/radius^4$), any inherent narrowing of the airway may be severely accentuated by mucous or oedema superimposed during respiratory illness. The infant pharynx and supraglottic structures are more floppy, and the upper airway may more easily collapse during inspiratory efforts. The collapse may be dependent upon sleep stage and position. The high position of the infant's larynx, which allows for simultaneous sucking and nasal breathing, can make the infant vulnerable to nasopharyngeal obstruction and aspiration of food. Airway obstruction in the infant is also commonly associated with more frequent and severe gastro-oesophageal reflux. These anatomical and physiological differences between infants and adults are magnified in infants and children with CFAs.

The most common structural anatomical abnormalities in children with CFAs are nasal obstruction, malformation of the cranial base and midface, macroglossia, and hypoplasia of the lower jaw. These patients often present with SDB or sleep-related disturbance. In the neonate, nasal obstruction may be due to choanal atresia. These malformations can present as an isolated entity or may be associated with facial clefting as in Treacher–Collins syndrome (Fig. 10.1a). Nasopharyngeal hypoplasia can occur secondary to malformations

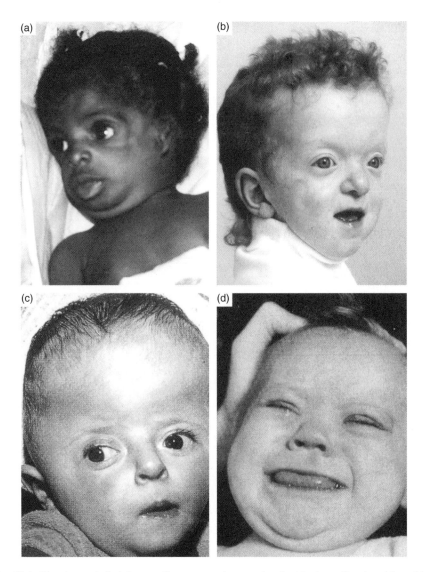

Fig. 10.1. Classic craniofacial anomalies commonly associated with sleep-disordered breathing: (a) infant with Treacher–Collins syndrome; (b) 4-year-old boy with Apert syndrome; (c) infant with Crouzon syndrome; (d) infant with Down syndrome.

of the cranial base or midface as seen in the Apert (Fig. 10.1b), Crouzon (Fig. 10.1c) and Down syndromes (Fig. 10.1d). The relatively small space resulting from hypoplasia is very vulnerable to obstruction even from normal adenotonsillar tissue. Hypoplasia of the lower jaw can compromise the upper airways, either because of retroglossia or by the intrusion of retromandibular structures. In addition to obstructive lesion, a central respiratory defect

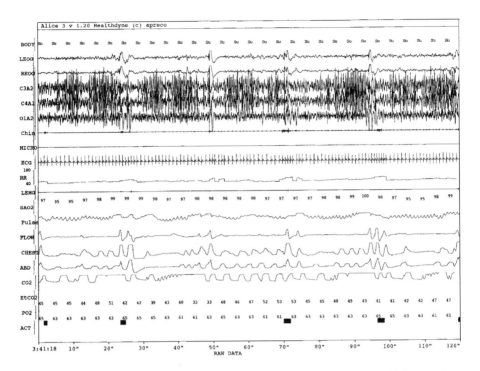

Fig. 10.2. Multichannel polysomnogram in 7-year-old girl with Down syndrome. This two-minute tracing reveals episodes of repetitive obstructive apnoea during stage 2 sleep associated with mild oxygen desaturation and hypoventilation. Notice that each of the apnoeic episodes is followed by an arousal.

may play an important role in these patients. Patients with craniofacial dysostosis frequently have associated hindbrain herniation that may lead to abnormalities of respiratory control. In infants and young children, the obstructive mechanism can lead to central apnoea. In obese children, central apnoea can be the result of low lung volume. The upper airway obstruction can lead to chronic alveolar hypoventilation that results in hypoxaemia or hypercarbia with respiratory acidosis. These gas exchange abnormalities may cause a constrictive response of the pulmonary vascular bed, resulting in increased right ventricular work and eventual cor pulmonale and heart failure. Severe obstructive sleep apnoea in a patient with achondroplasia was associated with absence of slow wave sleep and deficiency of overnight growth hormone secretion (Goldstein *et al.* 1987). Correction of apnoea by tracheostomy can improve growth rates postoperatively (Goldstein *et al.* 1985).

Characteristic sleep disorders
DOWN SYNDROME (see Chapter 8)
SDB is frequently seen in children with Down syndrome. Stebbens *et al.* (1991) reported that 30 per cent of patients with Down syndrome had sleep-related upper airway obstruction. Marcus *et al.* (1991) found abnormalities in overnight polysomnography studies in all

children with Down syndrome. They reported epochs of alveolar hypoventilation (80%), central (3%), obstructive (63%) and mixed apnoeas (4%), and oxygen desaturation (56%). The factors that predispose infants and children with Down syndrome to SDB include midfacial hypoplasia, relative macroglossia, and anatomical narrowing and hypotonia of the nasopharynx and oropharynx. No specific defect in central chemoreception has been reported to contribute to SDB in Down syndrome. Atlantoaxial subluxation may cause symptomatic spinal cord compression and may contribute to SDB. The incidence of SDB is not affected by age, obesity or the presence of congenital heart disease. Children who have both congenital heart disease and Down syndrome tend to have earlier onset and more severe pulmonary hypertension. It is speculated that nocturnal hypoxaemia secondary to SDB may contribute to the pulmonary hypertension seen in children with Down syndrome (Loughlin *et al.* 1981, Marcus *et al.* 1991). It is therefore important to evaluate children who have Down syndrome for SDB (Fig. 10.2), even in the absence of congenital heart disease.

CRANIOSYNOSTOSIS SYNDROMES
Craniosynostosis syndromes are characterized by premature closure of specific sutures in the bones of the cranial base, calvarium, orbit and maxilla. Orofacial manifestations of this disease include choanal and maxillary hypoplasia and prognathism. The two most commonly reported craniosynostosis syndromes with SDB are craniofacial dysostosis (Crouzon) and acrocephalosyndactyly (Apert). Patients with Apert syndrome may have airway abnormalities, *e.g.* laryngomalacia or tracheomalacia, which are more prominent in infants (Mixter *et al.* 1990). Obstructions in the upper airway have been reported secondary to septal deviation, midnasal and choanal abnormalities, and nasopharyngeal narrowing (McGill 1991).

Multiple factors predispose these patients to SDB including choanal stenosis, maxillary hypoplasia, posteriorly displaced tongue, lengthened soft palate and adenoid tissues, kyphosis of the cranial base resulting in a downward flexion of the clivus, depression of the sphenoid complex reducing both the anteroposterior dimension and the height of the nasopharynx, and marked narrowing of the transverse dimension of this space (Hui *et al.* 1998). Patients with craniosynostosis may have worsening of their SDB with growth due to failure of maxillary growth and increased growth of soft palate, soft tissue and adenoids (McGill 1991); serial polysomnography is therefore necessary to evaluate the presence and severity of SDB. Both central and obstructive apnoeas of varying severity during sleep have been reported in children with craniosynostosis. Upper airway compromise, obstructive sleep apnoea and cor pulmonale may result in early death in patients with Crouzon and Apert syndromes (Cohen and Kreiborg 1992).

MICROGNATHIA
Infants who have micrognathia, retrognathia and/or mandibular hypoplasia have increased risk of upper airway obstruction during sleep. Examples of micrognathia syndromes include glossoptosis–apnoea (Pierre Robin syndrome) and mandibulofacial dysostosis (Treacher–Collins syndrome, TCS). In Pierre Robin syndrome, upper airway obstruction is associated with episodes of repeated hypoxia that may result in cerebral impairment, failure to thrive

and cor pulmonale. SDB is manifested by snoring, obstructive sleep apnoea and disrupted sleep architecture, *e.g.* low percentage of REM sleep, which may not completely resolve after mandibular surgery (Spier *et al.* 1986). Dysmorphic features of TCS include anti-mongoloid slant to the palpebral fissures, colobomata of the eyelids and iris, hypoplasia of the malar and zygomatic bones, auricular atresia and extreme mandibular hypoplasia. Obstructive sleep apnoea has been reported in TCS (Johnston *et al.* 1981). It is manifested by daytime somnolence, behaviour problems and poor school performance. Surgical correction of the deformities can lead to resolution of sleep apnoea and improvement in performance and behaviour (Johnston *et al.* 1981). Significant pharyngeal narrowing was reported in seven of 11 children with TCS and probably contributed to upper airway obstruction during sleep and anaesthesia (Shprintzen *et al.* 1979).

ARNOLD–CHIARI MALFORMATION (ACM) (see also Chapter 19)
Structural abnormalities of the cranial base can also result in apnoea, the mechanisms of which are diverse and poorly understood. In ACM, the combination of a small posterior fossa and deformity of the craniocervical junction cause structural abnormalities of the cerebellum, brainstem and upper cervical spinal cord. ACM shares pathophysiological features of both neuromuscular and craniofacial disorders (see Chapter 17). A multitude of respiratory control disorders have been reported in ACM, *e.g.* stridor and obstructive apnoea secondary to bilateral abductor vocal cord paresis/palsy associated with increased intracranial pressure from hydrocephalus and/or hypoplasia of the central vagal nerves. In addition, central apnoea and central hypoventilation are frequently seen. Four types of ACM have been described, but obstructive sleep apnoea has been reported only in type II ACM. In contrast, compression of the brainstem in type I ACM is associated with central apnoea and hypersomnolence (Keefover *et al.* 1995). It has been speculated that downward displacement of the brainstem in type II ACM may lead to loss of pharyngeal sensation and incoordination of upper airway muscles, which may play an important role in SDB (Doherty *et al.* 1995). A recent study has reported polysomnographic findings of SDB in 63 per cent of patients with type II ACM (Waters *et al.* 1998). Risk factors for SDB in type II ACM include posterior fossa decompression, severe brainstem malformation and abnormal awake pulmonary functions (restrictive physiology) (Waters *et al.* 1998).

SKELETAL DISORDERS (see also Chapter 19)
The factors that contribute to SDB and other respiratory problems in children with chondrodystrophic skeletal disorders include chest wall deformity (thoracic dystrophy), upper airway obstruction, and small foramen magnum with brainstem and cervical spinal cord compression (Stokes *et al.* 1983). Achondroplasia (see also Chapter 19) is the prototype of generalized skeletal disorders that have respiratory control manifestations. Apnoea may be the sole manifestation of brainstem compression in achondroplasia (Fremion *et al.* 1984). Sudden unexpected death has been reported during infancy (Pauli *et al.* 1984). The most common form of SDB is sleep-related upper airway obstruction. Central apnoea and abnormal EMG of accessory muscles of respiration are reported during sleep (Waters *et al.* 1993) but there is no correlation between type and severity of apnoea and foramen

TABLE 10.1
Prototypical craniofacial disorders often associated with sleep-disordered breathing

Craniofacial abnormalities	Disorders	Sleep abnormalities*
Craniosynostosis	Crouzon syndrome	OA, CA
	Apert syndrome	
Mandibular hypoplasia	Pierre Robin syndrome	OA
	Treacher–Collins syndrome	
Skeletal disorders	Achondroplasia	Hypoventilation, CA, OA
Miscellaneous	Down syndrome	Hypoventilation, OA
	Arnold–Chiari malformation	Hypoventilation, OA, CA

*OA = obstructive apnoea, CA = central apnoea.

TABLE 10.2
Recommendations for baseline clinical assessment of children with craniofacial anomalies

Anatomical assessment	Posterior–anterior and lateral chest radiographs
	Lateral nasopharyngeal airway, fluoroscopy, cephalometry
	Tomography, MRI (brainstem)
	Flexible airway endoscopy
Physiological assessment	Pulmonary function
	Electrocardiography, echocardiography
	Serum bicarbonate and awake capillary blood gas
	Polysomonography

magnum stenosis (Zucconi *et al.* 1996). Nasal continuous positive airway pressure (CPAP) has been shown to improve SDB, sleep architecture and neurological function in achondroplasia (Waters *et al.* 1995). We refer the reader to Table 10.1, which lists the most common craniofacial syndromes associated with SDB.

Clinical assessment

Children with CFAs usually present with upper airway obstruction during wakefulness and sleep, which may lead to chronic respiratory failure. The signs and symptoms of SDB are similar to those seen in normal children who have obstructive sleep apnoea syndrome secondary to adenotonsillar enlargement, *viz.* loud snoring, difficulty breathing during sleep, breathing pauses, nocturnal enuresis, nocturnal sweating, restless sleep and frequent awakening. They may, however, differ in the frequency and severity of such signs and symptoms. In addition, morning headaches, failure to thrive, respiratory failure and cor pulmonale more frequently accompany SDB in children with CFAs. This places them at increased risk of morbidity and mortality especially following sedation or general anaesthesia for minor surgical procedures. Because of their higher risk status, it is imperative to anticipate a more serious potential respiratory complication.

Table 10.2 summarizes recommendations for baseline clinical assessment of children with CFAs.

Overnight polysomnography is considered to be the most objective physiological study in the baseline evaluation of SDB in children with CFA. Daytime polysomnographic studies (nap studies) in patients with Down syndrome, however, have been shown to underestimate the presence and severity of SDB (Marcus *et al.* 1991). Polysomnograms will quantify the severity of the problem and determine the need for further intervention. Chest and abdominal wall movement are recorded simultaneously, so that paradoxical inward movement of the chest can be documented during periods of partial airway obstruction. The study can objectively document the type of apnoea present, *i.e.* central, obstructive or mixed, their relationship to sleep stage, and body position during sleep. It also can reveal if there is hypopnoea, significant hypoxaemia or hypoventilation. Furthermore, the sleep study also provides valuable information in the follow-up treatment plan for these children.

Management

The underlying cause of SDB must be clearly defined before treatment recommendations are made. Central apnoea has been successfully treated with a number of medications, most commonly methylxanthines such as caffeine and theophylline. Another respiratory stimulant, acetazolamide, has been shown to improve SDB in some infants with ACM (Milerad *et al.* 1992). Protriptyline has been reported to benefit some patients who have Down syndrome and SDB (Clark *et al.* 1980). If the patient is obese, weight loss is also important in the management of SDB.

Any indications for surgical intervention of the airway should be based upon careful evaluation for anatomical and physiological abnormalities. Tonsillectomy and adenoidectomy (T&A) is the first-step surgical procedure for relief of the signs and symptoms of SDB in children. Patients with Down syndrome and SDB usually show partial benefit from T&A. However, complications of simple T&A in children with Down syndrome include hypernasality and nasal regurgitation which can sometimes result in translaryngeal aspiration. Some patients may have residual apnoea after T&A and may require second-stage surgery with uvulopalatopharyngoplasty (UPPP) and tongue reduction (Donaldson and Redmond 1988). Children with CFAs who have SDB, failure to thrive, chronic respiratory failure and cor pulmonale are at significant increased risk of prolonged intensive care stays and repeated endotracheal intubations postoperatively. Alternative management includes topical nasal decongestants, nasopharyngeal or oral airways, and nasal CPAP. This last is technically difficult to initiate under acute conditions in the young child. If these approaches fail or if prolonged endotracheal intubation is required, then tracheostomy may be necessary, particularly in the infant with CFA. Tracheostomy will immediately reduce airway resistance and anatomical dead space, ameliorate respiratory failure, and ultimately reverse cor pulmonale and promote growth. Experience has shown that reconstructive surgical airway management can allow successful decannulation in the young child with CFA (Sculerati *et al.* 1998). Reconstructive surgical approaches in children with CFA involve skeletal expansion in combination with soft tissue reduction, which can facilitate increase in the naso-oropharyngeal volumes (Cohen *et al.* 1998). Definitive reconstructive airway surgery, in the absence of a tracheostomy, is less likely to be successful in the infant with CFA and is associated with a greater incidence of complications (Januszkiewicz *et al.* 1997).

Successful use of noninvasive positive pressure ventilation through a nasal mask has been reported in children. Recent study has demonstrated that CPAP is safe, effective, and may reduce the number of operations done for children with craniofacial syndromes (Jarund *et al.* 1999). A problem with this therapy in any age-group, especially when psychomotor retardation is significant, is poor acceptance of the nasal mask by the patients. Follow-up polysomnography is needed to evaluate effectiveness of this treatment.

The care of children with CFA demands a multidisciplinary 'team' approach. Ideally, the team should comprise a paediatrician, geneticist, developmentalist–psychiatrist, ophthalmologist, otorhinolaryngologist, pulmonologist, maxillofacial and dental surgeons, and occupational, physical and speech therapists. Multidisciplinary assessment and treatment decreases morbidity and mortality in children with CFA (Bull *et al.* 1990). The most important role of team care is the organization and communication of a plan of care to the patient and family (Kaplan 1991). As implied at the start of this chapter, attention will need to be paid not only to the sleep disorders of physiological origin but also to those sleep problems of behavioural origin that can be expected in many cases.

REFERENCES

Bull, M.J., Givan, D.C., Sadove, A.M., Bixler, D., Hearn, D. (1990) 'Improved outcome in Pierre Robin sequence: effect of multidisciplinary evaluation and management.' *Pediatrics*, **86**, 294–301.

Clark, R.W., Schmidt, H.S., Schuller, D.E. (1980) 'Sleep-induced ventilatory dysfunction in Down's syndrome.' *Archives of Internal Medicine*, **140**, 45–50.

Cohen, M.M., Kreiborg, S. (1992) 'Upper and lower airway compromise in the Apert syndrome.' *American Journal of Medical Genetics*, **44**, 90–93.

Cohen, S.R., Ross, D.A., Burstein, F.D., Lefaivre, J.F., Riski, J.E., Simms, C. (1998) 'Skeletal expansion combined with soft-tissue reduction in the treatment of obstructive sleep apnea in children: Physiologic results.' *Otolaryngology – Head and Neck Surgery*, **119**, 476–485.

Doherty, M.J., Spence, D.P., Young, C., Calverley, P.M. (1995) 'Obstructive sleep apnoea with Arnold–Chiari malformation.' *Thorax*, **50**, 690–691.

Donaldson, J.D., Redmond, W.M. (1988) 'Surgical management of obstructive sleep apnea in children with Down syndrome.' *Journal of Otolaryngology*, **17**, 398–403.

Fremion, A.S., Garg, B.P., Kalsbeck, J. (1984) 'Apnea as the sole manifestation of cord compression in achondroplasia.' *Journal of Pediatrics*, **104**, 398–401.

Goldstein, S.J., Shprintzen, R.J., Wu, R.H., Thorpy, M.J., Hahm, S.Y., Marion, R.E., Sher, A.E., Saenger, P. (1985) 'Achondroplasia and obstructive sleep apnea: Correction of apnea and abnormal sleep-entrained growth hormone release by tracheostomy.' *Birth Defects Original Article Series*, **21**, 93–101.

—— Wu, R.H., Thorpy, M.J., Shprintzen, R.J., Marion, R.E., Saenger, P. (1987) 'Reversibility of deficient sleep entrained growth hormone secretion in a boy with achondroplasia and obstructive sleep apnea.' *Acta Endocrinologica*, **116**, 95–101.

Hui, S., Wing, Y.K., Kew, J., Chan, Y.L., Abdullah, V., Fok, T.F. (1998) 'Obstructive sleep apnea syndrome in a family with Crouzon's syndrome.' *Sleep*, **21**, 298–303.

Januszkiewicz, J.S., Cohen, S.R., Burstein, F.D., Simms, C. (1997) 'Age-related outcomes of sleep apnea surgery in infants and children.' *Annals of Plastic Surgery*, **38**, 465–477.

Jarund, M., Dellborg, C., Carlson, J., Lauritzen, C., Ejnell, H. (1999) 'Treatment of sleep apnoea with continuous positive airway pressure in children with craniofacial malformations.' *Scandinavian Journal of Plastic and Reconstructive Surgery and Hand Surgery*, **33**, 67–71.

Johnston, C., Taussig, L.M., Koopmann, C., Smith, P., Bjelland, J. (1981) 'Obstructive sleep apnea in Treacher–Collins syndrome.' *Cleft Palate Journal*, **18**, 39–44.

Kaplan, L.C. (1991) 'Clinical assessment and multispecialty management of Apert syndrome.' *Clinics in Plastic Surgery*, **18**, 217–225.

Keefover, R., Sam, M., Bodensteiner, J., Nicholson, A. (1995) 'Hypersomnolence and pure central sleep apnea

associated with the Chiari I malformation.' *Journal of Child Neurology*, **10**, 65–67.

Loughlin, G.M., Wynne, J.W., Victorica, B.E. (1981) 'Sleep apnea as a possible cause of pulmonary hypertension in Down syndrome.' *Journal of Pediatrics*, **98**, 435–437.

Marcus, C.L., Keens, T.G., Bautista, D.B., von Pechmann, W.S., Ward, S.L. (1991) 'Obstructive sleep apnea in children with Down syndrome.' *Pediatrics*, **88**, 132–139.

McGill, T. (1991) 'Otolaryngologic aspects of Apert syndrome.' *Clinics in Plastic Surgery*, **18**, 309–313.

Milerad, J., Lagercrantz, H., Johnson, P. (1992) 'Obstructive sleep apnea in Arnold–Chiari malformation treated with acetazolamide.' *Acta Paediatrica*, **81**, 609–612.

Mixter, R.C., David, D.J., Perloff, W.H., Green, C.G., Pauli, R.M., Popic, P.M. (1990) 'Obstructive sleep apnea in Apert's and Pfeiffer's syndromes: more than a craniofacial abnormality.' *Plastic and Reconstructive Surgery*, **86**, 457–463.

Pauli, R.M., Scott, C.I., Wassman, E.R., Gilbert, E.F., Leavitt, L.A., Ver, H.J., Hall, J.G., Partington, M.W., Jones, K.L., Sommer, A. (1984) 'Apnea and sudden unexpected death in infants with achondroplasia.' *Journal of Pediatrics*, **104**, 342–348.

Sculerati, N., Gottlieb, M.D., Zimbler, M.S., Chibbaro, P.D., McCarthy, J.G. (1998) 'Airway management in children with major craniofacial anomalies.' *Laryngoscope*, **108**, 1806–1812.

Shprintzen, R.J., Croft, C., Berkman, M.D., Rakoff, S.J. (1979) 'Pharyngeal hypoplasia in Treacher–Collins syndrome.' *Archives of Otolaryngology*, **105**, 127–131.

Spier, S., Rivlin, J., Rowe, R. D., Egan, T. (1986) 'Sleep in Pierre Robin syndrome.' *Chest*, **90**, 711–715.

Stebbens, V.A., Dennis, J., Samuels, M.P., Croft, C.B., Southall, D.P. (1991) 'Sleep related upper airway obstruction in a cohort with Down's syndrome.' *Archives of Disease in Childhood*, **66**, 1333–1338.

Stokes, D.C., Phillips, J.A., Leonard, C.O., Dorst, J.P., Kopits, S.E., Trojak, J.E., Brown, D.L. (1983) 'Respiratory complications of achondroplasia.' *Journal of Pediatrics*, **102**, 534–541.

Waters, K.A., Everett, F., Sillence, D., Fagan, E., Sullivan, C.E. (1993) 'Breathing abnormalities in sleep in achondroplasia.' *Archives of Disease in Childhood*, **69**, 191–196.

—— —— —— —— —— (1995) 'Treatment of obstructive sleep apnea in achondroplasia: Evaluation of sleep, breathing, and somatosensory-evoked potentials.' *American Journal of Medical Genetics*, **59**, 460–466.

—— Forbes, P., Morielli, A., Hum, C., O'Gorman, A.M., Vernet, O., Davis, G.M., Tewfik, T.L., Ducharme, F.M., Brouillette, R.T. (1998) 'Sleep-disordered breathing in children with myelomeningocele.' *Journal of Pediatrics*, **132**, 672–681.

Zucconi, M., Weber, G., Castronovo, V., Ferini-Strambi, L., Russo, F., Chiumello, G., Smirne, S. (1996) 'Sleep and upper airway obstruction in children with achondroplasia.' *Journal of Pediatrics*, **129**, 743–749.

11
SLEEP PROBLEMS IN CHILDREN WITH MUCOPOLYSACCHARIDOSIS

Gillian Colville and Martin Bax

The mucopolysaccharide disorders are a group of inherited lysosomal storage diseases, often with a degenerative course. (For a detailed description, see Brown 1999.)

Mucopolysaccharide disorders have both eponyms and numerical designations and comprise the following:
- Hurler (MPS IH), Scheie (MPS IS) and Hurler–Scheie (MPS IH/S) syndromes
- Hunter syndrome (MPS II)
- Sanfilippo syndrome types A, B, C and D (MPS IIIA, IIIB, IIIC, IIID)
- Morquio syndrome (MPS IVA) and variant Morquio (MPS IVB)
- Maroteaux–Lamy syndrome (MPS VI)
- Sly syndrome (MPS VII).

The Sanfilippo syndrome is the commonest disorder, with an incidence of 1 in 25,000 births, whereas Hunter and Hurler have an incidence of 1:100,000 and Morquio something between 1:200,000 and 1:300,000. The phenotype varies across the conditions, but, as a result of anatomical abnormalities of the upper airway, many children with mucopolysaccharidosis will have frequent ear and upper respiratory tract infections, and a sizeable proportion have a characteristically constant 'runny nose'.

The physical characteristics of the Hunter, Hurler and Morquio syndromes are such that these children are usually drawn to the attention of clinicians in the first year of life. Children with Hunter and Hurler syndromes have an accumulation of mucopolysaccharides in many tissues, which gives rise to dysmorphism, intellectual impairment and skeletal abnormalities. Hurler syndrome is the most severe, usually leading to death between the ages of 3 and 8 years (often from obstructive airway disease), whereas those affected by Hunter syndrome, and particularly the milder varieties, may survive into the second or third decade.

Morquio syndrome has a better life expectancy and milder intellectual impairment, but these children show dwarfism and problems associated with abnormalities of neck anatomy.

By contrast, children with the Sanfilippo syndrome have mild skeletal changes and may well initially be of normal appearance, although their hair and facies tend to coarsen over time. They tend to be diagnosed later than the other subtypes and to present initially with developmental delay and behaviour problems in the second to third year, with severe neurological degeneration occurring between 6 and 10 years of age.

Sleep problems

Sleep disturbance may be an early presenting behaviour problem, particularly in children with Sanfilippo syndrome (Leroy and Crocker 1966, Spranger 1972). It will not always be recognized as being associated with a disability, especially if the child is of preschool age, when sleep difficulties are not uncommon in children generally. However, it also often occurs subsequently, with high prevalence rates reported across all four main subtypes. Bax and Colville (1995) reported sleep disturbances in 29 of 49 children with Hurler syndrome (59%); 30 of 48 with Hunter syndrome (63%); 83 of 96 with Sanfilippo syndrome (86%); and 11 of 25 with Morquio syndrome (44%). Both van de Kamp (1981) and Nidiffer and Kelly (1983) have also reported high rates in Sanfilippo syndrome (56% and 86% respectively).

PRESENTATION

As in other children, sleeplessness (Chapter 4), notably settling and night-waking problems and short-duration sleep, features prominently in the reported sleep disturbances of children with mucopolysaccharidosis of whatever type.

Some unusual behaviours, summarized in Table 11.1, were reported by parents in a detailed study of the sleep habit patterns of 80 children with Sanfilippo syndrome (Colville *et al.* 1996). In addition to having settling difficulties and night waking, children were said to wander the house at night (one girl had started two fires by playing with gas appliances), chew bedclothes, laugh, sing or recite nursery rhymes. A significant number of children were in the habit of staying awake all night, and given the average age of the sample (mean = 10y 2mo; range = 4y 4mo to 25y 6mo) a surprisingly high proportion slept with parents. There was some evidence of variation in types of sleep problem across the Sanfilippo syndrome subtypes: those with type B had more night waking than those with type A and were reported more often to wake early in the morning.

It is clear that the various respiratory complications of the mucopolysaccharidoses include sleep-disordered breathing. This is likely to give rise not only to overtly respiratory symptoms during sleep, but also to the restlessness and quite possibly some of the unusual night-time behaviours just described [as mentioned in Chapters 5 and 6, parasomnias can be a manifestation of sleep-disordered breathing such as obstructive sleep apnoea (OSA)]. Eighty-nine per cent of the children studied by Semenza and Pyeritz (1988) had polysomnographically confirmed OSA. Mahowald *et al.* (1989) also described significant obstructive hyperventilation–obstructive apnoea, with severe sleep-related hypercapnoea (much worse during REM sleep) in the majority of a series of children mainly with Hurler or Hunter syndrome. Shapiro et al. (1985) considered that obstructive airway disease, including OSA, was a common cause of morbidity and death in the mucopolysaccharidoses. Belani *et al.* (1993) also reported a high rate of OSA.

AETIOLOGY AND ASSESSMENT

With such a wide range of sleep problems, the underlying causes are likely to be several and probably multiple in any one child.

TABLE 11.1
Types of sleep difficulty and night behaviours in 80
children with Sanfilippo syndrome*

	N	(%)
Settling difficulties	45	(56)
Night waking	47	(59)
Early waking	22	(28)
Sometimes awake all night	36	(45)
Crying out	30	(38)
Wandering around house	30	(38)
Entering parents' bed	24	(30)
Talking in sleep	18	(23)
Body rocking	14	(18)
Chewing bedclothes	20	(25)

*Reproduced by permission from Colville *et al.* (1996).

Parenting and other behavioural influences will be important in many instances in the ways described in earlier chapters. In this case, there will be scope for altering parenting practices or improving sleep patterns by other behavioural means based on a thorough assessment of the situation as described in Chapter 3.

In view of the prominence of sleep-related breathing problems in this group of children, routine assessment also needs to include careful clinical examination and evaluation of respiratory function during sleep (Chapters 3 and 5). A number of abnormalities might be found in children with mucopolysaccharidosis predisposing them to upper airway obstruction, namely anatomical abnormalities of the upper airway made worse by widespread mucopoly-saccharide deposits in the tongue, pharynx, trachea and bronchi. A short, thick neck and instability of the cervical spine also add to the risk. Semenza and Pyeritz (1988) reported high rates of upper airway narrowing, macroglossia, and enlarged tonsils, adenoids and mucous membranes in their series of children. Various degrees of skeletal abnormality affecting respiratory function (including scoliosis and thoracic hyperkyphosis) were usual. The chronic pulmonary disease of nearly all the patients in their series was considered to make them particularly prone to develop hypoxaemia and hypercarbia if upper airway obstruction was also present. Shapiro *et al.* (1985) described purulent rhinitis and chronic nasal congestion in four children with Hunter and Hurler syndromes and OSA.

In Sanfilippo syndrome, where obstructive problems are not so common, the disorganized sleep patterns may be attributed to the presence of abnormal levels of metabolite within the central nervous system (CNS). The overall prevalence of epilepsy (Chapter 15) in the sample reported by Colville *et al.* (1996) was 33 per cent (26/80). Some parents suggested that there was a temporal relationship between sleep difficulties and the onset of generalized convulsions. However, no significant association between presence of epilepsy and degree of sleep difficulty was found. Many authors have observed that in children with severe CNS damage, disruption is seen both in the structure and in the temporal organization of sleep, and there is evidence that the EEG in Sanfilippo syndrome is abnormal (Kriel *et al.* 1978).

MANAGEMENT

Clearly, management depends on the nature and cause of each child's sleep disorder.

Behavioural management

The diverse (even desperate) measures sometimes used are illustrated in the study by Colville *et al.* (1996). Parents reported using a number of strategies to deal with night waking. These included removing most of the furniture from the child's bedroom, leaving simply a mattress for him to lie on, and also removing the door handle or using a gate across the bedroom door in order to prevent him getting out. One family described enlarging the keyhole so that they could keep an eye on their child at night. Physical restraint with an elastic bed-belt was also mentioned, an unfortunate type of measure also reported by Cleary and Wraith (1993). A significant number of parents opted, albeit reluctantly, to keep the child in bed with them in the interests of his safety and to minimize disruption of the sleep of other family members. Some parents experimented with large teething rings in an effort to divert their children from chewing such things as their bedclothes.

Clearly, there is room for the use of more systematic behavioural approaches based on the established methods for treating sleeplessness that were reviewed in Chapter 4. It is important that child healthcare staff and parents know that such methods can be effective even for long-standing and severe sleep problems, including those of children with serious developmental disorders.

In a preliminary attempt to evaluate the usefulness of a behavioural approach in children with Sanfilippo syndrome, a small-scale intervention study was carried out with five families using established behaviour modification principles (Colville *et al.* 1996). This involved the collection of baseline data on the child's sleep pattern for two weeks and home visits by a clinical psychologist before and during intervention to negotiate and update the treatment plan. Weekly telephone contact was maintained throughout the six-week treatment period, with follow-up data available after four months for three of the five cases. The geographical scatter of the patients was such that a considerable amount of travelling was involved: one case was seen over 200 miles from the research base. There were clinically significant improvements in the sleep behaviour of all but one of the five children (Table 11.2).

Medication

Reservations about the use of drugs for treating most children's sleep disorders were expressed in the earlier chapters. Personal discussion with parents of children with Sanfilippo syndrome suggests that melatonin is being used by some of them, but there has been no controlled trial of the efficacy of this treatment. Some initial success has been reported anecdotally, but the effects have not been long-term. Other medications that have been tried include methylphenidate for overactivity in the hope that a more stable pattern of behaviour during the day might benefit sleep, but there seems little justification for this practice, based on systematic study. Two-thirds of children (52/80) in the study by Colville *et al.* (1996) had been given sleep medicine, but effects were mixed. In 22 cases the medicine was thought to have been useful as a last resort for short periods, but it was less effective over

TABLE 11.2
Results of brief behavioural intervention*

Case	Sex	Age (y:mo)	Sanfilippo subtype	Treatment goals	Goals achieved	Goals maintained at follow-up
1	F	6:10	A	1. Reduce settling time	Yes	No
				2. Decrease no. of night wakings	Yes	No
2	F	5:1	A	1. Decrease rate of early waking	Yes	No
				2. Reduce lengths of night waking	Yes	Yes
3	M	7:8	A	1. Reduce no. of night wakings	Yes	Yes
				2. Reduce disruption at night	Yes	Yes
4	M	6:7	B	1. Reduce settling time	No	NA
				2. Decrease no. of night wakings	No	NA
5	F	6:0	A	1. Decrease no. of night wakings	No	NA
				2. Reduce settling time	Yes	NA
				3. Move back into own room	Yes	NA

NA = not applicable.
*Reproduced by permission from Colville *et al.* (1996).

a long period of time. Many parents discontinued drug use because of side-effects, and sometimes they felt that, paradoxically, the child's arousal level had increased.

Surgical treatment
A variety of measures to relieve upper airway obstruction in children with mucopolysaccharidosis have been reported. Treatment is difficult because of the complicated and obstructive elements involved. In addition, obstruction may continue to occur because of persistent deposition of glycosaminoglycans in the tissues. Removal of tonsils and adenoids may not be helpful, and tracheostomy is sometimes required (Shapiro *et al.* 1985), Even this may be limited in effect in the presence of tracheomalacia and/or tracheal narrowing (Belani *et al.* 1993). Other measures that have been reported in different circumstances are bone marrow transplantation (Belani *et al.* 1993); nasal continuous positive airway pressure (CPAP) with supplemental oxygen (Ginzburg *et al.* 1990), although prior surgery may be necessary for CPAP to be effective (Orliaguet *et al.* 1999); and repeated laser excision of mucopolysaccharide deposits from the trachea (Adachi and Chole 1990).

Conclusion
The prevalence of sleep problems in children with mucopolysaccharidosis is high and

represents a considerable strain on families dealing with numerous other behaviour problems by day. As in other neurodevelopmental disorders there is a range of types of underlying factors in these children (some behavioural, others physical), probably operating in combination in many cases. By the same token, treatment programmes often need to be comprehensive and based on very careful evaluation of the nature of the underlying sleep disorders and their causes.

The fact that these conditions are rare often means that children are seen at specialized centres, often some distance from home, where, although general behavioural management advice may be given, the opportunities for intensive follow-up are limited. There is therefore clearly an argument for more involvement of local paediatricians and psychologists in these cases. Their proximity would allow greater focus on the day-to-day problems, such as sleep disturbance, that face these families, increasing the potential for their interventions to bring about significant improvements in the quality of life for both child and family.

REFERENCES

Adachi, K., Chole, R.A. (1990) 'Management of tracheal lesions in Hurler syndrome.' *Archives of Otolaryngology, Head and Neck Surgery*, **116**, 1205–1207.

Bax, M.C.O., Colville, G.A. (1995) 'Behaviour in mucopolysaccharide disorders.' *Archives of Disease in Childhood*, **73**, 77–81.

Belani, K.G., Krivit, W., Carpenter, B.L.M., Braunlin, E., Buckley, J.J., Liao, J.C., Floyd, T., Leonard, A.S., Summers, C.G., *et al.* (1993) 'Children with mucopolysaccharidosis: Perioperative care, morbidity, mortality and new findings.' *Journal of Pediatric Surgery*, **28**, 403–410.

Brown, M.B. (1999) 'The mucopolysaccharidoses.' *In:* Goldstein, S., Reynolds, C.R. (Eds.) *Handbook of Neurodevelopmental and Genetic Disorders in Children*. New York: Guilford Press, pp. 317–336.

Cleary, M.A., Wraith, J.E. (1993) 'Management of mucopolysaccharidosis type III.' *Archives of Disease in Childhood*, **69**, 403–406.

Colville, G.A., Watters, J.P., Yule, W., Bax, M.C.O. (1996) 'Sleep problems in children with Sanfilippo syndrome.' *Developmental Medicine and Child Neurology*, **38**, 538–544.

Ginzburg, A.S., Onal, E., Aronson, R.M., Schild, J.A., Mafee, M.F., Lopata, M. (1990) 'Successful use of nasal-CPAP for obstructive sleep apnea in Hunter syndrome with diffuse airway involvement.' *Chest*, **97**, 1496–1498.

Kriel, R.L., Hauser, W.A., Sung, J.H., Posalaky, Z. (1978) 'Neuroanatomical and electroencephalographic correlations in Sanfilippo syndrome type A.' *Archives of Neurology*, **35**, 838–843.

Leroy, J.G., Crocker, A.C. (1966) 'Clinical definition of the Hurler–Hunter phenotypes.' *American Journal of Diseases of Children*, **112**, 518–530.

Mahowald, M.W., Iber, C., Rosen, G.M., Krivett, W., Ramsay, N.K.C., Kersey, J.H., Belani, K., Whitley, C.B. (1989) 'Sleep disordered breathing in the mucopolysaccharidoses.' *Sleep Research*, **18**, 348. *(Abstract.)*

Nidiffer, F.D., Kelly, T.E. (1983) 'Developmental and degenerative patterns associated with cognitive, behavioural and motor difficulties in the Sanfilippo syndrome: an epidemiological study.' *Journal of Mental Deficiency Research*, **27**, 185–203.

Orliaguet, O., Pepin, J.L., Veale, D., Kelkel, E., Pinel, N., Levy, P. (1999) 'Hunter's syndrome and associated sleep apnoea cured by CPAP and surgery.' *European Respiratory Journal*, **13**, 1195–1197.

Semenza, G.L., Pyeritz, R.E. (1988) 'Respiratory complications of mucopolysaccharidosis storage disorders.' *Medicine*, **67**, 209–211.

Shapiro, J., Strome, M.S., Crocker, A.C. (1985) 'Airway obstruction and sleep apnea in Hurler and Hunter syndromes.' *Annals of Otology, Rhinology and Laryngology*, **94**, 458–461.

Spranger, J. (1972) 'The systemic mucopolysaccharidoses.' *Ergebnisse der Inneren Medizin und Kinderheilkunde*, **32**, 165–265.

van de Kamp, J.J.P., Niemeijer, M.F., von Figura, K., Giesberts, M.A.H. (1981) 'Genetic heterogeneity and clinical variability in the Sanfilippo syndrome (types A, B and C).' *Clinical Genetics*, **20**, 152–160.

12
SLEEP DISTURBANCES IN TUBEROUS SCLEROSIS COMPLEX

Paolo Curatolo and Stefano Seri

Tuberous sclerosis complex (TSC) is a multisystem genetic disorder with prominent signs and symptoms of CNS involvement. Its prevalence is 1.67 per 10,000 individuals. The condition has a remarkably high spontaneous mutation rate, with about 60 per cent of affected individuals having no family history of the disease, appearing to represent new mutations (Osborne *et al.* 1991). Recent genetic linkage studies have suggested that about one-half of cases are due to *TSC1* gene (9q34) and the other half to *TSC2* gene (16p13), with very similar clinical phenotypes (Povey *et al.* 1994). Neuropsychiatric symptoms in TSC patients are mainly characterized by a variable degree of mental retardation (50–60% of patients), epilepsy (92%) and autistic behaviour (60%), resulting in intellectual impairment and behavioural problems. The neuropathological background to the behavioural phenotype is a disruption in cell migration, proliferation and differentiation. This complex derange-ment results in heterotopias in the subcortical white matter, aggregates of dysplastic cortex (cortical tubers), and abnormal cell population in the germinal matrix zone (subependymal nodules). Cortical tubers are considered to be the hallmark of the syndrome, and their number and topography play a significant role in mental and behavioural outcome, as well as in seizure severity (Curatolo *et al.* 1991). Frontal lesions seem to be associated with refractory seizures as suggested by high time-resolution EEG studies (Seri *et al.* 1998). Autistic behaviour appears to have a strong relationship with presence of cortical tubers in the temporal lobes (Bolton and Griffiths 1997, Seri *et al.* 1999).

Characteristic sleep problems and aetiological factors

Only recently has attention been drawn to the prevalence of sleep disorders in children with TSC and data been collected from questionnaires and family interviews (Hunt and Stores 1994). The main sleep-related problems experienced by patients with TSC are settling difficulties (60%) and night waking (62%), and these can be exacerbated by parental stress and family problems. The only study on sleep structure in TSC patients showed significant abnormalities in the polygraphic recordings (Bruni *et al.* 1995). The main features were shorter total sleep time, reduced sleep efficiency, a high number of awakenings and stage transitions, an increased wake after sleep onset (WASO) and a decrease in REM sleep. Although the sample was relatively small (10 subjects), there was a clear tendency for children with seizures to show a more disturbed sleep architecture. A similar correlation was not evident for paroxysmal epileptiform activity density. By contrast, shorter awakenings

not related to epileptic seizures were not detected by the families, suggesting that the prevalence of sleep disorders in TSC patients is probably underestimated.

Special considerations for management

Frequent awakenings are not specific to TSC patients and have been previously reported in non-TSC patients with learning disorders (Petre-Quadens and Jouvet 1967) and with autism (Taira *et al.* 1998). In a recent polygraphic study of patients with learning disorders, autism and Down syndrome and with no history of epilepsy, abnormalities in the phasic components of sleep and the presence of REM sleep components in NREM sleep (undifferentiated sleep) were observed (Diomedi *et al.* 1999). The above-mentioned data highlight the fact that diagnosis and management of sleep problems in patients with TSC should be approached in an orderly manner due to the complexity of the underlying causes. Polysomnographic data have documented that the spectrum of sleep disturbances in children with TSC is wide. The high prevalence of seizures in this population requires the clinician to first rule out the possible epileptic nature of the episodes occurring during the night. Epilepsy is by far the most frequent cause of multiple awakenings in TSC patients, and careful history taking, associated with the use of home videos to record episodes, has proven to be very helpful. In selected cases, when a correct classification cannot be made or when the semiology of the ictal phenomena and of the associated EEG features is needed, polygraphic video–EEG recordings can be used. In the vast majority of cases, seizures occurring at night in TSC patients originate from the frontal lobe structures and are associated with complex motor phenomena (tonic posturing, clonic movement of one limb promptly bilateralizing), and require a careful clinico-neurophysiological assessment. This will result in more appropriate management of the epileptic condition and choice of the correct drug regimen.

In a significant number of patients, problems related to sleep onset can be associated with awakenings or present as an isolated sleep-related symptom. In these subjects melatonin given 20 minutes before bedtime has shown some promising results (O'Callaghan *et al.* 1999). The mechanisms underlying this effect are not fully understood. In normal subjects, the administration of melatonin can significantly reduce duration of sleep onset, increase spindle activity and reduce the amount of slow wave activity (Dijk and Cajochen 1997). The fact that melatonin does not exert any effect on sleep fragmentation leads us to believe that the main positive effect is in shortening sleep-onset latency and that it is more likely to be successful in those patients in whom frequent awakenings are not the main reported symptom. In Figure 12.1, polysomnograms of two patients are shown, suggesting that prolonged sleep latency (a) and frequent awakenings (b) due to epileptic seizures need to be differentiated.

Finally, sleep-related problems in TSC are part of a very complex clinical picture, and a comprehensive management strategy needs to take into account the wide comorbidity seen in these patients. This includes widespread psychiatric disturbances (including autism, discussed in Chapter 27), to which reference was made earlier and which can themselves produce sleep disruption to perhaps a severe degree (see Section Five). In the presence of such disorders, appropriate psychiatric help will need to be provided. Proper management

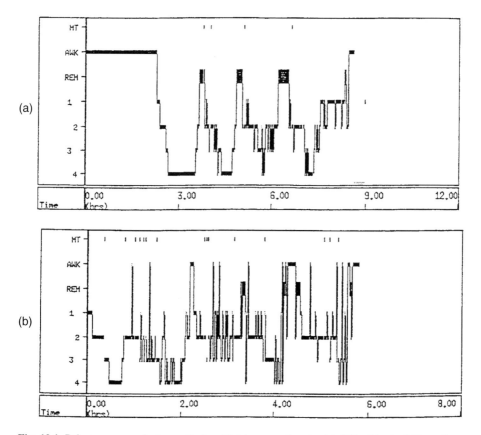

Fig. 12.1. Polysomnograms in two patients with tuberous sclerosis: (a) difficulties in falling asleep, well-controlled seizures; (b) frequent awakenings at night, nocturnal seizures characterized by tonic posturing of the upper limbs followed by generalized tonic–clonic manifestations (secondary bilateral synchrony).

of sleep disorders should also include extended counselling, with the aim of reducing the dramatic impact of sleep deprivation on the other members of the family.

REFERENCES

Bolton, P.F., Griffiths, P.D. (1997) 'Association of tuberous sclerosis of temporal lobes with autism and atypical autism.' *Lancet*, **349**, 392–395.

Bruni, O., Cortesi, F., Giannotti, F., Curatolo, P. (1995) 'Sleep disorders in tuberous sclerosis: a polysomnographic study.' *Brain and Development*, **17**, 52–56.

Curatolo, P., Cusmai, R., Cortesi, F., Jambaque, I., Chiron, C., Dulac, O. (1991) 'Neurological and psychiatric aspects of tuberous sclerosis.' *Annals of the New York Academy of Science*, **615**, 8–16.

Dijk, D.J., Cajochen, C. (1997) 'Melatonin and the circadian regulation of sleep initiation, consolidation, structure and sleep EEG.' *Journal of Biological Rhythms*, **12**, 627–635.

Diomedi, M., Curatolo, P., Scalise, A., Placidi, F., Caretto, F., Gigli, G.L. (1999) 'Sleep abnormalities in

mentally retarded autistic subjects: Down's syndrome with mental retardation and normal subjects.' *Brain and Development,* **21**, 548–553.

Hunt, A., Stores, G. (1994) 'Sleep disorder and epilepsy in children with tuberous sclerosis: a questionnaire-based study.' *Developmental Medicine and Child Neurology*, **36**, 108–115.

O'Callaghan, F.J.K., Clarke, A.A., Hancock, E., Hunt, A., Osborne, J.P. (1999) 'Use of melatonin to treat sleep disorders in tuberous sclerosis.' *Developmental Medicine and Child Neurology*, **41**, 123–126.

Osborne, J.P., Fryer, A., Webb, D. (1991) 'Epidemiology of tuberous sclerosis.' *Annals of the New York Academy of Science*, **615**, 125–127.

Petre-Quadens, O., Jouvet, M. (1967) 'Sleep in the mentally retarded.' *Journal of Neurological Sciences*, **4**, 354–357.

Povey, S., Burley, M.W., Attwood, J. (1994) 'Two loci for tuberous sclerosis: one on 9q34 and one on 16p13.' *Annals of Human Genetics*, **58**, 107–127.

Seri, S., Cerquiglini, A., Pascual Marqui, R.D., Michel, C., Pisani, F., Curatolo, P. (1998) 'Frontal lobe epilepsy associated with tuberous sclerosis: EEG-MRI fusioning.' *Journal of Child Neurology*, **13**, 33–38.

——— Pisani, F., Curatolo, P. (1999) 'Autism in tuberous sclerosis: evoked potential evidence for a deficit in auditory sensory processing.' *Clinical Neurophysiology*, **110**, 1825–1830.

Taira, M., Takase, M., Sasaki, H. (1998) 'Sleep disorders in children with autism.' *Psychiatry and Clinical Neurosciences*, **52**, 182–183.

13
SLEEP DISORDERS AND RETT SYNDROME

Henry S. Roane and Cathleen C. Piazza

Rett syndrome is a developmental disorder that affects approximately 1 in 15,000 females (Perry 1991), with very few cases in males. The disorder is associated with severe progressive intellectual and neurological impairments (including the development of epilepsy) and truncated development or regression of adaptive skills (*e.g.* locomotion, feeding or toileting skills). Midline stereotypic hand movements (*e.g.* hand wringing/washing or tapping/ clapping) are characteristic. In addition to these features, the disorder is associated with suppressed growth rate, microcephaly, loss of functional hand use, irregular breathing and a general dissociation from the surrounding environment. The progressive changes, from early signs of developmental abnormality between 6 and 18 months of age to a severe, multiple-disability syndrome years later, has been described in four stages (Hagberg and Witt-Engerström 1988). Sleep–wake disturbance of some description is a frequent feature at all stages although first becoming prominent in stage IV.

Characteristic sleep patterns
Sekul and Percy (1992) reported that over 80 per cent of Rett syndrome children develop multiple sleep problems. Irregular sleep–wake patterns are a common characteristic. These irregularities may be compounded by other inappropriate sleep-related behaviours including night-time screaming, crying and episodes of laughter. Coleman *et al.* (1988) surveyed the caregivers of individuals with Rett syndrome and found disturbed sleep in over 70 per cent of the sampled population, with 83 per cent demonstrating night-time emotional behaviour (*e.g.* laughing, crying or screaming). Sansom *et al.* (1993) noted that 75 per cent of a sample of individuals with Rett syndrome were reported to awaken early and that at least 50 per cent of the sample exhibited some type of night-time emotional behaviour.

The findings reported in those two studies were based on anecdotal caregiver reports. An alternative method of documenting sleep problems is to conduct direct observations of sleep–wake patterns. Piazza *et al.* (1990) utilized a direct observation measure of sleep dysfunction for individuals with the condition. Specifically, caregivers conducted brief observations of the participants at 30-minute intervals. During these observations, they recorded whether the participant was awake or asleep, and whether they were in or out of bed. Caregivers were instructed to use other behavioural indices (*e.g.* the occurrence of hand stereotypies) in determining wakefulness. Using this procedure, the investigators collected data on the sleep patterns of 20 girls with Rett syndrome, each of whom was observed for

an average of seven days. These data were compared to the developmental norms for children across a variety of age-groups. As a group the children with Rett syndrome had significantly less overnight sleep, more daytime sleep and more total sleep time. High rates of delayed sleep onset, night waking and early morning waking were also reported.

These findings suggest that sleep dysfunction (particularly excessive daytime sleep) may worsen as the individual with Rett syndrome ages. It is possible that excessive daytime sleep exacerbates the observed decreases in night-time sleep and contributes to the overall disruption of the sleep–wake cycle.

Aetiological factors

Given that the aetiology of Rett syndrome is not fully understood, it is not surprising that several hypotheses have been offered regarding the aetiology of sleep disturbances associated with the disorder. For example, Piazza *et al.* (1990) hypothesized that the presence of Rett syndrome causes sufficient damage to the central nervous system that the circadian rhythm is disrupted, thereby affecting the sleep–wake cycle. The findings of Challamel *et al.* (2000) are in keeping with the notion of a progressive loss of the circadian organization of sleep (*i.e.* progressive deterioration of nocturnal sleep accompanied by an increase in sleep during the day). The claimed success of melatonin in the treatment of sleep disturbances in individuals with Rett syndrome might be interpreted as implicating dysfunctional circadian rhythm (McArthur and Budden 1998), although the actions of melatonin in promoting sleep (where this happens) can be either through its hypnotic effect of promoting sleep onset or its sleep-phase shifting property (Kayumov *et al.* 2000).

Epilepsy (the potentially sleep-disruptive effects of which are discussed in Chapter 15) is said to develop in 70–80 per cent of cases, usually in stage II after about 2 years of age. Examination of the EEGs of patients with Rett syndrome suggests that abnormal brain function may be related to sleep disturbance. Basic brain activity gradually deteriorates as the disorder progresses (Segawa and Nomura 1992), including a paucity of sleep spindles (Espinar-Sierra *et al.* 1990). EEG patterns reviewed by Aldrich *et al.* (1990) showed increases in epileptiform spikes during sleep.

Although irregular breathing patterns (*e.g.* apnoea, irregular breathing rate) have been noted, breathing dysfunction does not appear to be related to sleep disturbance in this group (Elian and Rudolf 1989). The same conclusion was reached by Marcus *et al.* (1994) based on their findings from polysomnographic (PSG) studies of young persons with Rett syndrome compared to controls. Despite disordered breathing during wakefulness, both conventional PSG variables and measures of respiratory function during sleep were essentially normal in both groups.

Behavioural influences are highly likely in view of the serious effects of the disorder on the child's mental state and the impact of such an unfortunate condition on parents and other family members.

Considerations in management

Research has recently examined the use of pharmacological interventions in the treatment of sleep disturbances in individuals with Rett syndrome. For example, McArthur and

Budden (1998) monitored the sleep–wake patterns of nine individuals with Rett syndrome for a period of one week. All participants had irregular sleep and a long onset to sleep. Subsequently, trials of melatonin were conducted over a period of four weeks. Administration of the melatonin resulted in increased total sleep and a shorter delay to sleep onset. In a preliminary report by Miyamoto *et al.* (1999) melatonin was also found to be helpful long-term in two patients with Rett syndrome, though its effects on sleep varied. The sleep–wake cycle was improved in one patient, but a predominantly hypnotic effect was seen in the other.

Behavioural treatments have also been used in the regulation of sleep for individuals with Rett syndrome. Piazza *et al.* (1991) observed the sleep patterns of three girls with Rett syndrome. All participants experienced delayed sleep onset, daytime sleep and night awakenings. Following baseline, a fading procedure was implemented in which the participants' bedtimes were delayed by 30 minutes per day until a bedtime with rapid sleep onset (*i.e.* within 15 minutes) was achieved. In addition, a 'response cost' procedure was employed in which the participants were removed from their beds for periods of one hour if their sleep onset was not sufficiently brief (within 15 minutes). Finally, any daytime sleep that was not part of the regularly scheduled treatment (*i.e.* age-appropriate naps) was interrupted. Results of this intervention showed that the participants' sleep dysfunction decreased following treatment. The effectiveness of a behavioural intervention in the treatment of disordered sleep (frequently attributed to a neurological cause in the case of Rett syndrome) raises interesting issues concerning underlying aetiology of the sleep disturbance.

In summary, sleep disturbances affect the majority of individuals diagnosed with Rett syndrome. The aetiology of these disturbances is typically attributed to irregular fluctuations in brain activity that is inherent with the disorder. Previous research has demonstrated various successful approaches to the assessment and treatment of this problem. Both behavioural and pharmacological treatments (*i.e.* melatonin) have been demonstrated to improve to some extent the sleep of certain individuals with Rett syndrome.

REFERENCES

Aldrich, M.S., Garofalo, E.A., Drury, I. (1990) 'Epileptiform abnormalities during sleep in Rett syndrome.' *Electroencephalography and Clinical Neurophysiology*, **75**, 365–370.

Challamel, M.J., Nevsimalova, S., Pretl, M. (2000) 'Sleep in Rett and Willi–Prader syndromes.' *Presentation to the Satellite Meeting of the Development and Sleep Committee, 15th Congress of the European Sleep Research Society, Istanbul, September 2000.*

Coleman, M., Brubaker, J., Hunter, K., Smith, G. (1988) 'Rett syndrome: A survey of North American patients.' *Journal of Mental Deficiency Research*, **32**, 117–124.

Elian, M., Rudolf, N.M. (1989) 'Rett syndrome: Some behavioral aspects and an overview.' *Behavioural Neurology*, **2**, 211–218.

Espinar-Sierra, J. Toledano, M.A., Franco, C., Campos-Castello, J., Gonzalez-Hidalgo, M., Oliete, F., Garcia-Nart, M. (1990) 'Rett's syndrome: a neurophysiological study.' *Neurophysiologie Clinique*, **20**, 35–42.

Hagberg, B., Witt-Engerström, I. (1988) 'Clinical characteristics and differential diagnosis by stage.' *Journal of Child Neurology*, **3** (Suppl.), S13.

Kayumov, L., Zhdanova, I.V., Shapiro, C.M. (2000) 'Melatonin, sleep and circadian rhythm disorders.' *Seminars in Clinical Neuropsychiatry*, **5**, 44–55.

Marcus, C.L. Carroll, J.L., McCulley, S.A., Loughlin, G.M., Curtis, S., Pyzik, P., Naidu, S. (1994) 'Polysomnographic characteristics of patients with Rett syndrome.' *Journal of Pediatrics*, **125**, 218–224.

McArthur, A.J., Budden, S. (1998) 'Sleep dysfunction in Rett syndrome: a trial of exogenous melatonin treatment.' *Developmental Medicine and Child Neurology*, **40**, 186–192.

Miyamoto, A., Oki, J., Takahashi, S., Okuno, A. (1999) 'Serum melatonin kinetics and long-term melatonin treatments for sleep disorders in Rett syndrome.' *Brain and Development*, **21**, 59–62.

Perry, A. (1991) 'Rett syndrome: A comprehensive review of the literature.' *American Journal of Mental Retardation*, **96**, 275–290.

Piazza, C.C., Fisher, W.W., Kiesewetter, K., Bowman, L., Moser, H. (1990) 'Aberrant sleep patterns in children with Rett syndrome.' *Brain and Development*, **12**, 488–493.

—— —— Moser, H. (1991) 'Behavioral treatment of sleep dysfunction in patients with the Rett syndrome.' *Brain and Development*, **13**, 232–237.

Sansom, D., Krishnan, V.H.R., Corbett, J., Kerr, A. (1993) 'Emotional and behavioral aspects of Rett syndrome.' *Developmental Medicine and Child Neurology*, **35**, 340–345.

Segawa, M., Nomura, Y. (1992) 'Polysomnography in the Rett syndrome.' *Brain and Development*, **14** (Suppl.), S46–S54.

Sekul, E., Percy, A. (1992) 'Rett syndrome: clinical features, genetic considerations and the search for a biological marker.' *Current Neurology*, **12**, 173–200.

14
ASPECTS OF SLEEP IN OTHER NEURODEVELOPMENTAL DISORDERS

Gregory Stores

Details of the nature of the disorders considered in this chapter can be found in the relevant sections of O'Brien and Yule (1995) and Goldstein and Reynolds (1999).

Fragile X syndrome

Sleep problems are consistently reported as being a prominent part of the various behavioural disturbances in this relatively common condition, but the precise nature of these problems is unclear from the available published information. Similarly, the contributions to the sleep disturbance by associated conditions, such as attention deficit hyperactivity disorder (ADHD), autistic behaviour and epilepsy, need to be defined.

Polysomnographic differences have been described in preliminary studies of affected boys compared with controls (Musumeci *et al.* 1995), notably a reduction in total sleep time and in REM sleep, with an increase in REM latency (time between onset of sleep and the start of the first REM sleep period). Also, slow wave sleep was proportionately greater in the children with fragile X syndrome. The authors suggest that these findings might indicate a dysregulation of the cholinergic–monoaminergic system during sleep, but admit the need for more extensive investigation of this possibility.

At the clinical level, there has been a suggestion that children with fragile X syndrome are at particular risk for obstructive sleep apnoea (Tirosh and Borochowitz 1992), for which treatment by means of continuous positive airway pressure can be beneficial (Tirosh *et al.* 1995). However, normal respiratory function has been reported in other children (Musumeci *et al.* 1995).

Again, it is difficult to obtain a proper perspective on these possibilities because of the few cases reported, but, as in other neurodevelopmental disorders, both psychological and physical factors need to be considered in explaining the origins of sleep disturbance. The need to establish causal relationships in the individual child is further illustrated by the report by Hagerman *et al.* (1995) that clonidine often has a beneficial affect on the behaviour (including sleep patterns) of children with fragile X syndrome. As the children in the study had combinations of behavioural difficulties, it is difficult to judge whether the sleep improvement occurred due to a direct effect of the medication on sleep, or because it lessened the children's other problem behaviours.

Smith–Magenis syndrome (SMS)

Sleep disturbance is considered to be a major feature of this condition, which is associated

with a deletion of part of the short arm of chromosome 17. Reports that have included polysomnographic data have indicated low levels of REM sleep (*e.g.* Greenberg *et al.* 1996), but, as mentioned in Chapter 7, REM abnormalities are widely seen in people with intellectual impairment of different aetiologies. Various types of sleep disturbance have been reported in patients with SMS. Smith *et al.* (1998) described the sleep patterns of 39 patients ranging in age from 1.6 to 32 years (average 10.5 years), in the vast majority of whom sleep problems were reported by parents to be prominent. The problems included difficulty falling asleep, shortened sleep cycles, frequent and prolonged nocturnal wakings, and excessive daytime sleepiness, as well as snoring and bed-wetting at night. Medication was used in about 60 per cent of cases. Excessive daytime sleepiness (associated with fragmented nocturnal sleep) was prominent in three children described by Moldofsky *et al.* (1995), one of whom had obstructive sleep apnoea.

Again, these various sleep problems and symptoms are found in many people with an intellectual impairment. However, the reported nature of the night-time wakings is interesting, suggesting possible specificity for the syndrome, although, for lack of large-scale and detailed information, it is not yet possible to justify some of the 'behavioural phenotype' claims in this and other neurodevelopmental disorders (Flint 1996).

Colley *et al.* (1990) describe children in their small series who, from an early age, slept in short bursts (about two hours). Additional problems of early morning waking and disruptive behaviour when awake during the night were also reported in the refined sleep studies by De Leersnyder *et al.* (2000). They assessed 20 patients with SMS, aged 4–17 years, by means of combinations of sleep questionnaires, interviews, sleep diaries and nocturnal actometry. The characteristic sleep pattern was that the children went to bed early, usually woke repeatedly during the night, staying awake for about 30 minutes, and then remained awake from between 4 and 6 a.m., moving about in a hyperactive and hazardous way. The children tended to be sleepy during the day (including taking naps up to the age of 17 or older) and had frequent temper tantrums.

Eight of the children in this series underwent polysomnography and 24 hour monitoring of plasma and urinary melatonin and cortisol, and plasma growth hormone. The sleep recordings showed a reduction in slow wave sleep, disrupted REM sleep and frequent brief arousals. Awakenings longer than 15 minutes occurred in six of these eight children. In addition, abnormal basic EEG rhythms and spike discharges were often seen in rolandic areas. A major finding in the study was that, although cortisol and growth hormone patterns were normal, melatonin secretion was abnormal in a number of ways, indicating, in particular, a phase shift in keeping with the clinically advanced sleep phase.

The authors suggested that patients with SMS have an abnormality of the biological clock (possibly of genetic origin) that produces the abnormal sleep pattern by night and by day, with the behavioural consequences including difficult behaviour. This last suggestion is in keeping with the report by Dykens and Smith (1998) that sleep disturbance was the strongest predictor of maladaptive behaviour in the children and adolescents they studied.

Treatment possibilities depend again on the nature and cause of the sleep disturbance, with the likelihood that psychological (including parenting) factors will be involved to some extent. If melatonin abnormalities are confirmed, chronotherapeutic measures should

be helpful, including altering melatonin profiles. Clearly, the question of a fundamental circadian sleep–wake cycle deficit in SMS syndrome requires further investigation.

Angelman syndrome

This is a rare syndrome associated in the majority of cases with deletion of the proximal long arm of the maternally derived chromosome 15.

Sleep disturbance at some stage (especially between the ages of 2 and 6 years) was reported by Clayton-Smith (1993) in 90 per cent of her series of 82 patients between the ages of 17 months and 26 years with this disorder. More recent reports (*e.g.* Clarke and Marston 2000) have confirmed a high rate of disturbance, but the precise nature of the sleep problems, including their relationship to age, is unclear. Clayton-Smith referred to short sleep duration (five to six hours per night on average), but noted that the children's need for sleep increased with age and some adolescents slept longer than usual. She also reported that destruction of bedroom furniture during the night was common. However, the details of these behaviours and their cause is not described and, therefore, it is difficult to judge the likelihood of them being in any way associated specifically with the condition. The contributions of hyperactivity, other behavioural problems and epilepsy (all common features of Angelman syndrome) remain to be clarified.

In the meantime, treatment of the individual child's sleep disturbance, as usual, needs to be based on an understanding of the factors underlying the particular sleep problem. Clayton-Smith (1993) refers to the value of behaviour therapy and set routines in some cases. Similarly, Summers *et al.* (1992) described the successful use of a treatment regime that combined a behavioural approach and medication (diphenhydramine) for a sleep–wake cycle disorder in a child with Angelman syndrome.

On the other hand, Zhdanova *et al.* (1999) reported success in treating various sleep problems by means of a low dose (0.3 mg) of melatonin given shortly before bedtime. Their study involved 13 children (aged 2–10 years) whose parents described settling problems, prolonged night waking (with much restlessness when awake) and early morning waking. The short total sleep time and high levels of movement during sleep were confirmed by means of actigraphy.

No relationship was seen between melatonin patterns and sleep disturbance, but the administration of melatonin, producing a moderate increase in circulating melatonin levels, was usually followed by parental reports that their children fell asleep quicker and (in some cases) that their sleep was sounder. Actigraphy showed a decrease in motor activity during sleep. Overall, the results suggested to the authors that the beneficial effects of melatonin on sleep could have been the result of its acute promotion of sleep and changes in circadian sleep–wake cycle patterns. The study findings illustrate yet again the uncertainties associated with the use of melatonin in children's sleep disturbance and the need to explore further its basic modes of action.

Williams syndrome

This syndrome is linked to a small deletion on chromosome 7. Udwin and Yule (1990) reported that the high rates of behavioural disturbance in children with Williams syndrome included

frequent sleeping problems, possibly forming part of the behavioural phenotype of the condition. Prominent sleep problems have been reported in other series of children with the syndrome (Einfeld *et al.* 1997), but, as in other neurodevelopmental disorders, the reported nature of these problems has been mixed and generally nonspecific. Once again, it has been difficult to judge the aetiology of the sleep disturbance, in particular the relationship between it and associated features such as behavioural disorder of an ADHD type.

However, the study by Arens *et al.* (1998) is potentially very instructive about underlying biological factors. To explain possible physical causes of sleep disturbance (and, in turn, the effects of this disturbance on learning and behaviour), parents of 28 young children with Williams syndrome were questioned about their children's sleep including enquiries about possible sleep-disordered breathing and "movement arousal sleep disorder"(basically signs of restless or otherwise disrupted sleep). Features suggestive of respiratory dysfunction during sleep were recorded in a minority, but 16 children were reported to have frequent symptoms suggesting a movement arousal disorder. Of these, seven (age 1.8–7 years, average 3.9 years) agreed to have polysomnography, and the findings were compared with those from a group of 10 healthy children, matched for age. One of the patients was taking methylphenidate and another enalapril at the time of polysomnography.

The main finding was the prominence of periodic limb movements in sleep (PLMS) in all the children with Williams syndrome, associated with arousals and prolonged awakenings. All PLMS measures were greater in the patients than in the controls to a highly significant degree. The children with Williams syndrome also spent significantly more time awake during the night and more time in slow wave sleep but were overall no different in other aspects of sleep physiology (including respiratory variables) than the controls, although one showed evidence of upper airway obstruction. Parents of five of the children agreed to treatment with clonazepam at bedtime. This was reported to have promptly improved the child's sleep and daytime behaviour in four, and in three it was possible to demonstrate by repeat polysomnography a significant decrease in PLMS and arousals to levels that were similar to the control group.

These interesting findings are in keeping with other reports that PLMS are more common in children that previously supposed and that they might underlie daytime behavioural problems, including ADHD symptoms, because of their disruptive effect on sleep quality (Picchetti and Walters 1999). PLMS have also been associated with Tourette syndrome (Chapter 29) although their pathological significance in this condition is unclear. The same is true in the case of Williams syndrome, but, from a practical viewpoint, it seems important to consider their presence as a potentially treatable cause of sleep disturbance in children with the condition.

Miscellaneous neurodevelopmental disorders

There has been limited reference to sleep abnormalities in connection with a number of other neurodevelopmental disorders. The following conditions have been selected as illustrating more specific associations rather than nonspecific findings that probably simply reflect intellectual impairment.

Mizuno *et al.* (1979) reported that, compared to healthy controls, children with *Lesch–Nyhan syndrome* woke more often during the night and that self-mutilation could occur during any stage of sleep although it was least likely in slow wave sleep. Saito *et al.* (1998) conducted polysomnographic studies on three patients with the same condition. Two showed a reduction in both slow wave sleep and REM sleep as well in as other REM abnormalities. All three showed limb movements during sleep that the authors construed as abnormal. In a single case report of a child with Lesch–Nyhan syndrome, 5-hydroxytryptophan plus carbidopa appeared to improve sleep while having no effect on self-mutilating behaviour (Anders *et al.* 1978). The uncertainties surrounding the general relationship between self-injurious behaviours and sleep disturbance in intellectually impaired people, including the possibility of a common aetiology, have been discussed by Symons *et al.* (2000).

Children with *phenylketonuria* have been the subject of a number of polysomnographic studies, but with differing results. Early studies by Schulte *et al.* (1973) indicated little difference in sleep stages compared to controls, whether the affected children were treated with a low phenylalanine diet or not, although increased spindling (a nonspecific finding in intellectually impaired children) was evident. More recent investigations have shown a consistent delay in the early maturation of basic sleep EEG patterns, which might provide an indication of brain dysfunction in early infancy in children with this disorder (De Georgis *et al.* 1996).

A number of other preliminary reports suggest that certain types of sleep disturbance might be associated with some neurodevelopmental disorders in addition to sleep disturbance that might nonspecifically accompany the disorders, especially those of which intellectual impairment is usually a part. Sleep difficulties have been described as commonplace in adults with *neurofibromatosis* (Samuelsson and Riccardi 1989), and severe hypoventilation during sleep has been described in a child with this condition involving brainstem lesions (Sforza *et al.* 1994). Sleep-related breathing problems have also been described in *Joubert syndrome* (Andermann *et al.* 1999) and in *Rubenstein–Taybi syndrome* (Zucconi *et al.* 1993). Reference has been made to sleep disturbance as part of the behavioural phenotype of Smith–Lemli–Opitz syndrome (Tierney *et al.* 2000), Cornelia de Lange syndrome (Berney *et al.* 1999) and possibly Sotos syndrome (Rutter and Cole 1991). However, details of the sleep abnormalities and their origins remain unclear.

REFERENCES

Andermann, F., Andermann, E., Ptito, A., Fontaine, S., Joubert, M. (1999) 'History of Joubert syndrome and a 30 year follow up of the original proband.' *Journal of Child Neurology*, **14**, 565–569.

Anders, T.F., Cann, H.M., Ciaranello, R.D., Barcha, J.D., Berger, P.A. (1978) 'Further observations on the use of 5-hydroxytryptophan in a child with Lesch–Nyhan syndrome.' *Neuropädiatrie*, **9**, 157–166.

Arens, R., Wright, B., Elliott, J., Zhao, H., Wang, P.P., Brown, L.W., Namey, T., Kaplan, P. (1998) 'Periodic limb movement in sleep in children with Williams syndrome.' *Journal of Pediatrics*, **133**, 670–674.

Berney, T.P., Ireland, M., Burn, J. (1999) 'Behavioural phenotype of Cornelia de Lange syndrome.' *Archives of Disease in Childhood*, **81**, 333–336.

Clarke, D.J., Marston, G. (2000) 'Problem behaviors associated with 15q– Angelman syndrome.' *American Journal on Mental Retardation*, **105**, 25–31.

Clayton-Smith, J. (1993) 'Clinical research on Angelman syndrome in the United Kingdom: Observations on 82 affected individuals.' *American Journal of Medical Genetics*, **46**, 12–15.

Colley, A.F., Leversha, M.A., Voullaire, L.E., Rogers, J.G. (1990) 'Five cases demonstrating the distinctive behavioural features of chromosome deletion 17(p11.2 p11.2) (Smith–Magenis syndrome).' *Journal of Paediatrics and Child Health*, **26**, 17–21.

De Georgis, G.F., Nonnis, E., Crocioni, F., Gregori, P., Rosini, M.P., Leuzzi, V., Loizzo, A. (1996) 'Evolution of daytime quiet sleep components in early treated phenylketonuric infants.' *Brain and Development*, **18**, 201–206.

De Leersnyder, H., Munnich, A., de Blois, M.C., Claustrat, B. (2000) 'Sleep disturbance in Smith–Magenis syndrome.' *Presentation to the Satellite Meeting of the Development and Sleep Committee, 15th Congress of the European Sleep Research Society, Istanbul, September 2000.*

Dykens, E.M., Smith, A.C. (1998) 'Distinctiveness and correlates of maladaptive behaviour in children and adolescents with Smith–Magenis syndrome.' *Journal of Intellectual Disability Research*, **42**, 481–489.

Einfeld, S.L., Tonge, B.J., Florio, T. (1997) 'Behavioral and emotional disturbance in individuals with Williams syndrome.' *American Journal on Mental Retardation*, **102**, 45–53.

Flint, J. (1996) 'Behavioural phenotypes: a window into the biology of behaviour.' *Journal of Child Psychology and Psychiatry*, **37**, 355–367. *(Annotation.)*

Goldstein, S., Reynolds, C.R. (Eds.) (1999) *Handbook of Neurodevelopmental and Genetic Disorders in Children.* New York: Guilford Press.

Greenberg, F., Lewis, R.A., Potocki, L., Glaze, D., Parke, J., Killian, J., Murphy, M.A., Williamson, D., Brown, F., *et al.* (1996) 'Multidisciplinary clinical study of Smith–Magenis syndrome (deletion 17p11.2).' *American Journal of Medical Genetics*, **62**, 247–254.

Hagerman, R.J., Riddle, J.E., Roberts, L.S., Breese, K., Fulton, M. (1995) 'Survey of the efficacy of clonidine in fragile X syndrome.' *Developmental Brain Dysfunction*, **8**, 336–344.

Mizuno, T., Ohta, R., Kodama, K., Kitazumi, E., Minejima, N., Takeishi, M., Segawa, M. (1979) 'Self mutilation and sleep stage in the Lesch–Nyhan syndrome.' *Brain and Development*, **2**, 121–125.

Moldofsky, H., Blackman, A., MacFarlane, J.G., Costa, T., Feigenbaum, A. (1995) 'Abnormal REM and NREM sleep and excessive daytime somnolence in Smith–Magenis syndrome (deletion of 17p11.2).' *Sleep Research*, **24**, 406. *(Abstract.)*

Musumeci, S.A., Ferri, R., Elia, M., Del Gracco, S., Scuderi, C., Stefanini, M.C., Castano, A., Azan, G. (1995) 'Sleep neurophysiology in fragile X patients.' *Developmental Brain Dysfunction*, **8**, 218–222.

O'Brien, G., Yule, W. (Eds.) (1995) *Behavioural Phenotypes. Clinics in Developmental Medicine No. 138.* London: Mac Keith Press.

Picchetti, D.L., Walters, A.S. (1999) 'Moderate to severe periodic limb movement disorder in childhood and adolescence.' *Sleep*, **22**, 297–300.

Rutter, S.C., Cole, T.R.P. (1991) 'Psychological characteristics of Sotos syndrome.' *Developmental Medicine and Child Neurology*, **33**, 898–902.

Saito, Y., Hanaoka, S., Fukumizu, M., Morita, H., Ogawa, T., Takahashi, K., Ito, M., Hashimoto, T. (1998) 'Polysomnographic studies of Lesch–Nyhan syndrome.' *Brain and Development*, **20**, 579–585.

Samuelsson, B., Riccardi, V.M. (1989) 'Neurofibromatosis in Gothenburg, Sweden. III. Psychiatric and social aspects.' *Neurofibromatosis*, **2**, 84–106.

Schulte, F.J., Kaiser, H.J., Engelbart, S., Bell, E.F., Castell, R., Lenard, H.G. (1973) 'Sleep patterns in hyperphenylaninemia: A lesson on serotonin to be learned from phenylketonuria.' *Pediatric Research*, **7**, 588–599.

Sforza, E., Columaria, V., Lugaresi, E. (1994) 'Neurofibromatosis associated with central alveolar hypoventilation syndrome during sleep.' *Acta Paediatrica*, **83**, 794–796.

Smith, A.C.M., Dykens, E., Greenberg, F. (1998) 'Sleep disturbance in Smith–Magenis syndrome (del 17p11.2).' *American Journal of Medical Genetics, Neuropsychiatric Genetics*, **81**, 186–191.

Summers, J.A., Lynch, P.S., Harris, J.C., Burke, J.C., Allison, D.B., Sandler, L. (1992) 'A combined behavioral/pharmacological treatment of sleep–wake schedule disorder in Angelman syndrome.' *Journal of Developmental and Behavioral Pediatrics*, **13**, 284–287.

Symons, F.J., Davis, M.L., Thompson, T. (2000) 'Self-injurious behavior and sleep disturbance in adults with developmental disabilities.' *Research in Developmental Disabilities*, **21**, 115–123.

Tierney, E., Nwokoro, N.A., Kelley, R.I. (2000) 'Behavioral phenotype of RSH/Smith–Lemli–Opitz syndrome.' *Mental Retardation and Developmental Disabilities Research Reviews*, **6**, 131–134.

Tirosh, E., Borochowitz, Z. (1992) 'Sleep apnea in fragile X syndrome.' *American Journal of Medical Genetics*, **43**, 124–127.

—— Tal, Y., Jaffe, M. (1995) 'CPAP treatment of obstructive sleep apnoea and neurodevelopmental deficits.' *Acta Paediatrica*, **84**, 791–794.

Udwin, O., Yule, W. (1990) 'A cognitive and behavioural phenotype in Williams syndrome.' *Journal of Clinical and Experimental Neuropsychology*, **13**, 232–244.

Zhdanova, I.V., Wurtman, R.J., Wagstaff, J. (1999) 'Effects of a low dose of melatonin on sleep in children with Angelman syndrome.' *Journal of Pediatric Endocrinology and Medicine*, **12**, 57–67.

Zucconi, M., Ferini-Strambi, L, Erminio, C., Pestalozza, G., Smirne, S. (1993) 'Obstructive sleep apnoea in the Rubenstein–Taybi syndrome.' *Respiration*, **60**, 127–132.

SECTION THREE

OTHER NEUROLOGICAL CONDITIONS

15
SLEEP PATTERNS IN THE EPILEPSIES

Gregory Stores

Few generalizations about epilepsy are justified, because the term covers such a wide variety of conditions that differ in their cause, manifestations, natural history and consequences. Because of this diversity it is more appropriate to refer to the 'epilepsies' or 'epilepsy syndromes', of which many are described in the international classification system (Commission on Classification and Terminology of the International League Against Epilepsy 1989). Not surprisingly, the relationship to sleep varies from one type of epilepsy to another, as is evident from the informed discussions that have been published on the subject such as that concerning childhood epilepsies by Bourgeois (1996).

Disturbances of sleep physiology have been reported in various forms of epilepsy (Autret *et al.* 1999) and have been implicated in the behavioural disorders of some people with epilepsy (Verma *et al.* 1991), but the main clinically important ways in which epilepsy and sleep are connected are as follows.

- Sleep can induce or enhance the interictal EEG abnormalities associated with certain types of epilepsy. The enhancement of the centro-temporal discharges in benign rolandic epilepsy (Panayiotopoulos 1999) is an example. Use has been made of this diagnostically in clinical EEG by means of such activation techniques as recording during sleep occurring either naturally or following sleep deprivation (which itself can have an activating effect). Conversely, epileptic discharges may be suppressed in certain types of sleep. A striking illustration of this is the suppression during REM sleep of the generalized seizure discharge seen in NREM sleep in electrical status epilepticus in slow wave sleep or ESES (Tassinari *et al.* 1992).
- Sleep loss or disruption can increase the frequency of clinical seizures (Frucht *et al.* 2000).
- In some epilepsy syndromes seizures occur predominantly (and sometimes exclusively) during sleep. Examples include benign rolandic epilepsy and mesial frontal seizures (Stores *et al.* 1991). In other epilepsies, seizure occurrence is closely related to the sleep–wake cycle, *e.g.* juvenile myoclonic epilepsy, in which seizures occur on awakening in the morning (Timmings and Richens 1992).
- Seizures (especially those of a dramatic nature) in some forms of epilepsy may well be confused with other recurrent episodes of disturbed behaviour associated with sleep (Stores 1991) including primary parasomnias, particularly the arousal disorders (Lombroso 2000). Again, mesial frontal seizures and benign rolandic seizures are examples. In addition, nocturnal seizures and other secondary parasomnias (such as panic attacks) may be mistaken for each other.

- The possible confusions between epilepsy and sleep disorders go beyond the parasomnias. Excessive daytime sleepiness (Chapter 5) has many causes, overwhelmingly of a non-epileptic nature, but sometimes it is the result of antiepileptic medication or the seizures themselves, including nonconvulsive status epilepticus (Stores *et al.* 1995).
- Epilepsy and a primary sleep disorder may coexist and even interact. For example, seizures may be exacerbated by sleep apnoea and improve with treatment of the breathing disorder (Koh *et al.* 2000).
- For various reasons, many people with epilepsy are likely to be predisposed to clinical sleep disorders. It is this relatively little researched link between epilepsy and sleep that is the main subject of the present chapter.

Studies of clinical sleep disturbance in people with epilepsy
The number of published reports on sleep problems and disorders (as distinct from abnormalities of sleep physiology) in people with epilepsy is very limited. Interpreting the findings is made difficult by the fact that the types of epilepsy studied are mixed or incompletely defined. In addition, possible causes of the sleep disturbance are often difficult to disentangle, with comorbidity (including intellectual impairment) a recurrent issue. Nevertheless, collectively the published accounts strongly suggest that many patients have significant sleep disturbance of some form deserving attention in its own right.

The adult studies are instructive about the type of sleep disturbance that might be expected in children, and also the methodological issues involved in research on this topic. For some time clinicians have been mindful of sleep problems in people with epilepsy. For example, Passouant (1984) referred to their "poor sleep" and their need for long periods of sleep but his opinion seems to have been based on clinical impression, possibly of the more severe forms of epilepsy.

The empirical study by Hoeppner *et al.* (1984) involved the use of a self-report sleep questionnaire in 30 patients grouped according to their main seizure type, not the type of epilepsy (the two are not equivalent). The sleep enquiries were confined to time taken to fall asleep at night, frequent awakenings with difficulty returning to sleep, nightmares, night terrors (sleep terrors), sleepwalking and the restorative quality of overnight sleep. Few details were provided about the patients apart from their age (average 31 years, range 16–57 years), their sex (17 female, 13 male), and that they were "independently living" and maintained on at least one and usually two or three antiepileptic drugs. The same sleep information was collected on 23 control volunteers of similar age and sex. Patients with simple or complex partial seizures had significantly more overall sleep disturbance symptoms than the controls, but those with "generalized seizures" (details of this group were not provided) showed no difference from controls. Frequent night-time awakenings were the main disturbance in the partial seizure groups, while night terrors were said to be more common in all the epilepsy groups compared with controls. In general, more sleep symptoms were reported in those patients with frequent seizures (at least monthly). Age did not seem to be associated with sleep disturbance; possible medication effects were not considered.

Vaughn *et al.* (1996) also used a short sleep questionnaire (details not provided) in 154 adults with epilepsy (no details given), 84 of whom also completed the Epworth Sleepiness

Scale (ESS). The most frequent sleep complaint was excessive daytime sleepiness (61%), with 42 per cent describing their sleep as unrefreshing. The ESS results indicated that 31 per cent were moderately or highly likely to fall asleep when watching TV and 39 per cent to do so when sitting in a public place. Three per cent were likely to fall asleep during a conversation and 2 per cent while stopped in traffic. Nearly one-half of the series complained of difficulty getting off to sleep or staying asleep at night. The prevalence of sleep complaints was correlated with seizure frequency and, more specifically, patients with partial seizures complained most of difficulty getting to sleep or staying asleep, of unrefreshing sleep and of sleep problems interfering with their work. There was little or no relation between medication (types not specified) and sleep complaints.

A number of studies have taken excessive daytime sleepiness as their starting point. Manni *et al.* (1993a) assessed daytime sleepiness in 20 patients (mean age 22 years, range 18–30 years) who were well controlled on modest doses of either phenobarbitone or carbamazepine for their "primary generalized epilepsy" or "cryptogenic focal epilepsy" (details of both groups not specified). Various measures of sleepiness were used including a version of the Multiple Sleep Latency Test (see Chapter 3). Patients taking phenobarbitone were reported to be sleepier (and to perform less well on a test of mental speed and conceptual processing) than controls matched for age and "life style". Those taking carbamazepine showed no difference from controls. In a similar study by the same group comparing phenobarbitone and sodium valproate, phenobarbitone was again seen as a cause of excessive sleepiness (Manni *et al.* 1993b).

Antiepileptic medication was also implicated in a study by Salinsky *et al.* (1996) in which both subjective and objective sleepiness measures were taken in 30 patients (mean age 35 years, range 21–55 years), of whom 24 were taking a single drug for their epilepsy (carbamazepine, phenobarbitone, phenytoin or valproic acid), the remainder taking two of these drugs. Care was taken to exclude possible effects on level of alertness of antiepileptic drug toxicity, recent seizures, other medication, alcohol, other neurological or psychiatric disorder, and sleep–wake schedule disorders such as those caused by shift work. Comparisons were made with three control groups matched appropriately with the treated epilepsy group: healthy volunteers, medication-free epilepsy patients, and patients with multiple sclerosis. The essence of the findings was that, as a group, the epilepsy patients (on chronic stable antiepileptic medication) showed more sleepiness than the comparison groups, although prominent individual differences were seen. The design of the study did not allow other possible explanations to be convincingly excluded but the authors felt that the daytime sleepiness was likely to be at least partly caused by the chronic medication. The number of patients involved in the study precluded comparisons of the different antiepileptic drugs or blood levels.

Frost *et al.* (1996) published a brief account of their study of sleep disorders, assessed by means of a questionnaire, in 75 people with "partial or generalized seizures" (further details including the age of the patients not specified) compared with 25 controls of comparable age and sex. Significantly more of the epilepsy group (37%) than controls (8%) complained of sleepiness. In both groups equally, other sleep complaints raised the possibility of sleep disruption by sleep apnoea or restless legs and/or periodic limb movements

during sleep, which was confirmed by polysomnography (PSG) in two of the patients with epilepsy.

The study by Malow *et al.* (1997a) took a wide view of possible causes of sleepiness in adult patients with epilepsy by considering the relative contributions not only of antiepileptic medication but also of symptoms of sleep disorders as well as seizure frequency, other epilepsy variables and sedative medication. The ESS and a standardized 12-item self-report sleep apnoea scale were administered to 158 people with epilepsy (age range from teens to over 60 years) and 68 nonepileptic neurology patients as controls. Additional enquiries in both groups concerned age, sex, medications, average hours of sleep obtained at night, and the presence and severity of restless legs symptoms. The epilepsy group was also described in terms of a number of seizure variables including whether the epilepsy was partial or generalized, and the occurrence of seizures during sleep. PSG findings were available in a small number of the epilepsy patients. The main finding was that the significant predictors of elevated ESS scores in both the epilepsy and control groups were the sleep apnoea scores and reports of restless legs. In the epilepsy group, sleepiness was not associated with antiepileptic medication, seizure frequency, type of epilepsy or seizures during sleep. The authors admit that they could not claim to have definitively diagnosed sleep apnoea or the restless legs syndrome. However, they emphasize the need to consider coexisting sleep disorders as a cause of daytime sleepiness in people with epilepsy, rather than assume that it is the result of antiepileptic medication or uncontrolled seizures.

The potential diagnostic yield of PSG in patients with epilepsy is also illustrated in a review of findings in 63 adult patients in whom obstructive sleep apnoea and a variety of other sleep disorders were revealed (Malow *et al.* 1997b). The need to sometimes consider subtle aspects of sleep physiology to explain sleep problems was illustrated in a study by Zucconi *et al.* (2000) of a group of patients with autosomal dominant nocturnal frontal lobe epilepsy in whom instability at the microstructural level of sleep physiology (see discussion of sleep fragmentation in Chapter 2) was associated with complaints of daytime sleepiness.

Studies of sleep disorder in children with epilepsy are very few. In preliminary studies (Zaiwalla 1989, Zaiwalla and Stores 1989) parental questionnaires were used to assess sleep behaviour in 45 children (aged 7–14 years) with various forms of epilepsy and 34 control children of similar age, sex and intellectual level. All the children with epilepsy were of normal intelligence with seizures well controlled on either sodium valproate or carbamazepine in moderate dosage. Their parents reported a significantly higher rate of severe and persistent sleep problems than in the control group, especially sleeplessness, daytime lethargy and unrefreshing sleep. In both children with epilepsy and controls, sleep problems were significantly associated with overall behavioural disturbance. PSG was performed on the eight children with unrefreshing sleep. Two were shown to have unsuspected seizure discharge at night associated with frequent arousals. When the remaining six were compared with age- and sex-matched controls, no differences in conventional sleep variables were seen, but the children with epilepsy showed a different pattern of arousals with more sustained arousals later in the night.

Another preliminary report by Deray and Epstein (1991) concerned PSG findings in 43 patients (almost all children) with various forms of medication-resistant epilepsy some-

times combined with intellectual disability. The group's average age was 10 years (range 1.7–24 years). Medication and various other relevant details were not provided. Compared with 12 control children, the children with epilepsy showed abnormalities of their sleep architecture, especially those with "generalized or multifocal epilepsy" as distinct from the subgroups whose seizures were described as temporal or extratemporal in origin. Clinical sleep disorders were not considered in this study.

Sleep disorders were assessed in more detail by Stores *et al.* (1998) in their study of 79 children with relatively mild forms of epilepsy considered typical of cases under general paediatric care rather than those attending specialized epilepsy services. The children, aged 5–16 years with an average age of 10 years, were compared with healthy children from the general population matched for age and sex. Children in the epilepsy group were described by seizure type, age of onset and duration of their seizure disorder, seizure rate and antiepileptic medication. Intellectual impairment, behavioural disturbance and/or other physical disorder were identified in a small minority. The parental sleep questionnaire used was known to have satisfactory psychometric characteristics and covered a wide range of sleep disorder symptoms. These items were grouped into five clinical categories: poor quality (non-restorative) sleep, anxieties about sleep, episodic disturbances during sleep, disordered breathing during sleep, and short-duration sleep. The behaviour of children in both groups was assessed by means of the Conners Revised Parent Rating Scale, an established instrument for these purposes. Compared with their controls, the children with epilepsy showed significantly higher rates of sleep disorder symptoms, especially those suggesting poor quality sleep and sleep-related anxieties. Anxiety at night was associated with a higher seizure frequency. In the younger children with epilepsy, sleep problems (especially poor quality sleep) were associated with disturbed daytime behaviour.

Following earlier preliminary reports (Gianotti *et al.* 1994, 1996), Cortesi *et al.* (1999) described a detailed study in which sleep and behaviour were assessed in 89 children aged 6–13 years (average 9 years) diagnosed as having either a generalized or partial form of idiopathic epilepsy. Seizure frequency varied widely. All children were being treated with sodium valproate alone. The sleep of these children and of a control group of age- and sex-matched healthy children (including some sibling controls) was assessed by means of a parental questionnaire (the Sleep Behaviour Questionnaire) developed and psychometrically evaluated by the same researchers. The 29-item questionnaire covered a wide range of sleep disorder symptoms. Seizure variables were also assessed in some detail. Additional measures were the Child Behavior Checklist and the Malaise Inventory to assess mothers' emotional state. The main findings were that the children with epilepsy showed significantly more sleep problems than did controls (including siblings), in particular parasomnias other than epilepsy, sleep fragmentation, daytime drowsiness, bedtime difficulties and parent–child interactions during the night. The last two problems (and total number of sleep problems) were more common in younger patients. Current seizures were particularly associated with the sleep problems of the children with epilepsy, although other more complex associations were also seen regarding age and certain other seizure variables. Both child behavioural disturbance and maternal malaise were greater in the epilepsy group, the extent of the behavioural disturbance also being associated with their sleep problems.

Sleep problems in children with epilepsy, their aetiology and management

The above review of adult and child studies demonstrates how much further research is needed to clarify the various issues involved regarding sleep and its disorders in people with epilepsy. Nevertheless, certain basic conclusions can be drawn that are important for the care of those with epilepsy whether the epileptic disorder stands alone, or is an accompaniment or part of one of the developmental disorders considered in other sections of this book.

- Sleep problems are very commonly reported in both children and adults with epilepsy. This appears to be so not only in severe forms of the condition, but also in those groups more representative of the epilepsies in general.
- All three of the basic types of sleep complaint discussed in Chapters 4 to 6 are reported, namely sleeplessness, excessive daytime sleepiness and nonepileptic parasomnias.
- The underlying likely causes of these sleep problems or complaints are not well identified in the epilepsy literature. However, certain possibilities are raised that should be considered in explaining a person's sleep disturbance in the light of what is generally known about the aetiology of sleep loss or disruption. Systematic and comprehensive enquiries about the seizure disorder, the patient's sleep and related aspects of his condition and circumstances are important to explain the individual case because choice of treatment depends on which factors can be convincingly identified.

There are two main implications for clinical practice:

- It can be assumed that, in many cases, careful enquiry will reveal the presence of a sleep problem, the cause of which needs to be identified precisely. In children with epilepsy a range of possible explanations (physical and psychological) needs to be considered. Some are specific to epilepsy or its treatment; others are general in that they might be relevant to any child whose sleep is disturbed, although possibly the form of their expression is influenced by the nature of the child's epilepsy and family reactions to it. Each cause or combination of causes will require a particular type of help.
- The importance of effective treatment for the child's sleep disorder lies not only in alleviating the sleep problem itself but also in the fact that improved sleep may aid seizure control.

The following are examples of factors that might underlie the various forms of sleep disturbance.

SLEEPLESSNESS

The possible causes of sleeplessness discussed in Chapter 4, some of them related to age, should be considered in any child. Depending on the child's type of epilepsy and its severity, *difficulty getting off to sleep* caused by emotional factors may be prominent as part of the psychological upset that is a consequence in children with epilepsy. For example, separation from parents at bedtime might hold special fears, especially in children subject to nocturnal seizures of which they are aware. Emotional overdependency, associated with some forms of childhood epilepsy (Stores and Piran 1978), increases this likelihood. On the other hand, difficult behaviour at bedtime might be a reflection of parents' inability or reluctance to set limits to the child's behaviour as part of their general overpermissiveness.

Help for these problems consists of psychological support for the child or advice about parenting practices.

Recurrent and troublesome waking at night may again be the result of various factors encountered in children in general as discussed in Chapter 4. Alternatively, the episodes may be parasomnias of a type more specifically associated with epilepsy (see below).

The effects of *antiepileptic medication* on sleep have been little studied. The general impression is that successful treatment of seizures improves the quality of sleep (Rosen *et al.* 1982), but individual differences in response to medication are well known and sleep disturbance can be a side-effect in some patients. For example, a seemingly convincing association between lamotrigine and insomnia has been reported in a number of adult patients (Sadler 1999). Interestingly, although in the past phenobarbitone had a reputation for causing sleep disturbances (including night waking in children treated for febrile seizures) this has not always been confirmed (Hirtz *et al.* 1993).

EXCESSIVE DAYTIME SLEEPINESS
As discussed already, *antiepileptic medication* tends to be implicated when patients are somnolent during the day, and, indeed, this may be the explanation because of the direct action of certain drugs (either at modest dosage in some patients or at toxic blood levels) or because of interactions such as the tendency for sodium valproate to potentiate the sedative effect of other drugs. However, enquiries should be made about other possibilities including *sleep loss or disruption.*

Alternatively, sleep quality may be impaired because of the coexistence of a *sleep disorder.* In older children and adolescents in particular, abnormalities of the sleep–wake cycle (Chapter 5) are common in the general population and a potentially treatable cause of daytime sleepiness. To a lesser extent, the same is true of upper airway obstruction and periodic limb movements in sleep, both of which disrupt sleep continuity. *Illicit drug effects* have also to be considered in young people. *Poor sleep hygiene*, from whatever cause, may need to be corrected as part of overall management.

In the absence of an explanation in terms of the conditions already mentioned, the child's quality of sleep may be impaired by subtle *disruptive effects of seizure activity on sleep physiology*, detectable by PSG. If confirmed, adjustment of antiepileptic medication might be helpful, although this possibility has not been examined in any systematic way.

PARASOMNIAS
The characterization of paroxysmal disturbances at night in children with epilepsy can be a problem even when they include obvious clinical manifestations. In a study of sleep disorders in children with tuberous sclerosis (Hunt and Stores 1994), in which a high rate of such disorders was found (closely associated with current epilepsy), an incidental but important observation concerned diagnostic uncertainty about the children's night-time attacks. From the descriptions available, it was unclear in a third of cases whether the episodes were epileptic in nature or not. Especially if detailed accounts are not obtained, there is a risk that in children with undoubted daytime seizures, nocturnal episodes will also be considered to be epileptic (and antiepileptic medication increased) despite the many other possibilities.

A number of primary parasomnias may be misconstrued as epileptic, such as the different types of rhythmic movement disorder, arousal disorders or awakenings associated with obstructive sleep apnoea. Nonepileptic secondary parasomnias, such as panic attacks, may also be misdiagnosed as seizures. However, the opposite error can occur with the less well-known type of seizure, such as mesial frontal seizures, misdiagnosed for example as nightmares (Stores *et al.* 1991). Nocturnal epilepsy and other forms of parasomnia such as sleep terrors may coexist (Tassinari *et al.* 1972), and epilepsy during sleep may be simulated by patients who are actually awake (Thacker *et al.* 1993).

Distinctions between the different primary and secondary parasomnias should usually be possible by careful clinical enquiry, although physiological monitoring may be required in some cases. The value of such monitoring is greatest where nocturnal attacks are less than obvious, *e.g.* tonic seizures forming part of the Lennox–Gastaut syndrome (mixed seizure types associated with intellectual impairment), or in circumstances where accurate clinical descriptions are difficult to obtain.

Research needs

The number of issues concerning epilepsy and sleep that remain to be clarified is obvious from the above review. Main requirements for future research include detailed descriptions of the epilepsies concerned including their aetiology, severity, associated problems (including intellectual impairment) and treatment, and equally careful diagnosis of the underlying sleep disorder. This clinical refinement should be matched by additional measures used to assess sleep or the psychological consequences of the sleep disturbance. Some standardized instruments are available for these purposes but their further development is needed, especially for use with children. To avoid misleading generalizations, individual differences should not be overlooked, including the possibility of age and sex effects on the relationship between epilepsy and sleep.

The complexity of research in this area may seem daunting but should not act as a deterrent in view of the importance of the subject for the welfare of children with a seizure disorder, not least because of the likely harmful effects on daytime learning and behaviour of persistently disturbed sleep.

REFERENCES

Autret, A., de Toffol, B., Corcia, P.H., Hommet, C., Prunier-Levilion, C., Lucas, B. (1999) 'Sleep and epilepsy.' *Sleep Medicine Reviews*, **3**, 201–217.
Bourgeois, B. (1996) 'The relationship between sleep and epilepsy in children.' *Seminars in Pediatric Neurology*, **3**, 29–35.
Commission on Classification and Terminology of the International League Against Epilepsy (1989) 'Proposal for revised classification of epilepsies and epileptic syndromes.' *Epilepsia*, **30**, 389–399.
Cortesi, F., Giannotti, F., Ottaviano, S. (1999) 'Sleep problems and daytime behaviour in childhood idiopathic epilepsy.' *Epilepsia*, **40**, 1557–1565.
Deray, M.J., Epstein, M.A. (1991) 'Sleep abnormalities in children with intractable epilepsy.' *Sleep Research*, **20**, 98. *(Abstract.)*
Frost, M., Malow, B., Aldrich, M. (1996) 'A survey of sleep disorders in epilepsy patients.' *Neurology*, **46**, A120. *(Abstract.)*
Frucht, M.M., Quigg, M., Schwaner, C., Fountain, N.B. (2000) 'Distribution of seizure precipitants among epilepsy syndromes.' *Epilepsia*, **41**, 1534–1539.

Gianotti, F., Cortesi, F., Bruni, O. (1994) 'Sleep habits in children with idiopathic epilepsy.' *Sleep Research*, **23**, 361. *(Abstract.)*

—————— Marotta, A. (1996) 'Sleep problems in childhood epilepsy: a questionnaire based study.' *Neurology*, **46**, A121. *(Abstract.)*

Hirtz, D.G., Chen, T.C., Nelson, K.B., Sulzbacher, S., Farwell, J.R., Ellenberg, J.H. (1993) 'Does phenobarbital used for febrile seizures cause sleep disturbances?' *Pediatric Neurology*, **9**, 94–100.

Hoeppner, J.B., Garron, D.C., Cartwright, R.D. (1984) 'Self-reported sleep disorder symptoms in epilepsy.' *Epilepsia*, **25**, 434–437.

Hunt, A., Stores, G. (1994) 'Sleep disorder and epilepsy in children with tuberous sclerosis: a questionnaire-based study.' *Developmental Medicine and Child Neurology*, **36**, 108–115.

Koh, S., Ward, S.L., Lin, M., Chen, L.S. (2000) 'Sleep apnea treatment improves seizure control in children with neurodevelopmental disorders.' *Pediatric Neurology*, **22**, 36–39.

Lombroso, C.T. (2000) 'Pavor nocturnus of proven epileptic origin.' *Epilepsia*, **41**, 1221–1226.

Malow, B.A., Bowes, R.J., Lin, X. (1997a) 'Predictors of sleepiness in epilepsy patients.' *Sleep*, **20**, 1105–1110.

—— Fromes, G., Aldrich, M. (1997b) 'Usefulness of polysomnography in epilepsy patients.' *Neurology*, **48**, 1389–1394.

Manni, R., Ratti, M.T., Galimberti, C.A., Morini, R., Perucca, E., Tartara, A. (1993a) 'Daytime sleepiness in epileptic patients on long-term monotherapy: MSLT, clinical and psychometric assessment.' *Neurophysiologie Clinique*, **23**, 71–76.

—— —— Perucca, E., Galimberti, C.A., Tartara, A. (1993b) 'A multiparametric investigation of daytime sleepiness and psychomotor functions in epileptic patients treated with phenobarbital and sodium valproate: a comparative controlled study.' *Electroencephalography and Clinical Neurophysiology*, **86**, 322–328.

Panayiotopoulos, C.P. (1999) 'Benign childhood epilepsy with centrotemporal spikes or Rolandic seizures.' *In: Benign Childhood Partial Seizures and Related Epileptic Syndromes.* London: John Libbey, pp. 33–70.

Passouant, P. (1984) 'Historical aspects of sleep and epilepsy.' *In:* Degen, R., Niedermeyer, E. (Eds.) *Epilepsy, Sleep and Sleep Deprivation.* Amsterdam: Elsevier, pp. 67–73.

Rosen, I., Blennow, G., Risberg, A.M., Ingvar, D.H. (1982) 'Quantitative evaluation of nocturnal sleep in epileptic children.' *In:* Sterman, M.B., Shouse, M.N., Passouant, P. (Eds.) *Sleep and Epilepsy.* New York: Academic Press, pp. 397–409.

Sadler, M. (1999) 'Lamotrigine associated with insomnia.' *Epilepsia*, **40**, 322–325.

Salinsky, M.C., Oken, B.S., Binder, L.M. (1996) 'Assessment of drowsiness in epilepsy patients receiving chronic antiepileptic drug therapy.' *Epilepsia*, **37**, 181–187.

Stores, G. (1991) 'Confusions concerning sleep disorders and the epilepsies in children and adolescents.' *British Journal of Psychiatry*, **158**, 1–7.

—— Piran, N. (1978) 'Dependency of different types in schoolchildren with epilepsy.' *Psychological Medicine*, **8**, 441–445.

—— Zaiwalla, Z., Bergel, N. (1991) 'Frontal lobe complex partial seizures in children: a form of epilepsy at particular risk of misdiagnosis.' *Developmental Medicine and Child Neurology*, **33**, 998–1009.

—— —— Styles, E., Hoshika, A. (1995) 'Nonconvulsive status epilepticus.' *Archives of Disease in Childhood*, **73**, 106–111.

—— Wiggs, L., Campling, G. (1998) 'Sleep disorders and their relationship to psychological disturbance in children with epilepsy.' *Child: Care, Health and Development*, **24**, 5–19.

Tassinari, C.A., Mancia, D., Bernadina, B., Gastaut, H. (1972) 'Pavor nocturnus of nonepileptic nature in epileptic children.' *Electroencephalography and Clinical Neurophysiology*, **33**, 603–607.

—— Bureau, M., Dravet, C., Dalla Bernadina, B., Roger, J. (1992) 'Epilepsy with continuous spikes and waves during slow sleep – otherwise described as ESES (epilepsy with electrical status-epilepticus during slow sleep).' *In:* Roger J., Bureau, M., Dravet, C., Dreifuss, F.E., Perret, A., Wolf, P. (Eds.) *Epileptic Syndromes in Infancy, Childhood and Adolescence, 2nd Edn.* London: John Libbey, pp. 245–256.

Thacker, K., Devinsky, O., Perrine, K., Alper, K., Luciano, D. (1993) 'Nonepileptic seizures during apparent sleep.' *Annals of Neurology*, **33**, 414–418.

Timmings, P.L., Richens, A. (1992) 'Juvenile myoclonic epilepsy.' *British Medical Journal*, **305**, 4–5.

Vaughn, B.V., Miller, M.T., D'Cruzo, O.F., Messenheimer, J.A. (1996) 'Prevalence of sleep complaints in patients with epilepsy: application of the Epworth Sleepiness Scale.' *Sleep Research*, **24**, 453. *(Abstract.)*

Verma, N.P., Policherla, H., Kapen, S., McKee, D., Williams, L., Yusko, M. (1991) 'Are behavioural disorders and sleep disruption in complex partial seizures related?' *Journal of Epilepsy*, **4**, 217–223.

Zaiwalla, Z. (1989) 'Sleep abnormalities in children with epilepsy.' *Electroencephalography and Clinical Neurophysiology*, **72**, 29. *(Abstract.)*

—— Stores, G. (1989) 'Sleep and arousal disorders in childhood epilepsy.' *Sleep Research*, **18**, 129. *(Abstract.)*

Zucconi, M., Oldani, A., Smirne, S., Ferini-Strambi, L. (2000) 'The macrostructure and microstructure of sleep in patients with autosomal dominant frontal lobe epilepsy.' *Journal of Clinical Neurophysiology*, **17**, 77–86.

16
SLEEP ABNORMALITIES AND CEREBRAL PALSY

Suresh Kotagal

Cerebral palsy is a static encephalopathy resulting from an insult to the developing brain that may be acquired in the pre-, peri- or postnatal period, generally with consequent alterations in muscle tone, mobility and posture, epilepsy, and impaired cognition, vision or communication. The incidence is approximately 1.2 per 1000 (Irie 1999), and the prevalence 2.1 to 2.5 per 1000 (Pharoah *et al.* 1998, Robertson *et al.* 1998). There is no entirely satisfactory classification that takes into account the aetiology, clinical features and extent of functional disability, but a clinical classification based on the nature of the neurological deficit (Table 16.1) seems to be the most useful. Spastic cerebral palsy is the most common form.

While clinical experience suggests that cerebral palsy is associated with disturbed sleep, the literature in this field is sparse and anecdotal. Also, longitudinal data are lacking. This chapter summarizes the key sleep–wake disturbances in this population. As the literature is composed largely of cases of severe spastic or athetoid cerebral palsy, one must be cautious in generalizing the available information to cerebral palsy of all types and levels of severity.

Characteristic sleep problems
Table 16.2 summarizes the commonly experienced sleep problems in cerebral palsy.

SLEEP-RELATED BREATHING DISTURBANCES
Kotagal et al. (1994) found that, compared to age-matched controls, children with severe cerebral palsy (n=9) had more apnoeas and hypopnoeas per hour of sleep, with fewer body position changes during sleep at night, thus being unable to compensate for the respiratory events by shifting from the supine into the lateral decubitus. Pharyngeal obstruction from macroglossia, glossoptosis, and aspiration consequent to gastro-oesophageal reflux may impair respiration during sleep. The clinical manifestations of obstructive sleep apnoea include irritability, habitual snoring, increased nocturnal awakenings, mouth breathing, opisthotonic posturing and observed apnoea. The respiratory disturbance may be refractory to conventional medical treatment with artificial airway devices and continuous positive airway pressure breathing (Cohen et al. 1997). A component of central apnoea may also coexist.

CIRCADIAN RHYTHM ABNORMALITIES
The suprachiasmatic nucleus of the hypothalamus is the circadian timekeeper. It receives

TABLE 16.1
The clinical classification of cerebral palsy

Spastic
    Diplegic (predominately involving the lower extremities)
    Hemiplegic
    Tetraplegic
Dystonic
Hypotonic
Ataxic
Mixed (spastic–dystonic)

TABLE 16.2
Anatomical sites and their relationship to sleep disturbances in cerebral palsy

Cerebrum
Seizures leading to arousals
Anticonvulsant medications leading to arousals
Circadian rhythm abnormalities (advanced sleep phase syndrome, delayed sleep phase syndrome,
    irregular sleep–wake rhythms)
Central, mixed or obstructive sleep apnoea

Upper airway
Obstructive or mixed sleep apnoea from macroglossia, glossoptosis, adenotonsillar hypertrophy

Gastrointestinal
Gastro-oesophageal reflux

Pulmonary
Recurrent aspiration pneumonia

Musculoskeletal
Decreased ability to change body position, thus provoking arousals

illumination-dependent impulses from the retina, and is essential to signalling the time of sleep onset. Patients with cerebral palsy who are blind from lesions in the anterior visual pathway, *e.g.* those with chorioretinitis or septo-optic dysplasia, may experience a delay in the secretion of the initial surge of nocturnal melatonin, which plays a role in both sleep induction and maintenance. This can impact the timing (phase delay) and length of their sleep. In a study of eight functionally blind and learning-disabled children or young adults, Palm *et al.* (1997) found a non-24-hour sleep–wake syndrome. Diurnal variations in serum and urinary melatonin were out of phase relative to sleep and melatonin secretion in five of these patients, who thus exhibited internal resynchronization. Administration of melatonin in the evening dramatically improved sleep continuity in all eight subjects.

SLEEP AND EPILEPSY
Subclinical epileptiform discharges and clinical seizures are most common during stages I and II of non-REM (NREM) sleep (Bourgeois 1996). Both types of paroxysmal events provoke excessive arousals. The most consistent abnormalities consequent to seizures are prolonged sleep latency (time taken to fall asleep after lights are turned off), increased

stage I and II NREM sleep, decreased stage III and IV NREM sleep and REM sleep, and an overall decrease in the total amount of sleep per 24 hours (Besset 1982, Bourgeois 1996). Anticonvulsant medications generally decrease sleep latency and improve sleep continuity, although phenobarbitone and the benzodiazepines have been known to suppress REM sleep. Some of the newer anticonvulsants like lamotrigine, gabapentin and topiramate do not significantly impact sleep architecture. Felbamate may trigger insomnia. Other relationships between epilepsy and sleep are discussed in Chapter 15.

PRIMARY ALTERATIONS IN SLEEP ARCHITECTURE
Besides the above disorders, a primary disturbance in sleep organization consequent to brainstem dysfunction may also occur. Hayashi *et al.* (1990) reported that in a series of 10 athetoid cerebral palsy patients, there was a marked decrease in the number of rapid eye movements along with a decreased rate of twitch and gross body movements during periods of REM sleep.

EFFECTS OF PSYCHOLOGICAL DISTURBANCE ON SLEEP
The lives of children with cerebral palsy and their parents are frequently complicated by the child's disturbed behaviour. Studies concentrating on hemiplegic cerebral palsy have demonstrated that many children (of all ages and both sexes) with this condition are affected in this way. Psychological disturbance is seen to a severe degree in about 50 per cent of hemiplegic children compared with at most 15 per cent of children in the general population (Goodman and Graham 1996). In addition, such disturbance has been shown to persist for more than four years in 70 per cent of cases, with new disorders developing over the same period in another 30 per cent who were not psychologically disturbed at the start of that period (Goodman 1998). The main psychological difficulties described have been irritability and other difficult behaviour, anxiety, low mood, overactivity and poor attention. These features are very similar to those described in children in general with persistent sleep disturbance (Chapter 1). The poor sleep of children with cerebral palsy for the reasons and in the ways already mentioned might well contribute to these psychological difficulties (a possibility not yet investigated). Conversely, the various types of psychological disturbance caused by factors other than disturbed sleep (including rejection by other children, poor self-esteem or maternal depression) are likely to cause or worsen the children's sleep disturbance. The same is true of intellectual impairment (Chapter 7), which sometimes accompanies cerebral palsy.

Special considerations of management
Sleep logs and actigraphy (Sadeh *et al.* 1995) are helpful in the study of patients with sleep-onset insomnia and suspected circadian rhythm abnormalities. Those with consequent sleep-onset insomnia may benefit from the administration of 1–3 mg of melatonin, 30–60 minutes before their bedtime. Bright light exposure in the early morning hours may also help reset circadian rhythms.

Nocturnal polysomnography is essential in evaluating sleep maintenance difficulties. The EEG segment of the polysomnogram is helpful in determining whether the arousals

are epileptic or nonepileptic (secondary to sleep apnoea, gastro-oesophageal reflux, etc.). Therapeutic doses of appropriate anticonvulsants may reduce sleep fragmentation from epilepsy.

Patients with *obstructive sleep apnoea* should undergo an otolaryngological evaluation in order to assess for surgically correctable lesions like enlarged tonsils or adenoids, macroglossia and mandibular recession. If the surgery fails to improve sleep, a trial of continuous positive airway pressure breathing is recommended. Tracheotomy is indicated only in rare instances when other therapeutic options have been exhausted.

As in any group of children with a chronic disorder, psychological evaluation of each affected child (and the effects of the disorder on the family) should be assessed routinely and help provided as appropriate to minimize adverse consequences on the child's sleep and the well-being of the family as a whole (Eiser 1993).

REFERENCES

Besset, A. (1982) 'Influence of generalized seizures on sleep organization.' *In:* Sterman, M.B., Shouse, M.N., Passouant, P. (Eds.) *Sleep and Epilepsy.* New York, Academic Press, pp. 339–346.

Bourgeois, B. (1996) 'The relationship between sleep and epilepsy in children.' *Seminars in Pediatric Neurology*, **3**, 29–35.

Cohen, S.R., Lefaivre, J.F., Burstein, F.D., Simms, C., Kattos, A.V, Scott, P.H., Montgomery, G.L., Graham, L. (1997) 'Surgical treatment of obstructive sleep apnea in neurologically compromised patients.' *Plastic and Reconstructive Surgery*, **99**, 638–646.

Eiser, C. (1993) *Growing Up With A Chronic Disease: the Impact on Children and their Families.* London: Jessica Kingsley.

Goodman, R (1998) 'The longitudinal stability of psychiatric problems in children with hemiplegia.' *Journal of Child Psychology and Psychiatry*, **39**, 347–354.

—— Graham, P. (1996) 'Psychiatric problems in children with hemiplegia: cross sectional epidemiological survey.' *British Medical Journal*, **312**, 1065–1069.

Hayashi, M., Inoue Y., Iwakawa, Y., Saski, H. (1990) 'REM sleep abnormalities in severe athetoid cerebral palsy.' *Brain Development*, **12**, 494–497.

Irie, N. (1999) 'A study on incidence of developmental disabilities in Higashi-Osaka City, Japan, 1988–1992.' *No To Hattatsu*, **31**, 32–37.

Kotagal, S., Gibbons, V.P., Stith, J.A. (1994) 'Sleep abnormalities in patients with severe cerebral palsy.' *Developmental Medicine and Child Neurology*, **36**, 304–311.

Palm, L., Blennow. G., Wetterberg, L. (1997) 'Long-term melatonin treatment in blind children and young adults with circadian rhythm disorders.' *Developmental Medicine and Child Neurology*, **39**, 319–325.

Pharoah, P.O., Cooke, T., Johnson, M.A., King, R., Mutch, L. (1998) 'Epidemiology of cerebral palsy in England and Scotland.' *Archives of Disease in Childhood, Fetal and Neonatal Edition*, **79**, F21–F25.

Robertson, C.M., Svenson, L.W., Joffres, M.R. (1998) 'Prevalence of cerebral palsy in Alberta.' *Canadian Journal of Neurological Sciences*, **25**, 117–122.

Sadeh, A., Hauri, P.J., Kripke, D.F., Lavie, P. (1995) 'The role of actigraphy in the evaluation of sleep disorders.' *Sleep*, **18**, 288–302.

17
SLEEP DISORDERS AND NEUROMUSCULAR DISEASES

Narong Simakajornboon and Robert Beckerman

Cardiorespiratory failure is the most common cause of morbidity and mortality in children who have neuromuscular disease (NMD). Respiratory insufficiency may present acutely, or can develop insidiously as a result of progressive respiratory muscle weakness. Physiological changes during sleep place a high demand on the respiratory muscles and may exaggerate awake abnormalities in respiratory function. In fact, respiratory disturbances during sleep such as sleep-disordered breathing (SDB) and progressive alveolar hypoventilation may be the first evidence of respiratory muscle weakness and can even occur in the face of minimal neuromuscular functional disability (Heckmatt *et al.* 1989). Successful management of sleep-related respiratory disturbances in children with NMD has been facilitated in recent years by the introduction of both noninvasive negative and positive pressure ventilation. In this chapter, we will review the pathophysiology, characteristic sleep abnormalities, clinical assessment and management of SDB in children with static and progressive NMD. Since a complete discussion of respiratory control aspects of all childhood NMD is beyond the scope of this chapter, we will limit our remarks to prototypical NMD. The likelihood of additional behaviourally determined sleep problems, caused by the psychological effects of the basic condition on the child and parents (see opening chapters), also needs to be considered in overall diagnosis and care.

Pathophysiology (aetiological factors)
Sleep-related respiratory dysfunction in children with NMD is primarily caused by the abnormalities in the respiratory muscle 'pump' (chest wall and diaphragm). However, other factors predispose children with NMD to manifest signs and symptoms of SDB as follows.
- *Physiological changes in respiratory mechanics during sleep* include decreases in tidal volume, minute ventilation and functional residual capacity (FRC), mild alveolar hypoventilation, and variable fluctuations in cardiorespiratory rate and rhythm with sleep stage change. These normal physiological responses are accentuated by baseline awake abnormalities in respiratory muscle and lung function.
- *Upper airway and intercostal muscle hypotonia* caused by a loss of tonic activity of the pharyngeal and laryngeal muscle dilators during sleep may result in an increase in upper airway resistance (Hudgel and Robertson 1984). Hypotonia during non-REM (NREM) and atonia during REM sleep of intercostal muscles can lead to further decrease in FRC (Hudgel and Devadatta 1984). Children with NMD may also have selective bulbar

111

involvement that results in additional hypotonia of the upper airway muscles and reduction in protective reflexes that can lead to aspiration of upper airway secretion during sleep. Hypotonia of the upper airway and intercostal muscles in infants with NMD is associated with an increased chest-wall compliance, rib-cage deformability and reduced FRC (Papastamelos *et al.* 1996).

- *Diaphragmatic involvement.* Although the diaphragm maintains normal tonic activity during NREM sleep, it decreases in activity during REM sleep. Since atonia of intercostal muscles occurs during REM sleep, ventilation is almost completely dependent on preserved diaphragmatic function. Certain NMDs, *e.g.* spinal muscular atrophy (SMA) and Duchenne muscular dystrophy (DMD), can involve the diaphragm, which predisposes them to significant hypoxaemia or hypoventilation during REM sleep. In fact, patients with bilateral diaphragmatic paralysis have been reported to have profound oxygen desaturation and hypoventilation during REM sleep (Skatrud *et al.* 1980). Infants, who have a high percentage of active or REM sleep, are particularly vulnerable to unsuspected respiratory failure. The reduction in FRC (20–30%) during sleep is accentuated in the supine position and after meals because of hydrostatic fluid pressure from abdominal contents on the weakened diaphragm.
- *Control of ventilation.* Respiratory control dysfunction during sleep in NMD is usually secondary to respiratory muscle failure and not to a primary decrease in respiratory drive. Patients with progressive NMD and chronic hypercarbia may sometimes develop a secondary reduction in hypoxic and hypercarbic response (Riley *et al.* 1977). It is difficult, however, to differentiate a primary reduction in respiratory drive from a change in chest wall and lung mechanical properties caused by muscle weakness. Most published studies in NMD have failed to demonstrate true primary abnormalities in respiratory control (Begin *et al.* 1980, Newsom-Davis 1980). To the contrary, some studies suggest that central respiratory drive is intact and may be increased to overcome abnormal respiratory mechanics (Baydur 1991).
- *Secondary scoliosis.* Most children with NMD, especially those who are wheelchair dependent, eventually develop progressive thoracolumbar scoliosis, which further compromises lung volumes, respiratory mechanics and pulmonary clearance, which may lead to atelectasis and pneumonia.

Characteristic sleep disorders and prototypical neuromuscular diseases
SDB can occur in a variety of childhood NMDs at different stages of the illness. Examples are DMD, SMA, myotonic dystrophy, infantile familial myasthenia gravis, poliomyelitis, nonprogressive NMDs including nemaline myopathy, cerebral palsy (CP) and acute spinal cord injuries.

CEREBRAL PALSY (see also Chapter 16)
Infants and children with CP are at risk of developing obstructive sleep apnoea and hypoventilation. In these patients, muscles of the upper airway including tongue, soft palate, pharynx and larynx may have varying degrees of spasticity during wakefulness. However, hypotonia of these muscle groups may occur during sleep. The common types of apnoea

are obstructive and mixed apnoea, associated with partial obstruction, hypopnoea, oxygen desaturation and alveolar hypoventilation. SDB in these patients can be managed by nasal ventilation; some patients may require tracheostomy for stabilization of the airway. Certain patients may benefit from other alternative surgical management such as tonsillectomy and adenoidectomy, turbinectomy, uvulopalatoplasty or mandibular advancement (Cohen *et al.* 1997). In patients with athetoid cerebral palsy, abnormalities of REM sleep have been observed. Hayashi *et al.* (1990) reported an abnormal distribution of body movements during REM sleep including increased chin muscle tone, decreased phasic muscle twitches and decreased REM.

SPINAL MUSCULAR ATROPHY

SMA is an autosomal recessive disease of anterior horn cells characterized by weakness and atrophy of the distal muscles. The phrenic nerves, however, are typically intact until the late stages of the disease (Kuzuhara and Chou 1981). SMA type I (Werdnig–Hoffmann disease) usually presents with marked hypotonia soon after birth, and patients will develop respiratory failure and die during early childhood unless mechanical ventilatory support is initiated. In SMA type II, the muscle weakness manifests later on and with partial involvement of respiratory muscles. These children may have unrecognized nocturnal hypoxaemia and hypoventilation early in life leading to acute respiratory insufficiency during episodes of respiratory infection (Bach and Wang 1995). Nocturnal polysomnography can detect silent SDB in these patients without any predisposing factor and with normal awake blood gas. Polysomnography in these patients may reveal prolonged central apnoea, mixed apnoea, hypopnoea, REM-related oxygen desaturation and hypoventilation (Fig. 17.1) (Manni *et al.* 1993). Nocturnal ventilation has been shown to improve rib-cage development, lung growth and daytime ventilation.

DUCHENNE MUSCULAR DYSTROPHY

The sleep complaints in DMD patients are usually related to respiratory disturbance during sleep. Symptoms of SDB can present early in life and the severity cannot be predicted from daytime pulmonary function tests (Smith *et al.* 1988). Manifestations of SDB in DMD include obstructive apnoea, central apnoea, paradoxical breathing, nocturnal hypoventilation and nonapnoeic oxygen desaturation (Khan and Heckmatt 1994). The most common and early abnormality is obstructive apnoea, which is often accompanied by hypercapnia, although central apnoea can develop in advanced cases. SDB in these patients is often associated with frequent arousals and sleep fragmentation.

MYOTONIC DYSTROPHY

Congenital myotonic dystrophy is a fairly common neonatal muscle disorder. Infants can present with hypotonia, facial diplegia and limb contractures, and have problems sucking and swallowing that predispose them to recurrent aspiration pneumonia. Steinert's myotonic dystrophy, on the other hand, is a myopathic disorder of the adolescent and adults.

Polysomnographic studies in these patients may reveal the presence of central apnoea, mixed apnoea, obstructive apnoea, REM-sleep-related hypoxaemia, alveolar hypoventilation

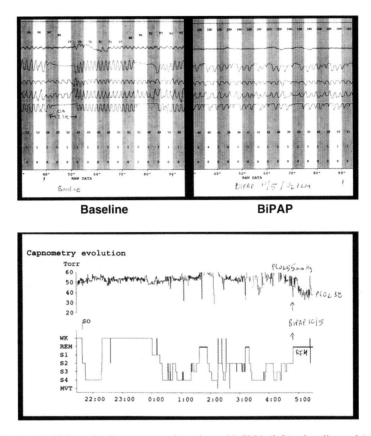

Fig. 17.1. *(Top)* Multichannel polysomnogram in patient with SMA *(left)* at baseline and *(right)* after initiation of noninvasive positive pressure ventilation with nasal bilevel positive airway pressure (BiPAP). The recording revealed only respiratory channels; from top to bottom: pulse oximetry, pulse waveform, nasal thermister, thoracic and abdominal movements, end-tidal CO_2, transcutaneous pO_2 and pCO_2. Patient had episodes of obstructive apnoea with SpO_2 (oxygen desaturation) and alveolar hypoventilation that resolved after BiPAP.

(Bottom) Capnometry (pCO_2) revealed significant nocturnal hypoventilation. After initiation of BiPAP, a decrease in end-tidal pCO_2 was associated with REM rebound.

and periodic breathing (Coccagna *et al.* 1975, Guilleminault *et al.* 1978). There are reports of some patients with myotonic dystrophy who presented with hypersomnolence and had sleep-onset REM episodes on multiple sleep latency test (MSLT—Park and Radtke 1995). Excessive daytime sleepiness in these patients often occurs in the absence of sleep apnoea. Furthermore, correction of hypoventilation does not always improve this symptom (Coccagna *et al.* 1982). It is postulated that sleep-onset REM episodes and excessive daytime sleepiness may be related to primary CNS abnormality. This symptom may respond to treatment with methylphenidate. Table 17.1 summarizes pulmonary function, sleep and ventilatory control abnormalities in prototypical NMDs.

TABLE 17.1
Pulmonary function, sleep and ventilatory control abnormalities in prototypical neuromuscular diseases

Disease	Pulmonary function	Sleep abnormalities	Ventilatory control
Cerebral palsy	No data available	OA, MA>CA, hypopnoea, alveolar hypoventilation, abnormal REM	No data available
Spinal muscular atrophy	↓TLC, FRC ↓MIP, MEP	CA, MA, hypopnoea, alveolar hypoventilation	↑Occlusion pressure
Duchenne muscular dystrophy	↓TLC, FRC ↓MIP, MEP	OA, MA, CA, paradoxical breathing, hypoventilation, nonapnoeic hypoxaemia	↓Hypoxic and hypercapnic response; N or ↑occlusion pressure
Myotonic dystrophy	N or ↓FRC, ↓MIP, MEP	CA>OA, MA, periodic breathing, REM-related hypoxaemia and hypoventilation, EDS, sleep-onset REM	↓Hypoxic and hypercapnic response; N or ↑occlusion pressure

Abbreviations: N= normal; OA = obstructive apnoea; CA = central apnoea; MA = mixed apnoea; TLC = total lung capacity; FRC = functional residual capacity; MIP = maximal inspiratory pressure; MEP = maximal expiratory pressure; EDS = excessive daytime sleepiness.

Clinical assessment

SDB in NMD may be asymptomatic or may present with complaints of morning headaches, fatigue, exertional dyspnoea, irritability, hyperactivity, impaired learning, vomiting, difficulty tolerating supine position, and restlessness during sleep (Heckmatt *et al.* 1989, Labanowski *et al.* 1996). In children, excessive daytime sleepiness is an uncommon complaint, and some children may report frequent awakening or insomnia. Other less common symptoms include failure to thrive, nocturnal sweating, delayed developmental milestones, and cor pulmonale (Beckerman and Hunt 1992). These symptoms may be erroneously attributed to the neuromuscular disease rather than SDB (Gozal 2000). It is imperative that specific questions regarding the quality of sleep are directed to the patients and parents. Nonrestorative sleep or daytime somnolence may be the early signs of SDB. Physical examination may reveal a bell-shaped chest, tachypnoea, use of accessory muscles and paradoxical breathing. However, these symptoms or signs are neither sensitive nor specific and are poor predictors of SDB. Even patients with mild symptoms may have unrecognized significant SDB (Labanowski *et al.* 1996).

Pulmonary function testing (PFT) should be performed periodically to prospectively evaluate respiratory muscle weakness. PFT includes simple spirometry, lung volumes and assessment of respiratory muscle strength at least annually. When lung volume drops below 60 per cent of normal, more frequent PFT may be needed (Gozal 2000). Reductions in all the subdivisions of lung volume, especially vital capacity, functional residual capacity (FRC) and expiratory reserve volume exemplify the restrictive physiology seen in NMD. Several studies have demonstrated that PFT during wakefulness may not be predictive of

SDB (Smith *et al.* 1988, Heckmatt *et al.* 1989, Manni *et al.* 1989, White *et al.* 1995). Factors other than abnormal PFT that may contribute to SDB are upper-airway, intercostal and diaphragm muscle hypotonia, poor airway clearance, pulmonary atelectasis, abdominal distension after eating, gastro-oesophageal reflux, pulmonary aspiration and progressive malnutrition or obesity (Givan 2000).

Even though most children with NMD do not have a primary decrease in ventilatory drive, those with chronic hypercapnia and hypoventilation may develop a secondary reduction in hypercapnic and/or hypoxic ventilatory response (Riley *et al.* 1977, Begin *et al.* 1980). The precise measurement of ventilatory drive is confounded by the contribution of respiratory muscle weakness. Studies such as fluoroscopy and EMG of the diaphragm and serum bicarbonate may be helpful in supporting a clinical diagnosis of hypoventilation but cannot differentiate between central and neuromuscular causes.

Polysomnography (PSG) is an essential tool in the evaluation of SDB. The American Thoracic Society (1996) has published consensus recommendations regarding the indications for PSG in paediatric NMD. These include impaired pulmonary function, snoring, cor pulmonale, morning headaches, and other symptoms and signs of SDB disproportionate to the degree of neurological impairment, polycythaemia or elevated serum bicarbonate.

PSG is also important for planning and implementation of elective nocturnal assisted ventilation, assessment of the adequacy of respiratory support, and evaluation of preoperative and postoperative status of patients with NMD (American Thoracic Society 1996).

A measurement of noninvasive ventilation such as end-tidal or transcutaneous CO_2 is essential in evaluation of SDB in children with NMD. In addition to apnoea of any type, it is important to quantify sleep disruption, paradoxical movement of the chest wall and diaphragm, and nocturnal alveolar hypoventilation. Nocturnal hypoventialtion (raised CO_2) may be documented in the absence of significant oxygen desaturation. REM-related oxygen desaturation correlates with diaphragm weakness and the need to initiate ventilatory support (White *et al.* 1995). Later, hypoventilation and hypoxia will occur at all sleep stages. If polysomnography is normal, repeat studies should be performed annually.

Management

The importance of general supportive care in the management of SDB in NMD cannot be overemphasized. These measures include adequate hydration, nutritional support and airway clearance techniques. It is important to assess the caloric need since obesity can develop insidiously in patients with significant disability caused by muscle weakness. Correction and spinal stabilization procedures for paralytic scoliosis should be performed before significant loss of lung function occurs.

A variety of modalities have been attempted to improve sleep-related respiratory disturbance. Nocturnal use of supplemental oxygen has been shown to alleviate the REM-related oxygen desaturation associated with respiratory muscle weakness in patients with DMD. However, the total sleep time, the sleep stage distribution, and the frequency and duration of arousals are not different between control and oxygen-treated groups, and supplementation may prolong the duration of apnoea and hypopnoea (Smith *et al.* 1989a). Protriptyline, a tricyclic antidepressant, has been shown to decrease sleep-related episodes

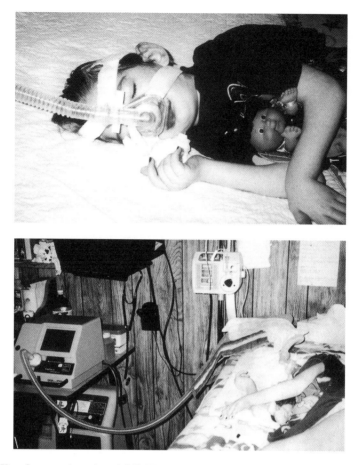

Fig. 17.2. Use of nocturnal nasal mask BiPAP over five years was successful in reducing frequency of episodes of acute respiratory failure in this 7-year-old girl with Werdnig–Hoffman disease.

of oxygen desaturation in some patients with DMD; however, a significant anticholinergic effect may limit its usefulness in regular practice (Smith *et al.* 1989b). Simple elevation of the upper body in bed can increase FRC and may prevent dependent airway closure and atelectasis. A rocking bed may have the same effect as body positioning but may also help drain secretions from the lower airways. Furthermore, this form of therapy may ameliorate daytime hypercapnia and subjective sleepiness by inhibition of arousal associated with phasic accessory muscle activation and improvement in sleep fragmentation (Iber *et al.* 1989).

Mechanical ventilatory support remains the mainstay treatment for SDB in children with NMD. Negative pressure ventilation (NPV) may be suitable in some patients. These devices include plexiglass lung, cuirass shell and pulmowrap. The NPV replaces the bellow function of failing respiratory muscles by artificially generating subatmospheric pressure around the chest. However, the use of NPV in these children is often associated with

increased frequency of SDB caused by collapse of upper airway muscles (Levy *et al.* 1989, Hill *et al.* 1992b). Although positive pressure ventilation via tracheotomy is the most effective mode of long-term assisted ventilation, it is not easily accepted as first-line therapy by patients and parents. Nasal mask ventilation has become the preferred and effective method of nocturnal ventilation because it may obviate the need for tracheotomy tube (Fig. 17.2). Nasal mask ventilation can be provided by continuous positive airway pressure (CPAP) or by nocturnal intermittent positive pressure ventilation (NIPPV), either through bilevel positive airway pressure (BiPAP) or conventional ventilator. Long-term nasal ventilation by any of these methods has been shown to normalize gas exchange and alleviate symptoms of hypercapnia (Heckmatt *et al.* 1990, Hill *et al.* 1992a). It is also been shown to stabilize declining lung function and prolong life expectancy of patients with DMD (Vianello *et al.* 1994). The decision to initiate positive pressure ventilation in children is a major one for the patients and their families. When the patients and caretakers accept this and are properly educated, then they can be active participants in this critical decision (Gilgoff *et al.* 1989). These decisions and the individual prognosis should be discussed with the patients and parents before the point of respiratory failure is reached.

REFERENCES

American Thoracic Society (1996) 'Standards and indications for cardiopulmonary sleep studies in children.' *American Journal of Respiratory and Critical Care Medicine*, **153**, 866–878.

Bach, J.R., Wang, T.G. (1995) 'Noninvasive long-term ventilatory support for individuals with spinal muscular atrophy and functional bulbar musculature.' *Archives of Physical Medicine and Rehabilitation*, **76**, 213–217.

Baydur, A. (1991) 'Respiratory muscle strength and control of ventilation in patients with neuromuscular disease.' *Chest*, **99**, 330–338.

Beckerman, R.C., Hunt, C.E. (1992) 'Neuromuscular diseases.' *In:* Beckerman, R.C., Brouillette, R.T., Hunt, C.E. (Eds.) *Respiratory Control Disorders in Infants and Children.* Baltimore: Williams & Wilkins, pp. 251–270.

Begin, R., Bureau, M.A., Lupien, L., Lemieux, B. (1980) 'Control and modulation of respiration in Steinert's myotonic dystrophy.' *American Review of Respiratory Disease*, **121**, 281–289.

Coccagna, G., Mantovani, M., Parchi, C., Mironi, F., Lugaresi, E. (1975) 'Alveolar hypoventilation and hypersomnia in myotonic dystrophy.' *Journal of Neurology, Neurosurgery and Psychiatry*, **38**, 977–984.

—— Martinelli, P., Lugaresi, E. (1982) 'Sleep and alveolar hypoventilation in myotonic dystrophy.' *Acta Neurologica Belgica*, **82**, 185–194.

Cohen, S.R., Lefaivre, J.F., Burstein, F.D., Simms, C., Kattos, A.V., Scott, P.H., Montgomery, G.L., Graham, L. (1997) 'Surgical treatment of obstructive sleep apnea in neurologically compromised patients.' *Plastic and Reconstructive Surgery*, **99**, 638–646.

Gilgoff, I., Prentice, W., Baydur, A. (1989) 'Patient and family participation in the management of respiratory failure in Duchenne's muscular dystrophy.' *Chest*, **95**, 519–524.

Givan, D.C. (2000) 'Sleep and breathing in children with neuromuscular disease' *In:* Loughlin, G.M., Carroll, J.L., Marcus, C.L. (Eds.) *Sleep and Breathing in Children: A Developmental Approach.* New York: Marcel Dekker, pp. 691–795.

Gozal, D. (2000) 'Pulmonary manifestations of neuromuscular disease with special reference to Duchenne muscular dystrophy and spinal muscular atrophy.' *Pediatric Pulmonology*, **29**, 141–150.

Guilleminault, C., Cummiskey, J., Motta, J., Lynne-Davies, P. (1978) 'Respiratory and hemodynamic study during wakefulness and sleep in myotonic dystrophy.' *Sleep*, **1**, 19–31.

Hayashi, M., Inoue, Y., Iwakawa, Y., Sasaki, H. (1990) 'REM sleep abnormalities in severe athetoid cerebral palsy.' *Brain and Development*, **12**, 494–497.

Heckmatt, J.Z., Loh, L., Dubowitz, V. (1989) 'Nocturnal hypoventilation in children with nonprogressive neuromuscular disease.' *Pediatrics*, **83**, 250–255.

———— ———— (1990) 'Night-time nasal ventilation in neuromuscular disease.' *Lancet*, **335**, 579–582.

Hill, N.S., Eveloff, S.E., Carlisle, C.C., Goff, S.G. (1992a) 'Efficacy of nocturnal nasal ventilation in patients with restrictive thoracic disease.' *American Review of Respiratory Disease*, **145**, 365–371.

———— Redline, S., Carskadon, M.A., Curran, F.J., Millman, R.P. (1992b) 'Sleep-disordered breathing in patients with Duchenne muscular dystrophy using negative pressure ventilators.' *Chest*, **102**, 1656–1662.

Hudgel, D.W., Devadatta, P. (1984) 'Decrease in functional residual capacity during sleep in normal humans.' *Journal of Applied Physiology*, **57**, 1319–1322.

———— Robertson, D.W. (1984) 'Nasal resistance during wakefulness and sleep in normal man.' *Acta Oto-laryngologica*, **98**, 130–135.

Iber, C., Davies, S.F., Mahowald, M.W. (1989) 'Nocturnal rocking bed therapy: Improvement in sleep fragmentation in patients with respiratory muscle weakness.' *Sleep*, **12**, 405–412.

Khan, Y., Heckmatt, J.Z. (1994) 'Obstructive apnoeas in Duchenne muscular dystrophy.' *Thorax*, **49**, 157–161.

Kuzuhara, S., Chou, S.M. (1981) 'Preservation of the phrenic motoneurons in Werdnig–Hoffmann disease.' *Annals of Neurology*, **9**, 506–510.

Labanowski, M., Schmidt-Nowara, W., Guilleminault, C. (1996) 'Sleep and neuromuscular disease: frequency of sleep-disordered breathing in a neuromuscular disease clinic population.' *Neurology*, **47**, 1173–1180.

Levy, R.D., Bradley, T.D., Newman, S.L., Macklem, P.T., Martin, J.G. (1989) 'Negative pressure ventilation. Effects on ventilation during sleep in normal subjects.' *Chest*, **95**, 95–99.

Manni, R., Ottolini, A., Cerveri, I., Bruschi, C., Zoia, M. C., Lanzi, G., Tartara, A. (1989) 'Breathing patterns and HbSaO$_2$ changes during nocturnal sleep in patients with Duchenne muscular dystrophy.' *Journal of Neurology*, **236**, 391–394.

———— Cerveri, I., Ottolini, A., Fanfulla, F., Zoia, M.C., Lanzi, G., Tartara, A. (1993) 'Sleep related breathing patterns in patients with spinal muscular atrophy.' *Italian Journal of Neurological Sciences*, **14**, 565–569.

Newsom-Davis, J. (1980) 'The respiratory system in muscular dystrophy.' *British Medical Bulletin*, **36**, 135–138.

Papastamelos, C., Panitch, H.B., Allen, J.L. (1996) 'Chest wall compliance in infants and children with neuromuscular disease.' *American Journal of Respiratory and Critical Care Medicine*, **154**, 1045–1048.

Park, J.D., Radtke, R.A. (1995) 'Hypersomnolence in myotonic dystrophy: demonstration of sleep onset REM sleep.' *Journal of Neurology, Neurosurgery and Psychiatry*, **58**, 512–513.

Riley, D.J., Santiago, T.V., Daniele, R.P., Schall, B., Edelman, N.H. (1977) 'Blunted respiratory drive in congenital myopathy.' *American Journal of Medicine*, **63**, 459–466.

Skatrud, J., Iber, C., McHugh, W., Rasmussen, H., Nichols, D. (1980) 'Determinants of hypoventilation during wakefulness and sleep in diaphragmatic paralysis.' *American Review of Respiratory Disease*, **121**, 587–593.

Smith, P.E., Calverley, P.M., Edwards, R.H. (1988) 'Hypoxemia during sleep in Duchenne muscular dystrophy.' *American Review of Respiratory Disease*, **137**, 884–888.

———— Edwards, R.H., Calverley, P.M. (1989a) 'Oxygen treatment of sleep hypoxaemia in Duchenne muscular dystrophy.' *Thorax*, **44**, 997–1001.

———— ———— ———— (1989b) 'Protriptyline treatment of sleep hypoxaemia in Duchenne muscular dystrophy.' *Thorax*, **44**, 1002–1005.

Vianello, A., Bevilacqua, M., Salvador, V., Cardaioli, C., Vincenti, E. (1994) 'Long-term nasal intermittent positive pressure ventilation in advanced Duchenne's muscular dystrophy.' *Chest*, **105**, 445–448.

White, J.E., Drinnan, M.J., Smithson, A.J., Griffiths, C.J., Gibson, G.J. (1995) 'Respiratory muscle activity and oxygenation during sleep in patients with muscle weakness.' *European Respiratory Journal*, **8**, 807–814.

18
VISUAL IMPAIRMENT AND ASSOCIATED SLEEP ABNORMALITIES

Gregory Stores

'Visually impaired children' refers to a very broad category that is heterogeneous in a number of ways.

- The degree of impairment ranges between slight defects in visual activity to the total absence of light perception. 'Blindness' implies the most severe degrees of impairment.
- Aetiology is very varied, with different ages of onset. In Britain the main causes of severe impairment are congenital cataract, cerebral cortical abnormality, optic atrophy, retinal disorders and congenital ocular abnormalities (Rahi and Dezateux 1998).
- At least half of all visually impaired children have other disabilities such as hearing loss, cerebral palsy and intellectual impairment.

This heterogeneity means that the nature, cause and severity of any sleep disturbance are likely to vary from one subgroup to another. Much of the research on sleep and visual impairment has been conducted on adults, in whom high rates of sleep disturbance have been reported consistently (Tabandeh *et al.* 1998). The limited published research on children (other than clinical impressions) has largely concerned the more severely visually affected and consists of a number of reports about individual children or small groups and just a few other accounts of larger groups.

Sleep problems

Reports of individual cases and short series have emphasized *sleep–wake cycle disorders* (Chapter 5) in children with a visual impairment. Meier *et al.* (1975) described four blind, brain-damaged children with what appeared to be an irregular sleep–wake cycle disorder. Four congenitally blind children aged 4 to 12 years with severe to moderate intellectual impairment were shown by Okawa *et al.* (1987) to have either this same type of sleep disorder or a non-24-hour ('free running') sleep–wake cycle disorder. Palm *et al.* (1991) and Lapierre and Dumont (1995) each described the use of melatonin in a non-24-hour cycle disorder in a blind, intellectually impaired child. The same type of sleep disorder in a 12-year-old boy with anophthalmia was treated effectively by Mindell *et al.* (1994), who introduced a schedule that strictly regulated all the child's sleep and awake behaviours. The improvement was considered to have had widespread benefits for the family as a whole. An irregular sleep–wake cycle disorder was implicated by Sadeh *et al.* (1995) as at least a contributory factor in the severely aggressive and destructive behaviour of a 16-year-old

blind and intellectually impaired boy. However, it seems that treatment for the sleep disorder was not possible because of opposition from his parents.

These case descriptions are instructive about the nature and management of the sleep problems concerned, but other reports provide a more balanced view of the various ways in which the sleep of visually impaired children can be affected. Overall, *difficulties getting to sleep and staying asleep* appear to be common. *Daytime sleepiness* in mentioned in some reports.

Jan *et al.* (1977) assessed the sleep of 85 visually impaired patients, aged between infancy and late adolescence, and 85 controls matched for age, sex and residential locality. Comparability in terms of intellectual level is difficult to judge from the information available. Sleep problems over a past 12-week period were assessed in general terms (without the underlying cause being ascertained) by means of several questions. Difficulty falling asleep was the only significantly more common problem in the blind children (20% vs 5.9%), with nonsignificant trends towards more night waking and restless sleep. Total sleep time was the same in both groups.

Kitzinger and Hunt (1985) questioned the parents of 20 blind 2- to 5-year-olds (most with additional intellectual or physical disabilities) and found that 40 per cent had frequent settling difficulties and 20 per cent had frequent night-waking problems. No comparisons with other children were made.

High rates of settling and night-waking problems were reported by Tröster *et al.* (1996) in their large study of 265 visually impaired 1- to 6-year-olds compared with 67 non-impaired children of the same age. The degree of visual impairment, its cause, and the presence of other disabilities varied widely in this study. Most of the assessments (including those of many of the visual impairment variables) were based on parental opinion. Sleep assessment was confined to the occurrence of settling and night waking, again without regard to the cause of these problems. The main findings were that sleep problems (combined or separate) were significantly more often reported in the visually impaired group than in the control group (42.6% vs 20.9%) but that additional disabilities (*e.g.* intellectual impairment, epilepsy, speech or hearing defects) were closely associated with the presence of a sleep problem whatever the degree of visual impairment, although sleep problems were greatest in the more severely visually impaired children.

The findings of a number of more recent studies indicate that various types of sleep disturbance are common in children who are visually impaired. Mindell and De Marco (1997) used the comprehensive Sleep Habits Questionnaire for parents to compare 28 blind children aged 4 to 36 months (average 20 months) with a group of sighted children of comparable age, sex and family socioeconomic level. The aetiology of the blindness varied but associated physical or psychological problems were not stated. Compared to the sighted children, the blind children had significantly more sleep problems at bedtime and during the night and less overall sleep (apparently they went to bed later and were awake longer during the night). The authors make the point that, in this group of children, the relationship between parental reports and objective measures of their children's sleep is uncertain. The distinction is important, as a disparity between the two has been reported in connection with other children with a developmental disorder (Wiggs and Stores 1998).

121

Leger *et al.* (1999) compared 77 blind children aged 3 to 18 years (average 12 years) with control children matched for age, sex, academic level and socioeconomic background. Details of the causes of blindness were not provided but about three-quarters of the children were considered totally blind from birth. None had any other chronic illness or disorder. A 42-item questionnaire for parents and children was used, covering several aspects of sleep and wakefulness. The blind children had significantly more sleep complaints overall than the sighted children (often in combinations), the main problems being difficulty getting off to sleep, waking up early, non-restorative sleep and excessive daytime sleepiness. The authors considered that these problems could be explained in terms of a sleep–wake cycle disorder in only a small proportion of cases. They raised anxiety as a possible alternative explanation in some cases.

Returning to the main theme in the individual case reports or small series mentioned earlier of circadian sleep–wake cycle disorder, there have been a few studies highlighting this type of sleep disorder in larger series of blind children. Tzischinsky *et al.* (1991) investigated 11 children (mean age 15.2 ± 2.3 years) the cause of whose blindness was mainly congenital. Sleep was assessed both subjectively and by actometry. The main finding was that the common complaints in this group of insomnia and daytime sleepiness were associated with delayed peaks in melatonin secretion.

In a brief report of a survey of sleep in 73 adolescents (age range 13–18 years), apparently with various degrees of severe visual impairment of diverse aetiology, their complaints (which seemed to include late sleep onset and daytime sleepiness) were attributed to either the delayed sleep phase syndrome or a non-24-hour sleep–wake syndrome (Sasaki *et al.* 1992).

More recently, Davitt *et al.* (1997) studied a group of 13 blind children (average age 4.5 years, range 1–11 years) with bilateral congenital anophthalmia and/or microphthalmia. Parents were questioned about sleep problems, wider aspects of their child's condition and family circumstances, in a (limited) attempt to explain any sleep disturbance that was present. In fact, none of the children was reported to have any significant additional medical or psychiatric disorder. Ten of the 13 children were said to suffer from a sleep disturbance in the form of frequent or prolonged early morning waking (or both) and excessive daytime sleepiness. The siblings of nine of the children were said to sleep normally. No other aspect of the visually impaired children's condition, or any of the family factors recorded, was related to the sleep problem. Treatment, in the form of 'a strict daily schedule' (details not provided) to entrain the children's sleep–wake rhythm, was said to have produced significant improvement in all cases.

Obviously, these reports vary considerably in their scope and sophistication but there is consistent evidence that children with severe degrees of visual impairment have high rates of sleep disturbance according to their parents. This corresponds with the many sleep problems reported in blind adults. The rates for visually impaired children are higher than i.1 the general population where about 20 to 30 per cent are thought to have a significant sleep problem at some stage (Mindell 1993).

For lack of information, it is difficult to judge the sleep problems in children with lesser degrees of visual impairment.

Aetiological factors

Sleep–wake cycle disorders occur that are directly attributable to severe visual impairment. However, other sleep disorders are also described, as can be expected in any group of children, especially those suffering from a condition likely to have a serious impact on the child and the family as a whole. Indeed, behavioural factors may well underlie some of the sleep–wake cycle disorders that respond to strict daily and night-time routines. These 'behavioural' sleep disorders are not consistently acknowledged in the literature. In general, there has been insufficient attempt to explain the nature of the sleep disorders underlying the problems of sleeplessness and excessive sleepiness in children with a visual impairment.

Even in severely visually impaired children, various explanations for the sleep disturbance should be considered in addition to the possibility of a sleep–wake cycle disorder caused essentially by lack of light perception. Other factors that might be responsible include:

- parental attitudes and practices such as over-permissiveness, inability to set limits, or inconsistency, all of which are potent influences on the sleep habits of children in general (Chapter 4)
- the effect of coexisting intellectual impairment with which sleep problems are closely associated (Chapter 7)
- associated physical disorders such as epilepsy (Chapter 15), physical deformity or immobility causing discomfort at night, speech and language difficulties interfering with communication with parents, or hearing deficits with which sleep disturbance is also associated although in ways that have yet to be clarified (Chapter 21)
- psychiatric disorder in the child or parent (Section Five). In the multivariate analysis by Moseley *et al.* (1996), depression was a strong predictor of sleep disturbance in blind adults.

Of course, these various influences may well occur in combination. Where the sleep problem is fundamentally caused by a sleep–wake cycle disorder, its nature needs to be determined as there are several types to which blind people are prone, *i.e.* delayed sleep phase, advanced sleep phase, irregular or non-24-hour sleep–wake cycle (Lockley *et al.* 1999).

Special considerations of management

The available evidence justifies the view that close attention should be paid to the sleep–wake pattern of any visually impaired child whether problems in this area are volunteered by parents or not. At least in the more severely impaired children, parents are likely to highlight sleep abnormalities as a major problem. In any case, the nature of the problem should be described in detail and the underlying sleep disorder identified as far as possible.

It follows from the range of possible explanations that there is no one treatment prescription for the sleep disturbance. Different forms of help are needed depending on the sleep disorder. The earlier that help is provided the better.

- Conventional behavioural treatments are likely to be effective where the problem arises from inappropriate bedtime parenting practices (Chapter 4). Such techniques include establishing consistent daytime and bedtime routines, not allowing delaying tactics at bedtime, and discouraging the child's need for his parents to be present for him to get to sleep.
- Chronobiological approaches are required for sleep–wake cycle disorders, the particular procedure depending on the type of disorder. Strict daily schedules can help to entrain

sleep–wake patterns, at least in some children. Emphasis on secondary time cues, such as mealtimes and social contacts, is important in children without any useful vision. Exposure to bright light at key times of night or day can also be an adjunctive measure in correcting sleep–wake cycle disorders (Guilleminault *et al.* 1993). Some blind patients still seem to be sensitive to light cues for setting of their sleep–wake cycles, presumably because of functioning collateral visual pathways from the retina to the suprachiasmatic nuclei (Czeisler *et al.* 1995).

• As illustrated by some of the case reports mentioned earlier, melatonin has been used for sleep–wake cycle disorders including those in blind children (Espezel *et al.* 1996, Palm *et al.* 1997). Its use has a good theoretical foundation, at least where melatonin secretion is known to be abnormal (Zhdanova 2000) and in view of adult studies linking sleep–wake cycle disorders with abnormal melatonin rhythms (Lockley *et al.* 1999). However, not all children benefit from melatonin (perhaps especially where behavioural factors are prominent) and much needs to be clarified about fundamental aspects of its use including dosage and timing. Possible consequences of long-term use, such as effects on reproductive physiology, also need to be assessed. At present, melatonin should probably be used only short-term in children where behavioural factors are obviously not the cause of the sleep disturbance, and where other forms of treatment have failed. Another approach in need of further evaluation is the use of vitamin B_{12} in the treatment of sleep–wake cycle disorders (Okawa *et al.* 1990).

• Other aspects of treatment include (as required) attention to the psychiatric needs of child or parent.

Research

The need for further research on the sleep problems of visually impaired children is clear, especially in view of the serious effects on learning and behaviour (and on the family as a whole) of persistent sleep disturbance. In order to clarify the relationships involved, and to promote better care, there is a need for studies of more circumscribed subgroups of visually impaired children, defined in terms of, for example, severity of the visual defect, aetiology, age of onset and comorbid conditions. Response rates to invitations to take part in the studies (not always high or not commented on at all in the studies reviewed) need to be good to achieve a balanced view. Age, sex and family variables may also be relevant to the nature and extent of the sleep problem. The sleep disturbance should be defined as precisely as possible with an attempt to specify the underlying sleep disorder, especially distinguishing between the relative contribution of physical and psychological factors. Treatments chosen on the basis of the diagnosis need to be evaluated systematically for both their short- and long-term effects.

REFERENCES

Czeisler, C.A., Shanahan, T.L., Klerman, E.B., Martens, H., Brotman, D.J., Emens, J.S., Klein, T., Rizzo, J.F. (1995) 'Suppression of melatonin in some blind patients by exposure to bright light.' *New England Journal of Medicine*, **332**, 6–11.
Davitt, B.V., Morgan, C., Cruz, O.A. (1997) 'Sleep disorders in children with congenital anophthalmia and

microphthalmia.' *Journal of the American Association for Pediatric Ophthalmology and Strabismus*, **2**, 151–153.

Espezel, H., Jan, J.E., O'Donnell, M.E., Milner, R. (1996) 'The use of melatonin to treat sleep–wake rhythm disorders in children who are visually impaired.' *Journal of Visual Impairment and Blindness*, **1**, 43–50.

Guilleminault, C., Crowe McCann, C., Quera-Salva, M., Cetel, M. (1993) 'Light therapy as treatment of dyschronosis in brain impaired children.' *European Journal of Pediatrics*, **152**, 754–759.

Jan, J.E., Freeman, R.D., Scott, E. (Eds.) (1977) *Visual Impairment in Children and Adolescents.* New York: Grune & Stratton.

Kitzinger, M., Hunt, H. (1985) 'The effect of residential setting on sleep and behaviour patterns of young visually-handicapped children.' *In:* Stephenson, J.E. (Ed.) *Recent Research in Developmental Psychopathology.* Oxford: Pergamon Press, pp. 73–80.

Lapierre, O., Dumont, M. (1995) 'Melatonin treatment of a non-24-hour sleep–wake cycle in a blind retarded child.' *Biological Psychiatry*, **38**, 119–122.

Leger, D., Prevot, E., Philip, P., Yence, C., Labaye, N., Paillard, M., Guilleminault, C. (1999) 'Sleep disorders in children with blindness.' *Annals of Neurology*, **46**, 648–651.

Lockley, S.W., Skene, D.J., Butler, L.J., Arendt, J. (1999) 'Sleep and activity rhythms are related to circadian phase in the blind.' *Sleep*, **22**, 616–623.

Meier, K.A., Mikschiczek, D., Riemensperger, T. (1975) 'Schlafstorungen blinder Kinder.' *Fortschritte der Medizin*, **93**, 1173–1176.

Mindell, J.A. (1993) 'Sleep disorders in children.' *Health Psychology*, **12**, 151–162.

—— De Marco, C.M. (1997) 'Sleep problems of young blind children.' *Journal of Visual Impairment and Blindness*, **1**, 33–39.

—— Goldberg, R., Fry, J.M. (1994) 'Treatment of a circadian rhythm disorder in a blind 2 year old.' *Sleep Research*, **23**, 101. *(Abstract.)*

Moseley, M.J., Fouladi, M., Jones, H.S., Tobin, M.J. (1996) 'Sleep disturbance and blindness.' *Lancet*, **348**, 1514–1515.

Okawa, M., Nanami, T., Wada, S., Shimizu, T., Hishikawa, Y., Sasaki, H., Nagamine, H., Takahashi, K. (1987) 'Four congenitally blind children with circadian sleep–wake rhythm disorder.' *Sleep*, **10**, 101–110.

—— Mishima, K., Nanami, T., Shimizu, T., Iijima, S., Hishakawa, Y., Takahashi, K. (1990) 'Vitamin B-12 treatment for sleep wake cycle disorders.' *Sleep*, **13**, 15–23.

Palm, L., Blennow, G., Wetterberg, L. (1991) 'Correction of a non-24-hour sleep/wake cycle by melatonin in a blind retarded boy.' *Annals of Neurology*, **29**, 336–339.

—— —— (1997) 'Long-term melatonin treatment in blind children and young adults with circadian sleep–wake disturbances.' *Developmental Medicine and Child Neurology*, **39**, 319–325.

Rahi, J.S., Dezateux, C. (1998) 'Epidemiology of visual impairment in Britain.' *Archives of Disease in Childhood*, **78**, 381–386.

Sadeh, A., Klitzke, M., Anders, T.F., Acebo, C. (1995) 'Case study: Sleep and aggressive behavior in a blind retarded adolescent. A concomitant schedule disorder?' *Journal of the American Academy of Child and Adolescent Psychiatry*, **34**, 820–824.

Sasaki, H., Nakata, H., Murakami, S., Uesugi, R., Harada, S., Teranishi, M. (1992) 'Circadian sleep–wake rhythm disturbance in blind adolescents.' *Japanese Journal of Psychiatry and Neurology*, **46**, 209. *(Abstract.)*

Tabandeh, H., Lockley, S.W., Buttery, R., Skene, D.J., Defrance, R., Arendt, J., Bird, A.C. (1998) 'Disturbance of sleep in blindness'. *American Journal of Ophthalmology*, **126**, 707–712.

Tröster, H., Brambring, M., Van Der Berg, J. (1996) 'Daily routines and sleep disorders in visually impaired children.' *Early Child Development and Care*, **119**, 1–14.

Tzischinsky, O., Skene, D., Epstein, R., Lavie, P. (1991) 'Circadian rhythms in 6-sulphatoxymelatonin and nocturnal sleep in blind children.' *Chronobiology International*, **8**, 168–175.

Wiggs, L., Stores, G. (1998) 'Behaviour treatment for sleep problems in children with severe learning disabilities and challenging daytime behaviour: effect on sleep patterns of mother and child.' *Journal of Sleep Research*, **7**, 119–126.

Zhdanova, I.V. (2000) 'The role of melatonin in sleep and sleep disorders.' *In:* Culebras, A. (Ed.) *Sleep Disorders and Neurological Disease.* New York: Marcel Dekker, pp. 137–157.

19
DISORDERED SLEEP IN OTHER NEUROLOGICAL CONDITIONS

Gregory Stores

Myelodysplasia and associated conditions

Although abnormal respiratory function during sleep in children with myelodysplasia (with or without symptoms of apnoea or hypoventilation) was described some time ago, the extent and details of the problem have not been described until recently.

Waters and colleagues (1998) surveyed 107 children with the condition (98% of a clinic population) of whom 83 underwent overnight polysomnography. Breathing during sleep was considered normal in 37 per cent of the children, mildly abnormal in 42 per cent and moderately to severely abnormal in 20 per cent. Of the moderately to severely affected group (17 children), 12 had predominantly central and five predominantly obstructive apnoea. Patients more likely to have moderately or severely abnormal breathing during sleep were those with thoracic or thoracolumbar myelomeningocele, those who had previously undergone posterior fossa decompression, those with the more severe brainstem malformations and those with other respiratory abnormalities.

The importance of testing for sleep-disordered breathing in children with spina bifida/myelomeningocele was emphasized by Kirk *et al.* (1999). Having also identified moderate to severe sleep-disordered breathing in 20 per cent of their own clinic population, they surveyed 212 spina bifida clinics of which 41 per cent provided information on a total of 13,349 patients. Sleep studies had been performed on only 7.5 per cent of the children despite the availability of such investigations in 67 per cent of the responding centres.

Whatever their origin (in addition, that is, to their association with myelomeningocele), *Chiari malformation* (Chapter 10) and *hydrocephalus* can cause sleep-related breathing disorders because of disruption of brainstem mechanisms involved in the control of respiration. Brainstem compression in the Chiari malformation can produce both central apnoea (Keefover *et al.* 1995) and obstructive sleep apnoea including that caused by vocal chord paralysis (Ruff *et al.* 1987). The same problems are associated with syringobulbia and syringomyelia even in the absence of sleep-related symptoms (Encabo *et al.* 1987), which, in severe form, carry a risk of sudden death during sleep (Nogues *et al.* 1992).

The details and uncertainties of treating myelomeningocele and associated disorders have been discussed by Keens and Davidson-Ward (2000).

Head injury

Although relatively little studied, sleep disturbance related to head injury has been reported

consistently in adults, even following minor head injury. For example, Deb *et al.* (1998) found that sleep disturbance was one of the most common behavioural problems persisting one year after the injury, occurring in 29 per cent of 148 patients. An earlier report (Parsons and Ver-Beek 1982) discussed in some detail the changes in sleep–wake patterns before and after minor head injury in 75 young patients. Main significant changes described after the injury were increased awakenings at night, early morning waking, impaired performance after waking, and an apparently reduced quality of sleep.

Not surprisingly, more severe forms of brain injury are associated with particularly high rates of sleep disturbance. Cohen *et al.* (1992) reported that 16 of 22 patients in hospital had sleep problems (mainly difficulty getting to or staying asleep) and that 52 per cent of 77 discharged patients were troubled mainly by excessive sleepiness. Other evidence that sleep problems are common in adults with traumatic brain damage has been reviewed by Clinchot *et al.* (1998), who themselves reported high rates of insomnia and daytime sleepiness in such patients persisting a year after discharge from hospital. Long-term sleep complaints are common in adults with the chronic postconcussion syndrome (Perlis *et al.* 1997).

Some accounts describe specific types of sleep disorder, *e.g.* delayed sleep phase syndrome (Quinto *et al.* 2000), and there are a number of accounts (*e.g.* Lankford *et al.* 1994) of post-traumatic narcolepsy following closed head injury of various degrees of severity. It is generally felt that, similar to other forms of 'symptomatic narcolepsy' associated with various CNS lesions (Autret *et al.* 1994), genuine post-traumatic narcolepsy is a rarity. As illustrated by the series reported by Guilleminault *et al.* (1983), the excessive sleepiness following serious head injury is more usually attributable to other conditions such as (in their series) sleep-related breathing disorders. The posterior hypothalamus, third ventricle and posterior fossa are said to be the most often implicated sites of injury leading to post-traumatic hypersomnia (American Sleep Disorders Association 1997).

There is no reason, in principle, why sleep disturbance, with an equally wide range of sleep disorders, is not also a common consequence of severe head injury in young patients. However, there are few published reports. Sleep problems (sometimes persistent) were said by Nakayama *et al.* (1990) to be common after bicycle-related injuries (mostly to the head and causing injury of different degrees of severity) in children aged 2 to 15 years. Various forms of sleeplessness and excessive daytime sleepiness, persisting several years after severe head injury, were described by Bouldin *et al.* (1992) in a small group of children between 1 and 6 years of age. Post-traumatic central sleep apnoea in a child was reported by Quera-Salva and Guilleminault (1987), and Will *et al.* (1988) described the Kleine–Levin syndrome in two individuals (aged 14 and 16 years), apparently precipitated by head trauma. Insomnia caused by the delayed sleep phase syndrome following closed head injury was described by Patten and Lauderdale (1992) in a 13-year-old patient, and by Drake (1986) in a 16-year-old with severe brain dysfunction and head-banging.

Sleep disturbance is consistently included as one of the behavioural problems that are described as common following minor head injury in children and adolescents, although pre- and post-injury comparisons are sometimes difficult to judge from reports. The findings of Farmer *et al.* (1987) suggest that this might be a nonspecific result of a traumatic experience (rather than a neurological effect) and that the symptoms are short-lived.

Nevertheless, explanation and support for the parents is appropriate to help them cope with the problems, especially as the long-term psychosocial outcome for head-injured children is closely related to the degree of stress within their families (Rivara *et al.* 1996).

The origins of the sleep problems in severely brain-injured patients are likely to be diverse. Neurological factors can be expected to predominate in more severe injury, including post-traumatic epilepsy, which may add to the difficulties in the ways discussed in Chapter 15. Emotional consequences of the injury on the child and the parents will probably be particularly influential. Cognitive impairment in serious cases may add to a child's difficulties in re-establishing good sleep habits.

This likely multifactorial origin of both short-term and persistent sleep problems clearly indicates the need for careful analysis of the causal and maintaining factors underlying the child's sleep disturbance in order to define appropriate treatment strategies. The much-needed further research in this field should go beyond reporting of sleep problems by identifying precisely the underlying sleep disorders in order to understand the pathogenesis of the sleep disturbance and the exact treatment required.

Headaches including migraine

Sahota and Dexter (1990) listed a number of interesting and clinically important ways in which sleep and headache syndrome are associated. These include headache occurring during or after sleep; headache caused by lack of sleep, excessive sleep or disrupted sleep; headache relieved by sleep; headache occurring as part of a sleep disorder; and effects of headache on sleep. Their account is based essentially on adult headache sufferers, and because of the few studies in children, it is difficult to know the extent to which these relationships apply in children. Still less are the mechanisms involved understood, as illustrated by the report by Aaltonen *et al.* (2000) that younger children in particular often fall asleep during even severe migraine attacks with resolution of the headache during the period of sleep.

According to the findings of Bruni *et al.* (1997), children and adolescents share the high rate of sleep disturbance reported in adults with chronic headache. Parental information about their children's sleep was collected for 164 children and adolescents with migraine and 119 with "tension type headache" for comparison with healthy controls. Significantly higher rates of various sleep problems including night-wakings and daytime sleepiness were described in both headache groups equally, but with more sleep-related breathing disorder symptoms and parasomnias in the migraine group. The same research group has described significant improvements in childhood migraine with the use of sleep hygiene methods (Bruni *et al.* 1999). Cluster headaches and chronic paroxysmal hemicrania (both linked with REM sleep in contrast to migraine) are rare in children but may disrupt sleep during the night.

The high rate of parasomnias described in the study by Bruni *et al.* echoes earlier reports that sleepwalking in particular is associated with migraine. This included the study by Barabas *et al.* (1983) who considered that the link may arise from an underlying serotonin abnormality causing increased slow wave sleep and, as a result, liability to both arousal disorders and migraine. Dexter (1986) then extended the link with migraine to sleep terrors and also nocturnal enuresis (at that time thought to also be an arousal disorder).

Dexter (1984) was also instrumental in identifying headache as a possible symptom of obstructive sleep apnoea. Headache on awakening is often listed as one of the daytime manifestations of the obstructive sleep apnoea syndrome, although how characteristic it is seems debatable (Carroll and Loughlin 1995). It can also occur in association with other conditions including bruxism (Bader and Lavigne 2000). In adults, morning (or nocturnal) headaches have been described in association with various physical causes that might occur in young people (including substance abuse) as well as a number of sleep disorders (Paiva *et al*. 1995). Clinically, a complaint of headaches on waking should prompt enquiries to include sleep habits and symptoms.

The general aim in preventing sleep-related headaches is control of the underlying condition, avoiding potential triggering factors (including sleep loss or excessive sleep), and observing the principles of sleep hygiene (Culebras 2000).

Hearing impairment
Sleep problems in children with a hearing impairment hardly ever seem to be considered apart from anecdotal accounts by parents and some clinicians. The term 'hearing impairment' shares the characteristic of visual impairment in covering a very broad category of conditions regarding severity, cause, course (*i.e*. fluctuating or persistent) and comorbidity. Therefore, general statements rarely apply. However, at least the more severe forms of hearing impairment are likely to be associated with sleep problems for psychological reasons, if not also because of physical factors in some cases. High rates of psychiatric disorder have sometimes been quoted for children with hearing impairment, although the findings from different studies are inconsistent (Hindley 1997). In view of the strong relationship between child psychiatric disorder and sleep disturbance (Section Five), it is likely that sleep problems are common in at least the more severely hearing-impaired.

Some support for this view comes from the limited information on sleep problems of adults. This includes an early report of a small polysomnographic study of congenitally deaf young men who, compared to controls, were shown to spend significantly more time awake during the night and less time in NREM sleep (Robinson and Dawson 1975).

The majority of reports have concerned the apparently close relationship between tinnitus and sleep disturbance. Getting to sleep was the difficulty most frequently mentioned by a group of tinnitus sufferers (Tyler and Baker 1983). In a study by Alster *et al*. (1993) the main sleep complaints were difficulty getting to sleep, waking at night and daytime fatigue. Sleep disturbance was greater in the more severe cases of tinnitus and in the more depressed patients. Few of the patients had sought help for their sleep problems. Other more recent reports have confirmed that the distressing effects of tinnitus include sleep problems (Hallam 1996, Sanchez and Stephens 1997). Insomnia can be a persistent problem, despite routine counselling and advice, especially in patients with more severe degrees of tinnitus (Folmer and Griest 2000).

Clearly, there is a need for greater awareness of comparable problems in children and for assessment of the beneficial effects (including those concerning sleep) of cognitive–behavioural treatments such as those that have been used for adult tinnitus sufferers (Andersson and Lyttkens 1999). It is important to explore more widely the various types

of sleep disorder (and their causes) to which children with a hearing impairment might be subject. This is illustrated by the preliminary report of particularly high rates of circadian sleep–wake cycle disorders in hearing-impaired children, possibly because of the absence of sound as an important influence in the entrainment of sleep–wake rhythms (Oishibashi *et al.* 1993). Alternatively, the absence of sound when the child's hearing aid is removed at night might be sufficiently alarming to prevent him settling to sleep or being able to go back to sleep when he wakes in the night.

Additional neurological conditions
Children with a number of other neurological disorders are at risk for sleep-related breathing disorders.

The association of *achondroplasia* with obstructive sleep apnoea has been known for some time, but the various degrees of sleep-disordered breathing that can be associated with the condition were illustrated in a study by Mogayzel *et al.* (1998). Of the 88 children (age range 1 month to 12 years) nearly half had abnormalities demonstrated by overnight polysomnography. The most usual problem was hypoxaemia, but a substantial minority had significant obstructive or central apnoea. A number of aspects of achondroplasia may conspire to cause upper airway obstruction during sleep such as midfacial hypoplasia, structural abnormalities of the nasopharynx, and abnormalities of the base of the skull producing compression of the medullary and cervical cord and hydrocephalus. Respiratory function may be further compromised by restrictive lung disease caused by an abnormally shaped chest. Severe effects on respiratory function can result in failure to thrive and cor pulmonale. Because of the common occurrence of sleep-disordered breathing and its possibly relatively subtle clinical manifestations, sleep studies including respiratory monitoring are recommended in all children with achondroplasia (Carroll and Loughlin 1995).

Apnoeas and hypoventilation have also been described in *Leigh syndrome* (Keens and Davidson Ward 2000) and in *Riley–Day syndrome* (Guilleminault *et al.* 1992). A particularly wide range of sleep abnormalities (sleeplessness, various parasomnias, possible narcolepsy and respiratory problems) has been reported in *Moebius syndrome* (Parkes 1999).

Sleep disorders are also common and particularly troublesome in *neuronal ceroid-lipofuscinosis* (Santavuori *et al.* 1993), and sleep physiology is disrupted increasingly as the disease progresses (Kirveskari *et al.* 2000). In a series of studies, sleep–wake cycle disorders were shown to occur only in the later stages of the illness (Heikkilä *et al.* 1995), and melatonin was ineffective whatever the type of sleep disorder (Hätönen *et al.* 1999). The respective contributions of the various aspects of the disorder (especially brain damage, intellectual impairment, blindness and epilepsy) remain to be determined, although it appears that visual failure in these children is still compatible with regulation of sleep–wake rhythms by light (Hätönen *et al.* 1998). This is in keeping with reports of some blind adults by Czeisler *et al.* (1995) and presumably the result of intact collateral retino-hypothalamic pathways, as mentioned in Chapter 18.

Frequent waking with abnormal sleep architecture has been reported in association with *Menkes' kinky hair disease*. No improvement in sleep was seen following administration of copper in an attempt to overcome the deficit in copper absorption (Hashimoto *et al.* 1982).

Sleep abnormalities of various types (*e.g.* sleep fragmentation, circadian sleep–wake cycle disorders, respiratory disorders, and parasomnias including REM sleep behaviour disorder) are common and well documented in adult Parkinson's disease. A single case report was instructive about the possible origins of the excessive sleepiness, REM sleep behaviour disorder and daytime REM sleep onset in a teenager with *juvenile Parkinson's disease* (Rye *et al.* 1999). The authors argued that the sleep disturbance was likely to be the result of the dopamine and basal ganglia abnormalities intrinsic to the condition.

REFERENCES

Aaltonen, K., Hamalainen, M.L., Hoppu, K. (2000) 'Migraine attacks and sleep in children.' *Cephalalgia*, **20**, 580–584.

Alster, J., Shemesh, Z., Ornan, M., Attias, J. (1993) 'Sleep disturbance associated with tinnitus.' *Biological Psychiatry*, **34**, 84–90.

American Sleep Disorders Association (1997) *ICSD – International Classification of Sleep Disorders, Revised: Diagnostic and Coding Manual.* Rochester, MN: American Sleep Disorders Association.

Andersson, G., Lyttkens, L. (1999) 'A meta-analytic review of psychological treatments for tinnitus.' *British Journal of Audiology*, **33**, 201–210.

Autret, A., Lucas, B., Henry-Lebras, F., de Toffol, B. (1994) 'Symptomatic narcolepsies.' *Sleep*, **17**, Suppl. 8, S21–S24.

Bader, G., Lavigne, G. (2000) 'Sleep bruxism: an overview of an oromandibular sleep movement disorder.' *Sleep Medicine Reviews*, **4**, 27–43.

Barabas, G., Ferrari, M., Matthews, W.S. (1983) 'Childhood migraine and somnambulism.' *Neurology*, **33**, 948–949.

Bouldin, E.P, Kriel, R.L., Rosen, G.M., Mahowald, M.W., Krach, L.E. (1992) 'Pediatric head trauma and sleep disorders: follow up survey.' *Sleep Research*, **21**, 179. *(Abstract.)*

Bruni, O., Fabrizi, P., Ottoviano, S., Cortesi, F., Giannotti, F., Guidetti, V. (1997) 'Prevalence of sleep disorders in childhood and adolescence headache: a case-control study.' *Cephalalgia*, **17**, 492–498.

—— Galli, F., Guidetti, V. (1999) 'Sleep hygiene and migraine in children and adolescents.' *Cephalalgia*, **19**, Suppl. 25, 57–59.

Carroll, J.L., Loughlin, G.M. (1995) 'Obstructive sleep apnea syndrome in infants and children: Clinical features and pathophysiology.' *In:* Ferber, R., Kryger, M. (Eds.) *Principles and Practice of Sleep Medicine in the Child.* Philadelphia: W.B. Saunders, pp. 176–177.

Clinchot, D.M., Bogner, J., Mysiw, W.J., Fugate, L., Corrigan, J. (1998) 'Defining sleep disturbance after brain injury.' *American Journal of Physical Medicine and Rehabilitation*, **77**, 291–295.

Cohen, M., Oksenberg, A., Snir, D., Stern, M.J., Groswasser, Z. (1992) 'Temporally related changes of sleep complaints in traumatic brain injured patients.' *Journal of Neurology, Neurosurgery and Psychiatry*, **55**, 313–315.

Culebras, A. (2000) 'Headache disorders and sleep.' *In:* Culebras, A. (Ed.) *Sleep Disorders and Neurological Disease.* New York: Marcel Dekker, pp. 355–364.

Czeisler, C.A., Shanahan, T.L., Klerman, E.B., Martens, H., Brotman, D.J., Emens, J.S., Klein, T., Rizzo, J.F. (1995) 'Suppression of melatonin secretion in some blind patients by exposure to bright light.' *New Zealand Journal of Medicine*, **332**, 6–11.

Deb, S., Lyons, I., Koutzoukis, C. (1998) 'Neuropsychiatric sequelae one year after minor head injury.' *Journal of Neurology, Neurosurgery and Psychiatry*, **65**, 899–902.

Dexter, J.D. (1984) 'Headache as a presenting complaint of the sleep apnea syndrome.' *Headache*, **24**, 171. *(Abstract.)*

—— (1986) 'The relationship between disorders of arousal from sleep and migraine.' *Headache*, **26**, 322. *(Abstract.)*

Drake, M.E. (1986) 'Jactatio nocturia after head injury.' *Neurology*, **36**, 867–868.

Encabo, H., Gene, R., Nogues, M.A. (1987) 'Polysomnographic findings in syringomyelia and syringobulbia.' *Sleep Research*, **16**, 474. *(Abstract.)*

Farmer, M.Y., Singer, H.S., Mellits, E.D., Hall, D., Charney, E. (1987) 'Neurobehavioral sequelae of minor head injuries in children.' *Pediatric Neuroscience*, **13**, 304–308.

Folmer, R.L., Griest, S.E. (2000) 'Tinnitus and insomnia.' *American Journal of Otolaryngology*, **21**, 287–293.

Guilleminault, C., Faull, K.F., Miles, L., van den Hoed, J. (1983) 'Posttraumatic excessive daytime sleepiness: A review of 20 cases.' *Neurology*, **33**, 1584–1589.

—— Stoohs, R., Quera-Salva, M.A. (1992) 'Sleep-related obstructive and nonobstructive apnoeas and neurologic disorders.' *Neurology*, **42**, Suppl. 6, 53–60.

Hallam, R.S. (1996) 'Correlates of sleep disturbance in chronic distressing tinnitus.' *Scandinavian Audiology*, **25**, 263–266.

Hashimoto, T., Kawano, N., Hiura, K. (1982) 'Sleep polygraph studies of Menkes' kinky hair disease: effect of copper administration.' *Rinsho Noha*, **24**, 418–422.

Hätönen, T., Laakso, M-L., Heiskala, H., Alila-Johansson, A., Sainio, K., Santavuori, P. (1998) 'Bright light suppresses melatonin in blind patients with neuronal ceroid-lipofuscinosis.' *Neurology*, **50**, 1145–1450.

—— Kirveskari, E., Heiskala, H., Sainio, K., Laakso, M-L., Santavuori, P. (1999) 'Melatonin ineffective in neuronal ceroid lipofuscinosis patients with fragmented or normal motor activity rhythms recorded by wrist actigraphy.' *Molecular Genetics and Metabolism*, **66**, 401–406.

Heikkilä, E., Hätönen, T., Telekivi, T., Laakso, M-L., Heiskala, H., Salmi, T., Alila, A., Santavuori, P. (1995) 'Circadian rhythm studies in neuronal ceroid-lipofuscinosis (NCL).' *American Journal of Medical Genetics*, **57**, 229–234.

Hindley, P.A. (1997) 'Psychiatric aspects of hearing impairments.' *Journal of Child Psychology and Psychiatry*, **38**, 101–117.

Keefover, R., Sam, M., Bodensteiner, J., Nicholson, A. (1995) 'Hypersomnolence and pure central sleep apnea associated with the Chiari 1 malformation.' *Journal of Child Neurology*, **10**, 65–67.

Keens, T.G., Davidson Ward, S.L. (2000) 'Syndromes affecting respiratory control during sleep.' *In:* Loughlin, G.M., Carroll, J.L., Marcus, C.L. (Eds.) *Sleep and Breathing in Children. A Developmental Approach.* New York: Marcel Dekker, pp. 525–553.

Kirk, V.G., Morielli, A., Brouillette, R.T. (1999) 'Sleep disordered breathing in patients with myelomeningocele: the missed diagnosis.' *Developmental Medicine and Child Neurology*, **41**, 40–43.

Kirveskari, E., Partinen, M., Salmi, T., Sainio, K., Telekivi, T., Hamalainen, M., Larsen, A., Santavuori, P. (2000) 'Sleep alterations in juvenile neuronal ceroid-lipofuscinosis.' *Pediatric Neurology*, **22**, 347–354.

Lankford, D.A., Wellman, J.J., O'Hara, C. (1994) 'Posttraumatic narcolepsy in mild to moderate closed head injury.' *Sleep*, **17**, Suppl. 8, S25–S28.

Mogayzel, P.J., Carroll, J.L., Loughlin, G.M., Hurks, O., Francomano, C.A., Marcus, C.L. (1998) 'Sleep disordered breathing in children with achondroplasia.' *Journal of Pediatrics*, **132**, 667–671.

Nakayama, D.K., Gardner, M.J., Rogers, K.D. (1990) 'Disability from bicycle related injuries in children.' *Journal of Trauma*, **30**, 1390–1394.

Nogues, M.A., Gene, R., Encabo, H. (1992) 'Risk of sudden death during sleep in syringomyelia and syringobulbia.' *Journal of Neurology, Neurosurgery and Psychiatry*, **55**, 585–589.

Oishibashi, Y., Kakizawa, T., Otsuka, A., Kawama, K.N., Sato, Y., Suzuki, M., Sasaki, H. (1993) 'Disturbances of sleep and waking in handicapped children (II): trend of circadian rhythm disorders in deaf children.' *Japanese Journal of Psychiatry and Neurology*, **47**, 464–465.

Paiva, T., Batista, A., Martins, P., Martins, A. (1995) 'The relationship between headaches and sleep disturbance.' *Headache*, **35**, 590–596.

Parkes, J.D. (1999) 'Genetic factors in human sleep disorders with special reference to Norrie disease, Prader–Willi syndrome and Moebius syndrome.' *Journal of Sleep Research*, **8**, Suppl. 1, 14–22.

Parsons, L.C., Ver Beek, D. (1982) 'Sleep–awake patterns following cerebral concussion.' *Nursing Research*, **31**, 260–264.

Patten, S.D., Lauderdale, W.M. (1992) 'Delayed sleep phase disorder after traumatic brain injury.' *Journal of the American Academy of Child and Adolescent Psychiatry*, **31**, 100–102.

Perlis, M.L., Artiola, L., Giles, D.E. (1997) 'Sleep complaints in chronic postconcussion syndrome.' *Perceptual and Motor Skills*, **84**, 595–599.

Quera Salva, M.A., Guilleminault, C. (1987) 'Post-traumatic central sleep apnea in a child.' *Journal of Pediatrics*, **110**, 906–909.

Quinto, C., Gellido, C., Chokroverty, S., Masdeu, J. (2000) 'Posttraumatic delayed sleep phase syndrome.' *Neurology*, **54**, 250–252.

Rivara, J.B., Jaffe, K.M., Polissar, N.L., Fay, G.C., Liao, S., Martin, K.M. (1996) 'Predictors of family functioning and change 3 years after traumatic brain injury in children.' *Archives of Physical Medicine and Rehabilitation*, **77**, 754–764.

132

Robinson, L.D., Dawson, S.D. (1975) 'The EEG and REM sleep studies in deaf people.' *American Annals of the Deaf*, **210**, 387–390.

Ruff, M.E., Oakes, W.J., Fisher, S.R., Spock, A. (1987) 'Sleep apnea and vocal chord paralysis secondary to type 1 Arnold–Chiari malformation.' *Pediatrics*, **80**, 231–234.

Rye, D.B., Johnston, L.H., Watts, R.L., Bliwise, D.L. (1999) 'Juvenile Parkinson's disease with REM sleep behaviour disorder, sleepiness and daytime REM onset.' *Neurology*, **53**, 1868–1870.

Sahota, P.K., Dexter, J.D. (1990) 'Sleep and headache syndromes: a clinical review.' *Headache*, **30**, 80–84.

Sanchez, L., Stephens, D. (1997) 'A tinnitus problem questionnaire in a clinic population.' *Ear and Hearing*, **18**, 210–217.

Santavuori, P., Linnankivi, T., Jaeken, J., Vanhanen, S-L., Telakivi, T., Heiskala, H. (1993) 'Psychological symptoms and sleep disturbances in neuronal ceroid-lipofuscinosis (NCL).' *Journal of Inherited Metabolic Disease*, **16**, 245–248.

Waters, K.A., Forbes, P., Morielli, A., Hum, C., O'Gorman, A.M., Vernet, O., Davis, G.M., Tewfik, T.L., Ducharme, F.M., Brouillette, R.T. (1998) 'Sleep disordered breathing in children with myelomeningocele.' *Journal of Pediatrics*, **132**, 672–681.

Tyler, R.S., Baker, L.J. (1983) 'Difficulties experienced by tinnitus sufferers.' *Journal of Speech and Hearing Disorders*, **48**, 150–154.

Will, R.G., Young, J.P., Thomas, D.J. (1988) 'Kleine–Levin syndrome: report of two cases with onset of symptoms precipitated by head trauma.' *British Journal of Psychiatry*, **152**, 410–412.

SECTION FOUR

NON-NEUROLOGICAL
PAEDIATRIC DISORDERS

20
SLEEP DISORDERS AND CHILDHOOD ALLERGY

André Kahn, Marie José Mozin, José Groswasser, Martine Sottiaux, Bernard Dan,
Sonia Scaillet, Georges Casimir and Jean Duchâteau

The various types of sleep disorders, including aetiological factors at different ages, were reviewed in Chapters 4, 5 and 6.

Medical conditions are rarely responsible for sleep problems in children, accounting for less than 20 per cent of persistent insomnia that resists behavioral treatment. In children under 1 year, the most frequently reported medical conditions responsible for sleep disruptions include otitis, colic, severe gastro-oesophageal reflux, neurological impairment and seizures. Allergies must also be added to the list of medical conditions that induce or aggravate children's sleep problems.

Allergies and sleep disorders in children

The frequency of allergies in the general paediatric population is not known. The prevalence of cow's milk allergy could be as high as 7 per cent (Höst *et al.* 1988). Allergy to milk favours eczema, wheezing or gastrointestinal disturbances. Its association with sleep problems has rarely been reported in the literature, although paediatricians and practitioners have long been known to eliminate cow's milk from the diet of a cranky baby, particularly when there is a family history of atopy or other clinical manifestations of allergy.

RESPIRATORY, ENT, SKIN AND GASTROINTESTINAL SYMPTOMS OF ALLERGIES

Conditions associated with various forms of allergies may interfere with night-time sleep continuity. Awakenings can result from increased respiratory efforts during respiratory allergies, wheezing or asthma attacks (Chapter 21). Sleep may be disrupted by laborious mouth breathing and prolonged obstructive sleep apnoea due to thickening of the upper-airway mucosa (Guilleminault and Anders 1976). Night-time pain attacks may also result from middle-ear infections, recurrent skin itching and irritations, or abdominal ache due to gastro-oesophageal reflux, diarrhoea or colic (Jakobsson *et al.* 1989).

Settipane (1999) has drawn attention to the common condition of allergic rhinitis as a more serious cause of problems than often supposed. Poorly controlled symptoms may lead to sleep loss and its various adverse effects on daytime function and well-being. It may also contribute to a number of other abnormalities of the nasopharynx and related structures causing upper airway obstruction during the day and during sleep.

FOOD ALLERGIES

Insomnia due to food allergy usually begins in infancy, following the introduction of cow's milk into the diet (Kahn *et al.* 1985). It represents about 10 per cent of severe forms of insomnia resistant to behavioural or drug treatments. It is one of the most profound forms of sleep disturbance, with delayed sleep initiation (over 15 minutes), continuous restlessness, drenching night sweats, and repeated, prolonged night-time wakings and crying. Total sleep time is significantly decreased (under six hours per night). During daytime, the children are agitated, irritable and sleepy. There is usually a family history of allergy and repeated episodes of diarrhoea, wheezing, ENT infections or skin rashes. Parental interventions or drug treatments do not normalize sleep.

The direct link between food allergy and sleep problems is based on a series of observations. Children may show the presence of high titres of specific immunoglobulin E against milk proteins, such as beta-lactoglobulin antibodies. However, allergen testing, total eosinophil count and skin reactivity tests can be negative in children under 1 year of age. After the removal of dietary milk and the initiation of an exclusion diet, sleep improves or normalizes within three to four weeks. Relapses occur within one to four days after small amounts of milk proteins are reintroduced into the diet.

The treatment of food allergy insomnia requires the use of a formula containing no milk protein. Soya milk can be used, but in up to 50 per cent of cases the child will also develop intolerance to soya (John and Kernser 1997). A hypoallergenic hydrolyzed formula is usually recommended, based on enzymatically hydrolyzed cow's milk whey proteins. The dietary treatment must be followed with great care, as only small amounts of the offending food favour the reappearance of the sleep problems. The expertise of a dietician may be needed. The treatment can be interrupted when the child outgrows the sensitivity to milk proteins, usually by 4 years of age.

Severe insomnia due to milk allergies may also appear as repeated head banging or body rocking. The allergy is not responsible for the noisy body movements, but is significantly related to their repetition and duration during the night. We have shown that when sleep continuity is normalized with a milk-protein-free diet, the frequency of the parasomnias decreases (Kahn *et al.* 1991). In our study, after three years of follow-up, intolerant children were found to still have more frequent episodes of skin and respiratory atopy, longer sleep onset times, shorter total sleep time, and more frequent night-time awakenings than control children.

There is much debate about other food intolerances (*e.g.* to food additives) causing behavioural disturbances (including sleep problems) in children, but this explanation may apply in some children (Egger *et al.* 1992). The same may also apply to the provocation by certain foodstuffs of other conditions associated with sleep disturbance such as atopic eczema (Pike *et al.* 1989), epilepsy (Egger *et al.* 1989) and enuresis. However, alternative possibilities should be considered carefully before going for food intolerance as an explanation, which is best justified if a close relationship can be established between symptoms and ingestion of the foodstuff, including improvement when it is withheld.

There is occasional evidence that some adults suffer food allergy insomnia due to various allergens such as eggs or fish.

Conclusions

Most sleep problems in children are easily resolved by behavioural treatments. Resistance to treatments should suggest a clinical condition responsible for the insomnia. Allergies may directly or indirectly disturb night-time settling and sleep continuity. An allergic disorder should be considered as a cause of persistent sleeplessness when no other cause is apparent, especially when there is a family history of atopy. A medical history and physical examination contribute to establishing the diagnosis and permit adequate medical or dietary treatment.

REFERENCES

Egger, J., Carter, C.M., Soothill, J.F., Wilson, J. (1989) 'Oligoantigenic diet treatment of children with epilepsy and migraine.' *Journal of Pediatrics*, **114**, 51–58.
—— Stolla, A., McEwan, LM (1992) 'Controlled trial of hyposensitisation in children with food-induced hyperkinetic syndrome.' *Lancet*, **339**, 1150–1153.
Guilleminault, C., Anders, T.F. (1976) 'Sleep disorders in children.' *Advances in Pediatrics*, **22**,151–175.
Höst, A., Husby, S., Österballe, O. (1988) 'A prospective study of cow's milk allergy in exclusively breast-fed infants.' *Acta Paediatrica Scandinavica*, **77**, 663–670.
Jakobsson, I., Lindberg, T., Lothe, L. (1989) 'Cow's milk proteins as a cause of infantile colic.' *In:* Hamburger, R.N. (Ed.) *Food Intolerance in Infancy: Allergology, Immunology, and Gastroenterology.* New York: Raven Press, pp. 173–185.
John, A., Kernser, S. (1997) 'Use of infant formulas in preventing or postponing atopic manifestations.' *Journal of Gastroenterology and Nutrition*, **24**, 442–446.
Kahn, A., Mozin, M.J., Casimir, G., Montauk, L., Blum, D. (1985) 'Insomnia and cow's milk allergy in infants.' *Pediatrics*, **76**, 880–884.
—— —— Rebuffat, E., Sottiaux, M., Casimir, G., Duchâteau, J., Muller, M.F. (1991) 'Children intolerant to cow's milk may suffer from severe insomnia.' *In:* Peter, J.H. (Ed.) *Sleep and Health Risk.* Berlin: Springer-Verlag, pp. 458–467.
Pike, M.A., Carter, C.M., Boulton, P., Turner, M.W., Soothill, J.F., Atherton, D.J. (1989) 'Few food diets in the treatment of atopic eczema.' *Archives of Disease in Childhood*, **64**, 1691–1698.
Settipane, R.A. (1999) 'Complications of allergic rhinitis.' *Allergy and Asthma Proceedings*, **20**, 209–213.

21
SLEEP DISORDERS IN ASTHMA, BRONCHOPULMONARY DYSPLASIA AND CYSTIC FIBROSIS

Gerald Loughlin

Many paediatricians seem to have only a limited appreciation of how vulnerable children are during sleep and of the role that the changes in breathing that occur during sleep may play in the pathophysiology of respiratory disease in children. In infants and young children, sleep may occupy more than half the day. It is a period when the child is generally unobserved, yet also when the ability of the child to defend himself against dangerous respiratory situations is compromised. Changes in ventilation that occur when a child falls asleep are typically well tolerated by the child with normal control of breathing and lung function. However, in infants and children with chronic lung disease, these sleep-related changes in breathing may have profound effects on gas exchange. In addition, respiratory symptoms (cough, wheeze and dyspnoea) may disrupt normal sleep (Gaultier *et al.* 1985, Gaultier 1995).

Breathing during sleep
PaO_2 decreases and $PaCO_2$ increases secondary to decreases in functional residual capacity (FRC) and minute ventilation. Decreases in FRC result in diminished oxygen stores and altered ventilation/perfusion relationships, while the irregular breathing pattern and paradoxical inward ribcage movement (PIRCM) seen during REM sleep may decrease minute ventilation. The highly compliant chest wall of the infant, coupled with a lung compliance that is similar to an adults', results in a situation where, without intervention, FRC in the infant would be close to residual volume. This is an unacceptable situation because it compromises oxygen stores. In order to prevent this, infants determine FRC actively rather than passively. They do this by a combination of interrupting expiration with a premature initiation of inspiration and by apposition of the vocal cords at the end of expiration ('laryngeal braking'). This defence system may be compromised by ribcage destabilization as a result of inspiratory intercostal muscle inhibition associated with REM sleep, leading not only to lower FRC during REM sleep, but also to adverse affects on tidal volume breathing and minute ventilation (Gaultier 1995).

How the infant and child respond to respiratory challenges during sleep is also a concern. These include increased airway resistance and CO_2, and decreased O_2, as well as challenges to the airway from gastro-oesophageal reflux. Increase in airway hyperreactivity in the early morning hours also imposes a stress on the sleeping child, but this is controlled more

by circadian factors than sleep. In neonates, the response to hypoxia is biphasic (an initial increase in minute ventilation followed by a decrease), a reflection of an attempt to diminish oxygen consumption. This biphasic response is seen in both wakefulness and sleep, with a more sustained response during NREM sleep than in REM sleep. It is not known how older prepubertal children will respond, but it is unlikely that sex differences will exist. In children and adults, the response to CO_2 is decreased during sleep compared to when they are awake. Some studies in neonates have found a decreased response to CO_2 only during REM sleep. In neonates, the response to increased airway resistance is increased in NREM, but not in REM sleep. In young adults, a decrease in ventilatory response to both acute and sustained resistive load has been reported. It is not known how chronic hypoxia, hypercapnia and increased airway resistance associated with conditions such as bronchopulmonary dysplasia and cystic fibrosis will influence the maturation of these responses, but there is a suggestion that the responses may be blunted or delayed in development.

Bronchopulmonary dysplasia (BPD)

DEFINITION

Bronchopulmonary dysplasia is a chronic pulmonary disease that arises as a complication of both lung injury and its treatment. Typically, it is seen in preterm infants after treatment for hyaline membrane disease. Even in the age of surfactant replacement therapy and improvements in neonatal respiratory therapy, BPD is still a common cause of morbidity in preterm infants.

PATTERN AND AETIOLOGY OF SLEEP DISORDERS

Abnormal sleep and breathing patterns have been reported only in older infants. Infants with BPD demonstrate decreased REM sleep and sleep fragmentation. The cause of this sleep disruption is unknown, since infants had abnormal sleep patterns with baseline oxygen saturation above 90 per cent, and yet administration of supplemental oxygen increased total sleep time, as well as REM sleep time (Harris and Sullivan 1995, Fitzgerald *et al.* 1998).

Hypoxaemia during sleep has been reported in infants with BPD who had adequate oxygenation when awake (Garg *et al.* 1988a). The mechanism underlying hypoxaemia during sleep is not well established, but most likely is due in part to the loss of the active mechanism that defends FRC during REM sleep. This results in lower FRC and oxygen stores. The problem may be compounded by increases in airway resistance seen with hypoxaemia. Airway obstruction may worsen ventilation/perfusion ratios and also increase oxygen consumption. Although REM sleep exacerbates the problem, PIRCM is not merely REM related since paradoxical breathing is seen in infants with BPD during both REM and NREM sleep (Gaultier *et al.* 1987, Rome *et al.* 1987).

Sleep and PIRCM also affect cardiac function in infants with BPD (Praud *et al.* 1991). Decreased right (RV) and left ventricular (LV) ejection fractions during sleep, with a greater effect on RV function, have been reported. Abnormal LV function may affect oxygen delivery and may account for poor growth seen in infants with BPD. Heart rate variability has also been shown to be affected by chronic hypoxaemia during sleep, with abnormalities in autonomic control appearing to result from repeated episodes of hypoxaemia.

Increased mortality from sudden death during the first year of life has been reported among oxygen-dependent infants with BPD (Werthammer *et al.* 1982, Abman *et al.* 1989). These deaths are thought to be sleep related, since most often they occur during periods of presumed sleep. Despite early attempts to link these deaths to sudden infant death syndrome (SIDS), this association is not appropriate considering that the diagnosis of SIDS depends on an absence of either a history or post-mortem findings that could explain sudden death. Infants with BPD who have been weaned from supplemental oxygen have been shown to have a blunted response to subsequent hypoxic challenges when asleep (Garg *et al.* 1988b). Although the infants demonstrated an arousal from sleep in response to the challenge, it was an ineffective response and they required vigorous stimulation and supplemental oxygen in order to restore normal pre-study breathing patterns. Others have demonstrated that infants with BPD may have deficient peripheral chemoreceptor function that matures more slowly. The combination of unrecognized hypoxaemia during sleep and abnormal response to such challenges places the infant with BPD at increased risk for sudden death or other adverse outcomes.

MANAGEMENT OF SLEEP-RELATED ISSUES IN BPD
Since awake oxygen saturation does not predict what may be happening during sleep, oxygenation must be monitored during an extended period of sleep. Although pulse oximetry can provide noninvasive extended monitoring of oxygen saturation, it is subject to artefacts from movement, and in an unattended setting it may be difficult to get an uninterrupted monitoring period. If there is any question about associated obstructive apnoea or bradycardia without central apnoea, then polysomnography is indicated. Weaning supplemental oxygen should also be based on demonstration that the infant can maintain oxygen saturation above 92 per cent during all phases of sleep as well as when awake and with feeding (Garg *et al.* 1988a). Following discontinuation of supplemental oxygen, infants should be monitored for growth and development, polycythaemia, cor pulmonale and disturbance of sleep patterns. Cardiorespiratory monitoring during sleep is recommended both while the child is receiving supplemental oxygen and for at least a month after it is stopped.

Asthma
DEFINITION
Asthma is a form of chronic lung disease associated with airway inflammation resulting in obstruction from airway wall oedema, increased bronchoconstriction and secretions. Asthma is often reversible with therapy.

PATTERN AND AETIOLOGY OF DISORDERED SLEEP AND BREATHING
The occurrence of nocturnal asthma symptoms is a marker of poor control of asthma, as well as a reflection of baseline lung function when awake. Nocturnal symptoms are a common problem, yet often they go undetected and their clinical significance is unrecognized (Turner-Warnick 1988, National Institutes of Health 1995). Although an exacerbation of asthma at night is more likely to be secondary to circadian factors, certain changes in breathing that occur with sleep may contribute to the problem (McFadden 1988). Sleep may

augment changes in lung function such as increased airway resistance, and also affect the child's ability to compensate for circadian variability in lung function and for factors that may increase airway hyperreactivity. There has been increasing appreciation of the significance of nocturnal symptoms, not only in terms of their effects on daytime performance, but also as a risk factor for increased morbidity and mortality from asthma (Miller and Strunk 1989).

Lung function appears to vary throughout the day. The best function is seen at around 4 p.m. and the lowest values occur at around 4 a.m. In general, this diurnal variability is small, typically less than 10 per cent. These changes parallel changes in endogenous production of hormones known to affect airway function. Cyclic AMP levels decrease through the night, while cyclic GMP increases. Epinephrine and steroid levels are at their nadir around 4 a.m., while histamine levels are increased. Resting vagal tone also increases as the night progresses. Although lower endogenous steroid levels do not appear to play a role in the changes seen in airway function, they may do so in the heightened airway hyperreactivity seen as the night progresses (Martin *et al.* 1990). While circadian rhythms appear to play the major role, sleep itself is also a contributing factor. Sleep appears to augment the diurnal increase in airway resistance.

Variability in peak flow measurements of more than 50 per cent, some associated with desaturation, has been reported. Hypoxaemia during sleep in children with asthma occurs as both a lower baseline during sleep than seen in patients without asthma and as episodic desaturation. Hypoxaemia may also play a role in increasing airway obstruction and potentiating airway hyperreactivity.

In addition to circadian factors, exposure to environmental allergens and gastro-oesophageal reflux may play a role. The consequences of exposure to aeroallergens and reflux episodes may be magnified by the heightened airway reactivity seen as the night progresses. The dosing schedules and duration of effectiveness of many asthma drugs may compound this problem.

There are conflicting data regarding contribution of sleep state to triggering an asthma exacerbation. In a study of 10 children with asthma, reduced stage 4 sleep and increased awakenings and arousals compared to children without asthma were noted (Kales *et al.* 1970). More recently, Sadeh *et al.* (1998) compared sleep, assessed by subjective report and actometry, with subjective reports of nocturnal asthma symptoms and peak flow measures in 40 children with well-controlled stable asthma and 34 healthy controls, all children of school age. The children with asthma had "poorer quality sleep", with significantly more activity during sleep, and poor sleep was judged to be associated with reduced pulmonary function. However, in another group of children with moderate asthma that was under control, sleep architecture was considered normal despite the use of theophylline therapy (Avital *et al.* 1991). More data are needed in this area including the contribution that anti-asthma medications might make to sleep disruption. Theophylline has had this reputation, but the study by Avital *et al.* (1991) does not provide support and can be interpreted to mean that any direct sleep-disrupting effect might be outweighed by its beneficial action on respiratory function resulting in improved sleep. Studies need to focus on patients of different ages, the effects of different approaches to therapy, disease control and noninvasive measures of airway function.

Management

Comprehensive management of children with asthma must account for the diurnal variation in airway function that occurs at night. Assessment of patients with asthma must include questions about sleep patterns and sleep disturbance due to breathing difficulty. A diary may help parents keep track of nocturnal symptoms; and in patients who are old enough, recording peak flow rates in the morning and afternoon and if the patient wakes with symptoms, can provide invaluable information. Continuous recording of oximetry is rarely needed. However, recording of respiratory noises may offer a way to monitor asthma symptoms noninvasively. Current treatment plans that focus on reduction in airway inflammation typically will result in control of both daytime and nocturnal symptoms. Until control is achieved, treatment of nocturnal symptoms may require the addition of a long-acting beta agonist or theophylline. Environmental controls and treatment of reflux are also important components of nocturnal symptom control, especially those measures designed to reduce dust mite exposure.

The potential wide-ranging benefits of improved control of asthmatic symptoms at night are illustrated in a study by Stores *et al.* (1998). Subjective and polysomnographic evidence of sleep disturbance, respiratory function and daytime psychological function were studied in 21 school-age children with nocturnal asthma. Compared with matched controls, the children with nocturnal asthma had significantly more disturbed sleep in the form of frequent brief or longer awakenings, more psychological problems, and lower performance on some aspects of memory and concentration. Improvement of nocturnal asthma symptoms and respiratory function by changes of treatment were followed by improvements in sleep continuity and psychological function in subsequent weeks. In keeping with these results is the report by Diette *et al.* (2000) that awakenings in children with nocturnal asthma are associated with missed school, impaired educational performance and also parental absence from work.

The findings in both studies highlight the potential effects of asthma on sleep and its psychological consequences, as well as supporting the idea that these factors must be considered as part of overall care.

Cystic fibrosis (CF)

DEFINITION

CF is the most common cause of irreversible airway obstruction in children and adolescents. It is an inherited disorder secondary to a defect in the gene controlling water and electrolyte transport across epithelia (Davis *et al.* 1996).

PATTERN AND AETIOLOGY OF DISORDERED SLEEP AND BREATHING

Due to the chronic and progressive nature of the lung disease, most of the available information on the relationship between breathing during sleep and CF comes from older children with more established lung disease. In infants with early severe disease, it is likely that changes in respiration described in infants with BPD are applicable to children with CF. In one study, Stokes *et al.* (1985) reported that hypoxaemia during sleep, due in part to assumption of the recumbent position, was fairly common. Additional decreases in oxygen saturation

were seen in REM sleep and were felt to be a combination of worsening ventilation perfusion relationships and hypoventilation. Interestingly, the degree of hypoxaemia during sleep is not always associated with disease severity (Francis *et al.* 1980, Muller *et al.* 1980).

The quality of sleep can also be affected adversely by CF lung disease. Decreased sleep efficiency, more awakenings and sleep state changes have been reported in patients with CF (Spier *et al.* 1984). Coughing spells rather than hypoxaemia during sleep appears to be the major contributor to the sleep disturbance. In young adults with CF, arousals did not coincide with periods of hypoxaemia. Supplemental oxygen did not improve sleep quality despite controlling desaturation episodes (Boysen *et al.* 1979). Obstructive sleep apnoea is uncommon.

MANAGEMENT
The most effective way to improve sleep quality is to treat pulmonary infections and reduce coughing. Since the degree of oxygen desaturation during sleep cannot be predicted from awake pulmonary function, exercise testing or disease severity scores, oxygen levels must be assessed during nocturnal sleep. It is recommended that patients with CF who have awake PaO_2 below 70 mmHg or an equivalent oxygen saturation of less than 95 per cent during a stable period should be considered at increased risk for hypoxaemia during sleep and should have oxygen saturation monitored during sleep. This study should be obtained at least two weeks after treatment for an acute exacerbation (American Thoracic Society 1996). Even though oxygen may not improve sleep quality, patients receiving nocturnal supplemental oxygen, even for brief periods, were shown to have improved attendance at school and work, compared to a control group that did not receive supplemental oxygen (Zinman *et al.* 1989). There are insufficient data at this time to draw conclusions on the role of supplemental oxygen in preventing the development of cor pulmonale in patients with CF.

Conclusion
This is clearly an area in need of more research. Considering the amount of time that the average child spends asleep, it is essential that those caring for children with chronic lung disease be aware of the unique challenges that sleep poses for these patients. Furthermore, as with so many other conditions, it is not appropriate to apply sleep data from adults with lung disease to infants and children. Developmental status, age of onset of the disease and the natural history of the disease process must be accounted for when studying the influence of sleep and breathing during sleep on chronic respiratory disease in children.

REFERENCES

Abman, S.H., Burchell, M.F., Schaffer, M.S., Rosenberg, A.A. (1989) 'Late sudden unexpected deaths in hospitalized infants with bronchopulmonary dysplasia.' *American Journal of Diseases of Children*, **143**, 815–819.
American Thoracic Society (1996) 'Standards and indications for cardiopulmonary sleep studies in children.' *American Journal of Respiratory and Critical Care Medicine*, **153**, 866–878.
Avital, A., Steljes, G., Pasterkamp, H., Kryger, M., Sanchez, I, Chernick, V. (1991) 'Sleep quality in children with asthma treated with theophylline or cromolyn sodium.' *Journal of Pediatrics*, **119**, 979–984.
Boysen, P.G., Block, A.J., Wynne, J.W. (1979) 'Nocturnal pulmonary hypertension in patients with chronic obstructive pulmonary disease.' *Chest*, **76**, 536–540.

Davis, P.S., Drumm, M., Konstan, M.W. (1996) 'Cystic fibrosis.' *American Journal of Respiratory Critical Care Medicine*, **154**, 1229–1256.

Diette, G.B., Markson,L., Skinner, E.A., Nguyen, T.T., Algatt-Bergstrom, P., Wu, A.W. (2000) 'Nocturnal asthma in children affects school attendance, school performance, and parents' work attendance.' *Archives of Pediatrics and Adolescent Medicine*, **154**, 923–928.

Fitzgerald, D., Van Asperen, P., Leslie, G., Arnold, J., Sullivan, C.E. (1998) 'Higher SaO$_2$ in chronic neonatal lung disease: does it improve sleep?' *Pediatric Pulmonology*, **26**, 235–240.

Francis, P.W.J., Muller, N.J., Gurwitz, D., Milligan, D.W.A., Levison, H., Bryan, A.C. (1980) 'Hemoglobin desaturation: Its occurrence during sleep in patients with cystic fibrosis.' *American Journal of Diseases of Children*, **134**, 734–740.

Garg, M., Kurzner, S.I., Bautista, D.B., Keens, T.G. (1988a) 'Clinically unsuspected hypoxia during sleep and feeding in infants with bronchopulmonary dysplasia.' *Pediatrics*, **81**, 635–641.

—— —— —— —— (1988b) 'Hypoxic arousal responses in infants with bronchopulmonary dysplasia.' *Pediatrics*, **82**, 59–63.

Gaultier, C.L. (1995) 'Cardiorespiratory adaptation during sleep in infants and children.' *Pediatric Pulmonology*, **19**, 105–117.

—— Praud, J.P., Clement, A., Boule, M., Khiati, M., Tournier, G., Girard, F. (1985) 'Respiration during sleep in children with COPD.' *Chest*, **87**, 168–173.

—— —— Canet, E., Delaperche, M.F., D'Allest, A.M. (1987) 'Paradoxical inward rib cage motion during rapid eye movement sleep in infants and young children.' *Journal of Developmental Physiology*, **9**, 391–397.

Harris, M.A., Sullivan, C.E. (1995) 'Sleep pattern and supplementary oxygen requirements in infants with chronic neonatal lung disease.' *Lancet*, **345**, 831–832.

Kales, A., Kales, J.D., Sly, R.M., Scharf, M.B., Tan, T.L., Preston, T.A. (1970) 'Sleep patterns of asthmatic children: all-night electroencephalographic studies.' *Journal of Allergy*, **46**, 300–308.

Martin, R.J., Cicutto, L.C., Ballard, R.D. (1990) 'Factors related to the nocturnal worsening of asthma.' *American Review of Respiratory Disease*, **141**, 33–38.

McFadden, E.R. (1988) 'Circadian rhythms.' *American Journal of Medicine*, **85**, 2–5.

Miller, B.D., Strunk, R.C. (1989) 'Circumstances surrounding the deaths of children due to asthma.' *American Journal of Diseases of Children*, **143**, 1294–1299.

Muller, N.L., Francis, P.W., Gurwitz, D., Levison, H., Bryan, A.C. (1980) 'Mechanism of hemoglobin desaturation during rapid-eye-movement sleep in normal subjects and in patients with cystic fibrosis.' *American Review of Respiratory Disease*, **121**, 463–469.

National Institutes of Health (1995) *Global Initiative for Asthma: Global Strategy for Asthma Management and Prevention. NHLBI/WHO Workshop Report, March 1993.* Bethesda, MD: US Government. Publication No. 95-3659.

Praud, J.P., Cavailloles, F., Boulhadour, K., De Recondo, M., Guilleminault, C., Gaultier, C. (1991) 'Radionuclide evaluation of cardiac function during sleep in children with bronchopulmonary dysplasia.' *Chest*, **100**, 721–725.

Rome, E.S., Miller, M.J., Goldthwait, D.A., Osorio, I.O., Fanaroff, A.A., Martin, R.J. (1987) 'Effect of sleep state on chest wall movements and gas exchange in infants with resolving bronchopulmonary dysplasia.' *Pediatric Pulmonology*, **3**, 259–263.

Sadeh, A., Horowitz, I., Wolach-Benodis, L., Wolach, B. (1998) 'Sleep and pulmonary function in children with well-controlled, stable asthma.' *Sleep*, **21**, 379–384.

Spier, S., Rivlin, J., Hugues, D., Levison, H. (1984) 'The effect of oxygen on sleep, blood gases and ventilation in cystic fibrosis.' *American Review of Respiratory Disease*, **129**, 712–718.

Stokes, D.C., Wohl, M.E.B., Khaw, K.T., Strieder, D.J. (1985) 'Postural hypoxemia in cystic fibrosis.' *Chest*, **87**, 785–789.

Stores, G., Ellis, A.J., Wiggs, L., Crawford, C., Thomson, A. (1998) 'Sleep and psychological disturbance in nocturnal asthma.' *Archives of Disease in Childhood*, **78**, 413–419.

Turner-Warnick, M. (1988) 'Epidemiology of nocturnal asthma.' *American Journal of Medicine*, **85**, 6–8.

Werthammer, J., Brown, E.R., Neff, R.K., Taeusch, H.W. (1982) 'Sudden infant death syndrome in infants with bronchopulmonary dysplasia.' *Pediatrics*, **69**, 301–303.

Zinman, R., Corey, M., Coates, A.L., Canny, G.J., Connolly, J., Levison, H., Beaudry, P.H. (1989) 'Nocturnal home oxygen in the treatment of hypoxemic cystic fibrosis patients.' *Journal of Pediatrics*, **14**, 368–377.

22
ASPECTS OF SLEEP IN OTHER GENERAL PAEDIATRIC CONDITIONS

Gregory Stores

Sleep disturbances associated with various general medical disorders in adults have been reviewed by Chokroverty (1999). Some of the points made in that review are relevant to children, but a comparable account specifically concerning paediatric conditions is not available. However, there have been reports published sporadically about sleep problems and disorders in a number of childhood conditions in addition to those considered in the previous chapters. General issues relevant to paediatric practice, namely the effects on sleep of hospital admission or treatments, have also been discussed in the literature to some extent.

Painful and uncomfortable conditions
The vast majority of people with chronic pain complain of poor sleep (Smith *et al.* 2000). The various connections between sleep and pain in both adults and children include the direct effects of painful conditions on sleep duration and quality, effects on sleep of the distress of suffering a painful or frightening condition, and the significance of persistently disturbed sleep on a child's ability to cope with illness.

Obviously painful conditions that disturb sleep include *acute orthopaedic injury* (*e.g.* Selbst *et al.* 1999) and *post-surgical pain*. Sleep disturbance from night-time pain from *chronic middle-ear disease* may be misinterpreted as behavioural in origin. Other painful conditions in which sleep disturbance has been reported in children include *malignancy* (Miser *et al.* 1987), *juvenile rheumatoid arthritis* (Zamir *et al.* 1998), *sickle cell disease* (Shapiro *et al.* 1995), *haemophilia* (Walco and Varni 1991), *burn injury* (Lawrence *et al.* 1998), *juvenile fibromyalgia* (Siegel *et al.* 1998), and *abdominal pain* of diverse and sometimes obscure aetiology (Hyams 1997). The types of sleep disturbance in various rheumatological conditions (seen mainly in adults) have been reviewed by Mahowald and Mahowald (2000). In all of these, and other painful conditions, associated psychological upset will add to sleep disturbance.

The same can be said of other disorders in which discomfort rather than pain at night is a characteristic feature. *Deformity or physical disability* accompanying neurological disorder can cause difficulty in achieving or maintaining a comfortable sleeping position (Burton 1990). Similarly, irritating *skin conditions*, notably atopic dermatitis (Stores *et al.* 1998), cause sleep disruption to a serious degree because of scratching, although sleep may remain disturbed to some extent following clinical remission (Reuveni 1999). High rates

147

of sleep disruption have also been reported in young children with *gastro-oesophageal reflux* (Ghaem *et al.* 1998) but the explanation is unclear. The issue of serious effects of this condition on respiration during sleep remains contentious (Samuels 2000). *Nocturia*, of whatever cause, also disrupts sleep.

Medications that might be used in serious painful conditions and that are said to affect sleep are cytotoxic drugs, antiemetics, and also corticosteroids when used, for example, in the treatment of childhood leukaemia (Drigan *et al.* 1992) and other forms of cancer (Harris *et al.* 1986). Drug effects on children's sleep, however, are a little researched topic.

Lewin and Dahl (1999) have emphasized the ways in which sleep loss or disruption caused by painful conditions can add to children's perception of pain, and also to their difficulties in coping with their illness or disorder. The same applies to their parents if their sleep is seriously affected by the child's illness. Conversely, adequate sleep is highly beneficial not only psychologically but also because of the possible facilitating effects on physiological aspects of the healing process as mentioned in Chapter 1. For that reason, care of affected children needs to include, in addition to psychological help for the child and family, adequate pain relief by day and night, and the promotion of sleep by other means such as behavioural methods, which have been shown to be effective in adults with insomnia due to chronic pain (Currie *et al.* 2000). Short-term use of sedatives may be appropriate but their long-term use (and that of major analgesics) is known to have a deleterious effect on sleep as are various psychotropic drugs that might be prescribed to help ease distress (Schweitzer 2000).

Additional paediatric conditions associated with sleep disturbance

It is difficult to identify any acute or chronic physical disorder in which sleep disturbance is unlikely to be a complication, but there are some others in which sleep problems have been highlighted in published accounts.

Sleep-related breathing difficulty has been described in a miscellany of other childhood conditions in addition to those in which this form of sleep disturbance has already been discussed. One broad category is childhood *obesity*. The ways in which obesity can compromise respiratory function during sleep have been discussed by Mallory and Beckerman (1992), but only a minority of even very obese children have severe obstructive apnoea, the proportion varying somewhat in different studies (Mallory *et al.* 1989, Marcus *et al.* 1996). The likelihood of such problems is not related to degree of obesity in any simple way. In affected cases, adenotonsillectomy can be helpful even if the tonsils and adenoids are normal in size. This and other aspects of treatment are discussed by Keens and Davidson Ward (2000).

As already mentioned, children with *sickle cell disease* may sleep badly because of pain from vaso-occlusive crises and end-organ damage caused by sickling and occlusion of microvasculature. They are also at high risk of upper airway obstruction during sleep because of hyperplasia of tonsils and adenoids. The causes, consequences and management of this complication have been reviewed by Blaisdell (2000). Important points include the fact that oxygen desaturization during sleep might itself predispose the child to vaso-occlusive crises (which may be extremely serious, including stroke), and that desaturization

cannot be predicted from whether or not the child snores or has obviously enlarged tonsils. Polysomnography is required to confirm upper airway obstruction. Treatment consists principally of tonsillectomy with appropriate precautions against possible serious complications arising from the sickle cell disease itself.

A number of *other medical conditions have been associated with upper airway obstruction* during sleep caused in different ways according to the nature of the basic condition. Carroll and Loughlin (1995) mention case reports in which upper airway structures had been affected by *infiltrative diseases* or *granulomatous lesions, blockage by other lesions* and *hypothyroidism. Marfan syndrome* is also associated with a high rate of sleep-disordered breathing caused by structural abnormalities of the hard palate and maxilla (Cistulli *et al.* 1996). Of the many aetiological factors that have been suggested for the *sudden infant death syndrome* (SIDS), various abnormalities of sleep have been described including the involvement of upper airway obstruction in the terminal event. These sleep factors have been the subject of a number of reviews such as that by Glotzbach *et al.* (1995).

Disturbed sleep, especially excessive sleepiness and fatigue, is a prominent feature of various *infectious diseases* and their aftermath including some encountered in children (Jaffe 2000). These include *infectious mononucleosis* and *encephalitis* of bacterial or viral origin. *Human immunodeficiency virus* (HIV) infection in children is associated with prominent sleep–wake disturbances comparable to those described in affected adults (Franck *et al.* 1999).

In *other forms of chronic illness* (endocrine, renal or hepatic, for example) sleep is also disturbed as part of a general systemic upset. Inconsistently, abnormalities of sleep physiology have been reported in children and adolescents with insulin-dependant diabetes mellitus and nocturnal hypoglycaemia (Porter *et al.* 1996, Matyka *et al.* 2000). The implications of abnormal findings for daytime function are unclear but, if severe, the hypoglycaemia may trigger seizure activity at night.

Effects of treatments and hospital admission

Some forms of *medication*, in addition to those mentioned earlier in relation to the control of pain or discomfort, are thought to be capable of disrupting sleep, although this has been the subject of very little research. Theophylline, for example, has this reputation, which, however, has not been confirmed in children who have taken this medication for asthma (Avital *et al.* 1991). Any potential sleep-disrupting effect may well be outweighed by its beneficial respiratory action. The possible effects on sleep and wakefulness of antiepileptic medications were mentioned in Chapter 15. Other medications used for children and adolescents that might have adverse effects on sleep are stimulant drugs used for attention deficit hyperactivity disorder (Chapter 26) or narcolepsy (Chapter 5), antihistamines (causing sleepiness), and antidepressant drugs including selective serotonin reuptake inhibitors such as fluoxitine, which can cause insomnia and periodic limb movements in sleep (Sweitzer 2000).

Attendance at hospital, especially for uncomfortable or frightening diagnostic or treatment procedures, can cause concern and distress sufficient to affect a child's sleep patterns, sometimes severely. *Admission to hospital* is likely to add to the problem as indicated by

the high rate of sleep disturbance in children in hospital reported by White *et al.* (1990). There are likely to be many causes including the psychological effects of being ill and also being away from home. Other factors are the illness and its treatment, and aspects of the hospital environment including noise (Grumet 1993). Additional concerns have been expressed about the potentially traumatic experience of *paediatric intensive care* including serious sleep disturbances as reported by Cureton-Lane and Fontaine (1997), sometimes with persistence after discharge from hospital (Corser 1996). Hess *et al.* (1994) have also demonstrated a high rate of sleep disorders in young children after discharge from hospital following cardiac surgery. The psychological consequences of sleep deprivation in the paediatric intensive care unit have been discussed by Slota (1988), and Barndt-Maglio (1986) has recommended various measures to control psychological and environmental causes of sleep disruption in this setting to the advantage of the child during the period of admission and afterwards.

REFERENCES

Avital, A., Steljes, D.G., Pasterkamp, H., Kryger, M., Sanchez, I., Chernick, V. (1991) 'Sleep quality in children with asthma treated with theophylline or cromolyn sodium.' *Journal of Pediatrics*, **119**, 979–984.

Barndt-Maglio, B. (1986) 'Sleep pattern disturbance.' *Dimensions of Critical Care Nursing*, **5**, 342–349.

Blaisdell, C.J. (2000) 'Sickle cell disease and breathing during sleep.' *In:* Loughlin, G.M., Carroll, J.L., Marcus, C.L. (Eds.) *Sleep and Breathing in Children. A Developmental Approach*. New York: Marcel Dekker, pp. 755–763.

Burton, A. (1990) 'The management of sleep problems.' *In:* Hogg, J., Sebba, J., Lambe, I. (Eds.) *Profound Retardation and Multiple Impairment. Vol. 3. Medical and Physical Care and Management*. London: Chapman & Hall, pp. 274–284.

Carroll, J.L., Loughlin, G.M. (1995) 'Obstructive sleep apnea syndrome in infants and children: Clinical features and pathophysiology.' *In:* Ferber, R., Kryger, M. (Eds.) *Principles and Practice of Sleep Medicine in the Child*. Philadelphia: W.B. Saunders, pp. 163–191.

Chokroverty, S. (1999) 'Sleep disturbances in other medical disorders.' *In:* Chokroverty, S. (Ed.) *Sleep Disorders Medicine: Basic Science, Technical Considerations and Clinical Aspects. 2nd Edn*. Boston: Butterworth-Heinemann, pp. 587–617.

Cistulli, P.A., Richards, G.N., Palmisano, R.G., Unger, G., Berthon-Jones, M., Sullivan, C.E. (1996) 'Influence of maxillary construction on nasal resistance and sleep apnea severity in patients with Marfan's syndrome.' *Chest*, **110**, 1184–1188.

Corser, N.C. (1996) 'Sleep of 1- and 2- year-old children in intensive care.' *Issues in Comprehensive Pediatric Nursing*, **19**, 17–31.

Cureton-Lane, R.A., Fontaine, D.K. (1997) 'Sleep in the pediatric ICU: an empirical investigation.' *American Journal of Critical Care*, **6**, 56–63.

Currie, S.R., Wilson, K.G., Pontefract, A.J., Delaplante, L. (2000) 'Cognitive–behavioural treatment of insomnia secondary to chronic pain.' *Journal of Consulting and Clinical Psychology*, **68**, 407–416.

Drigan, R., Spirito, A., Gelber, R.D. (1992) 'Behavioral effects of corticosteroids in children with acute lymphoblastic leukemia.' *Medical and Pediatric Oncology*, **20**, 13–21.

Franck, L.S., Johnson, L.M., Lee, K., Hepner, C., Lambert, L., Passeri, M., Manio, E., Dorenbaum, A., Wara, D. (1999) 'Sleep disturbances in children with human immunodeficiency virus infection.' *Pediatrics*, **104**, e62.

Ghaem, M., Armstrong, K.L., Trocki, O., Cleghorn, G.J., Patrick, M.K., Shepherd, R.W. (1998) 'The sleep patterns of infants and young children with gastro-oesophageal reflux.' *Journal of Paediatrics and Child Health*, **34**, 160–163.

Glotzbach, S.F., Ariagno, R.L., Harper, R.M. (1995) 'Sleep and the sudden infant death syndrome.' *In:* Ferber, R., Kryger, M. (Eds.) *Principles and Practice of Sleep Medicine in the Child*. Philadelphia: W.B. Saunders, pp. 231–244.

Grumet, G.W. (1993) 'Pandemonium in the modern hospital.' *New England Journal of Medicine*, **328**, 433–437.

Harris, J.C., Carel, C.A., Rosenberg, L.A., Joshi, P. Leventhal, B.G. (1986) 'Intermittent high dose corticosteroid treatment in childhood cancer: Behavioural and emotional consequences.' *Journal of the American Academy of Child and Adolescent Psychiatry*, **25**, 120–124.

Hess, H.R., Kennedy, C., Lynch, M.E., Lee, K.A. (1994) 'Sleep behavior disorders in children after cardiac surgery.' *Sleep Research*, **23**, 367. *(Abstract.)*

Hyams, J.S. (1997) 'Recurrent abdominal pain and irritable bowel syndrome in children.' *Journal of Pediatric Gastroenterology and Nutrition*, **25** (Suppl. 1), S16–S17.

Jaffe, S.E. (2000) 'Sleep and infectious diseases.' *In:* Kryger, M.H., Roth, T., Dement, W.C. (Eds.) *Principles and Practice of Sleep Medicine, 3rd Edn.* Philadelphia: W.B. Saunders, pp. 1093–1102.

Keens, T.G., Davidson-Ward, S.L. (2000) 'Syndromes affecting respiratory control during sleep.' *In:* Loughlin, G.M., Carroll, J.L., Marcus, C.L. (Eds.). *Sleep and Breathing in Children. A Developmental Approach.* New York: Marcel Dekker, pp. 525–553.

Lawrence, J.W., Fauerbach, J., Endell, E., Ware, L., Munster, A. (1998) 'The 1998 Clinical Research Award. Sleep disturbance after burn injury: a frequent yet understudied complication.' *Journal of Burn Care and Rehabilitation*, **19**, 480–486.

Lewin, D.S., Dahl, R.E. (1999) 'Importance of sleep in the management of pediatric pain.' *Developmental and Behavioral Pediatrics*, **20**, 244–252.

Mahowald, M.L., Mahowald, M.W. (2000) 'Nighttime sleep and daytime functioning (sleepiness and fatigue) in well defined chronic rheumatic diseases.' *Sleep Medicine*, **1**, 179–193.

Mallory, G.B., Beckerman, R.C. (1992) 'Relationship between obesity and respiratory control abnormalities.' *In:* Beckerman, R.C., Brouillette, R.T., Hunt, C.E. (Eds.) *Respiratory Control Disorders in Infants and Children.* Baltimore: Williams & Wilkins, pp. 342–351.

—— Fiser, D.H., Jackson, R. (1989) 'Sleep-associated breathing disorders in morbidly obese children and adolescents.' *Journal of Pediatrics*, **115**, 892–897.

Marcus, C.L., Curtis, S., Koerner, C.B., Joffe, A., Serwint, J.R., Loughlin, G.M. (1996) 'Evaluation of pulmonary function and polysomnography in obese children and adolescents.' *Pediatric Pulmonology*, **21**, 176–183.

Matyka, K., Crawford, C., Wiggs, L., Dunger, D.B., Stores, G. (2000) 'Alterations in sleep physiology in young children with insulin dependant diabetes mellitus: Relationships to nocturnal hypoglycaemia.' *Journal of Pediatrics*, **137**, 233–238.

Miser, A.W., McCalla, J., Dothage, J.A., Wesley, M., Miser, J.A. (1987) 'Pain as a presenting symptom in children and young adults with newly diagnosed malignancy.' *Pain*, **29**, 85–90.

Porter, P.A., Byrne, G., Stick, S., Jones, T.W. (1996) 'Nocturnal hypoglycaemia and sleep disturbances in young teenagers with insulin dependant diabetes mellitus.' *Archives of Disease in Childhood*, **75**, 120–123.

Reuveni, H., Chapnick, G., Tal, A., Tarasiuk, A. (1999) 'Sleep fragmentation in children with atopic dermatitis.' *Archives of Pediatric and Adolescent Medicine*, **153**, 249–253.

Samuels, M.P. (2000) 'Apparent life-threatening events: Pathogenesis and management.' *In:* Loughlin, G.M., Carroll, J.L., Marcus, C.L. (Eds.) *Sleep and Breathing in Children.* New York: Marcell Dekker, pp. 423–441.

Schweitzer, P.K. (2000) 'Drugs that disturb sleep and wakefulness.' *In:* Kryger, M.H., Roth, T., Dement, W.C. (Eds.) *Principles and Practice of Sleep Medicine. 3rd Edn.* Philadelphia: W.B. Saunders, pp. 441–461.

Selbst, S.M., Lavelle, J.M., Soyupak, S.K., Markowitz, R.I. (1999) 'Back pain in children who present in the emergency department.' *Clinical Pediatrics*, **38**, 401–406.

Shapiro, B.S., Dinges, D.F., Orne, E.C., Bauer, N., Reilly, L.B., Whitehouse, W.G., Ohene-Fremponge, K., Orne, M.T. (1995) 'Home management of sickle cell-related pain in children and adolescents: natural history and impact on school attendance.' *Pain*, **61**, 139–144.

Siegel, D.M., Janeway, D., Baum, J. (1998) 'Fibromyalgia syndrome in children and adolescents: Clinical features at presentation and status at follow-up.' *Pediatrics*, **101**, 377–382.

Slota, M.C. (1988) 'Implications of sleep deprivation in the pediatric critical care unit.' *Focus on Critical Care*, **15**, 35–43.

Smith, M.T., Perlis, M.L., Smith, M.S., Giles, D.E., Curmody, T.P. (2000) 'Sleep quality and presleep arousal in chronic pain.' *Journal of Behavioral Medicine*, **23**, 1–13.

Stores, G., Burrows, A., Crawford, C. (1998) 'Physiological sleep disturbance in children with atopic dermatitis: a case control study.' *Pediatric Dermatology*, **15**, 264–268

Sweitzer, P.K. (2000) 'Drugs that disturb sleep and wakefulness.' *In:* Kryger, M.H., Roth, T., Dement, W.C. (Eds.) *Principles and Practice of Sleep Medicine, 3rd Edn.* Philadelphia: W.B. Saunders, pp. 441–461.

Walco, G.A., Varni, J.W. (1991) 'Chronic and recurrent pain: Hemophilia, juvenile rheumatoid arthritis and sickle cell disease.' *In:* Bush, H.S. (Ed.) *Children in Pain: Clinical and Research Issues from a Developmental Perspective.* New York: Springer-Verlag, pp. 297–336.

White, M.A., Williams, P.D., Alexander, D.J., Powell-Cope, G.M., Coulon, M. (1990) 'Sleep onset latency and distress in hospitalised children.' *Nursing Research*, **39**, 134–139.

Zamir, G., Press, J., Tal, A., Tarasiuk, A. (1998) 'Sleep fragmentation in children with rheumatoid arthritis.' *Journal of Rheumatology*, **25**, 1191–1197.

SECTION FIVE

PSYCHIATRIC DISORDERS

23
SLEEP DISTURBANCES IN ANXIOUS CHILDREN

E. Jane Garland

Anxiety disorders are among the most common psychiatric disorders found in epidemio-logical surveys of both adults and children. Prevalence ranges from 8.9 per cent in childhood populations up to 12.6 per cent in adolescent studies. Variations in reported prevalence are attributable in part to recent changes in diagnostic criteria; it is also common for children to have several comorbid anxiety disorders. Rates of subclinical anxiety are high, with 30 per cent of children reporting some overanxious symptoms and 15 per cent showing anxious temperament. Anxiety disorders tend to be chronic and recurrent. Anxious children and adolescents frequently have intrinsic sleep disorders, including psychophysiological insomnia and sleep terrors, and extrinsic sleep disorders related to chronically poor sleep hygiene and poor parental limit-setting.

Generalized anxiety disorder, formerly known as overanxious disorder, has a prevalence of 3–5 per cent. It is characterized by at least six months of excessive, difficult to control worry about many issues, with at least three associated symptoms including sleep disturbances, muscle tension, restlessness, difficulty concentrating, fatigue and irritability. In children only one associated symptom is required for diagnosis (American Psychiatric Association 1994), and the main complaint is usually insomnia.

Panic disorder is characterized by the occurrence of one or more panic attacks with at least four weeks of significant impairment due to avoidance or worry about attacks; many individuals become agoraphobic. A panic attack is an acute period of intense fear or discomfort, with four or more specific symptoms developing abruptly and reaching a peak within 10 minutes. Specific symptoms include palpitations, sweating, trembling, a choking sensation, chest pain, nausea or abdominal distress, dizziness, derealization (*i.e.* feelings of unreality), fear of losing control or going crazy, fear of dying, paraesthesias and chills or hot flushes. These episodes are highly aversive and can cause extremes of behavioural avoidance or acting out. Night-time panic attacks may occur.

Separation anxiety disorder is characterized by refusal to separate from parents, usually the mother, resulting in clinging behaviour, school avoidance and an insistence on co-sleeping. While more common in children, separation anxiety disorder can first present in the teen years, usually with associated panic attacks. Often, adults with panic disorder report a childhood history of separation anxiety.

Phobic disorders include social phobia and specific phobias. *Social phobia* is an intense and disabling fear of scrutiny by others in various social and performance situations; this

overlaps with extremes of shyness. Community studies report a prevalence of 7–8 per cent for current social phobia, and as high as 15 per cent for lifetime diagnosis. Children whose functioning is impaired by these symptoms were formerly diagnosed with avoidant disorder or elective mutism. Sleep complaints commonly relate to worry about school attendance and other upcoming social situations. *Specific phobias* may include fears of animals, the dark, enclosed spaces, insects, and other specific situations that produce anxiety at bedtime.

Obsessive–compulsive disorder, occurring in 1–2 per cent of children, is characterized by either obsessions or compulsions taking at least one hour daily and impairing psycho-social functioning. Transient subclinical obsessive–compulsive symptoms are common in early adolescence. Typical obsessions include intrusive unwanted thoughts such as violent or sexual imagery, fears of contamination, or repetitive words and phrases. Compulsions include rituals of counting, washing or checking, as well as sequences of activities that must be performed 'just so' or else 'something terrible' will happen. The child recognizes that these ideas are irrational, but the obsessions and compulsions seem uncontrollable. Prolonged checking or washing compulsions, anxiety about imperfectly performed rituals and obsessive thoughts may interfere with sleep onset.

Sleep disturbances associated with anxiety

In sleep laboratory investigations, consistent disturbances are observed in adults who suffer panic disorder, generalized anxiety disorder and social phobia (Mellman and Uhde 1990). This research supports the reports of anxious children and their parents regarding poor sleep quality. Typical findings are sleep onset latency, frequent awakenings, more sleep-associated movements, poor sleep efficiency, and sleep panic attacks. Children assessed at psychiatric clinics are found to have a particularly high rate of sleep complaints, including restless sleep (43%), night waking (47%) and a high incidence of sleep terrors (19%) (Simonds and Parraga 1984). In community studies of sleep symptoms, anxiety is associated with sleep-onset problems in children and poor sleep in adolescents. Adult studies report a high rate of depression and anxiety disorders in individuals assessed for sleep disturbance, especially sleep terrors. Panic attacks during sleep and sleep onset are also documented in both children and adults (Mellman and Uhde 1989), and can be difficult to distinguish from sleep terrors; the two disorders can co-occur (Garland 1995). Panic disorder patients who experience sleep panic attacks are more likely to have childhood onset, a chronic course, multiple comorbid anxiety disorders and depression.

Aetiology

Sleep disturbances in anxious children result from two factors: behavioural avoidance and heightened physiological arousal. As a result, both extrinsic and intrinsic sleep disorders may coexist in the same child. Because of the instinctive and aversive nature of the anxiety experience, the behavioural component can be difficult to extinguish.

Symptoms of anxiety develop from fundamental human survival responses, mediated by the serotonergic and noradrenergic systems, promoting harm avoidance, escape from danger, and assurance that helpless infants maintain close contact with adults. When this natural anxiety system is poorly regulated or its signals are misinterpreted, individuals will

react with a fight or flight response, instinctive avoidance of danger, and catastrophic worrying. Adrenergically based hyperarousal with behavioural inhibition is characteristic of anxious temperament, while serotonergic dysregulation characterizes obsessive–compulsive symptoms. There are strong genetic factors in anxious temperament and the vulnerability to anxiety disorders. Environmental stressors and developmental challenges may then trigger the clinical disorder.

Extrinsic sleep disorders such as inadequate sleep hygiene, limit-setting sleep disorder, and sleep onset association disorder develop as a result of chronic or recurrent anxiety symptoms. Anxious children dread bedtime. They know from experience that they have difficulty falling asleep and will be worrying about daytime problems and somatic symptoms; also, they often have fearful responses to being alone and in the dark. Hence, bedtime resistance problems can be extreme, and anxious parents often reinforce chronically poor sleep habits by capitulating to night-time demands for attention or co-sleeping.

Once children are settled to bed, heightened arousal interferes with sleep onset, and contributes to frequent and prolonged awakenings. The co-occurrence of parasomnias such as sleep terrors with anxiety disorders is postulated to reflect shared disturbances of arousal. Psychophysiologial insomnia may occur as a primary sleep disorder in children with anxious temperament, or secondary to a specific anxiety disorder such as panic disorder, generalized anxiety disorder or separation anxiety disorder. Furthermore, sleep deprivation will exacerbate anxiety symptoms and panic attacks.

Management of sleep disturbances in anxious children

ASSESSMENT

The context of the sleep complaint needs to be evaluated. A recent onset of sleep complaints in an anxious child may be a response to an acute stressor such as parental illness or marital conflict, school-related problems or a traumatic event. Psychosocial stressors are a common precipitant of panic attacks in panic-prone children. Diagnostic evaluation should also include enquiry about specific anxiety symptoms such as panic attacks, obsessions, compulsions, phobias, separation anxiety and uncontrollable worry.

Acute sleep problems may also reflect the development of a complicating major depressive episode, which occurs in up to one-half of anxious children and adolescents. Other indicators of depression include daytime sadness, decline in interest and motivation, social withdrawal, and changes in appetite and concentration. Treatment of the depressive episode will generally address the sleep problem as well.

PARENTAL EDUCATION AND BEHAVIOUR MANAGEMENT TRAINING

Anxious children with sleep problems are usually enmeshed with anxious parents who are unintentionally reinforcing the child's difficulty settling to bed or prolonging night awakenings. Children with separation anxiety become extremely oppositional in their desperation to maintain parental contact. Positive reinforcement with a prize in the morning, a star on a chart or accumulated points for 'bravery' can be given for appropriate behaviours such as staying in the bedroom all night. Parents will require tremendous support to be consistent when the child's behaviours escalate during the retraining phase. Creative solutions to help

both parent and child feel more comfortable include a night light, a ritualized bedtime routine, special toys or charms, and audio-tapes on which the parent has read the child's favourite stories in a soothing voice.

RELAXATION, SELF-HYPNOSIS AND COGNITIVE STRATEGIES
Relaxation or self-hypnosis strategies can help reduce bedtime hyperarousal and create distraction from worries. Self-hypnosis has been combined with educational strategies and pharmacological interventions to reduce the frequency of night terrors. Cognitive and behavioural therapy (CBT) is effective with panic, phobic and obsessive–compulsive disorders in children (Frances and Beidel 1995). CBT has been applied to night-time fears in separation anxiety disorder, combining self-control training with contingent reinforcement by parents (Ollendick et al. 1991). The fact that the reinforcement component was essential for significant improvement emphasizes the importance of concurrent parental behavioural training. Through CBT, children and adolescents are taught how physical anxiety symptoms and mental worries are mutually reinforcing. They learn to challenge negative thoughts, turning their 'talent' for worrying into creative problem-solving.

PHARMACOLOGICAL INTERVENTIONS
Because of the chronicity of anxiety, 'as needed' medication is of limited value. Sedative antihistamines such as diphenhydramine may be helpful in the context of acute stressors. One of the intermittent medications commonly used in clinical practice with anxious children is low-dose trazodone (25–50 mg), a serotonergic, antihistaminic and sedative antidepressant. Trazodone is effective for sleep disturbances in adults with insomnia and depression, reducing sleep latency, increasing total sleep time, increasing stage 4 sleep, and improving sleep efficiency with no REM suppression on polysomnographic evaluation (Scharf and Sachais 1990).

The tricylic antidepressant imipramine, which is both noradrenergic and serotonergic, is effective in adults with generalized anxiety disorder, panic disorder, depression, sleep panic attacks and night terrors. Imipramine has been reported to be effective in open studies in children with separation anxiety, panic disorder and night terrors (Garland 1995). At doses of 10–25 mg imipramine in young children, and 25–75 mg in older children, improvement in insomnia and sleep terrors occurs within one to two weeks. Due to the recommended electrocardiographic monitoring of tricyclics, they are reserved for children with comorbid conditions responsive to imipramine, such as enuresis and attention deficit hyperactivity disorder, or for those who have not responded to newer medications. Clomipramine is a sedative serotonergic tricyclic that is effective for obsessive–compulsive and panic disorders; hence it may be an option for insomnia in children with these conditions. The anticonvulsant carbamazepine has also been used for sleep panic and sudden sleep arousals or night terrors (Dantendorfer et al. 1996).

Specific serotonin reuptake inhibitors (SSRIs) are effective for childhood overanxious, socially anxious and obsessive–compulsive disorders (Kutcher et al. 1995). In adults, SSRIs are indicated for generalized anxiety, panic disorder, social phobia and obsessive–compulsive disorder. SSRIs have complex effects on sleep that do not suggest a hypnotic effect.

However, in an open trial, paroxetine has been shown to improve subjective sleep and daytime well-being in adults with primary insomnia even though this was associated with minimal improvement on polysomnography (Nowell *et al.* 1999). In anxious patients, improvement in psychophysiological insomnia would be predicted with SSRIs.

The more sedative SSRIs, paroxetine and fluvoxamine, are usually prescribed for anxious children with insomnia. Sleep may improve within days, while full anti-anxiety or antidepressant response may take two months. A low starting dose, 5–10 mg of paroxetine or 25 mg of fluvoxamine, is recommended in panic-prone patients, but up to 40 mg of paroxetine or 200 mg of fluvoxamine may be required for full remission. Side-effects of nausea, somnolence or insomnia are mild or respond to changes in dosing schedule. However, dose-related behavioural activation can be a limiting side-effect in some children. Because a discontinuation syndrome with insomnia and agitation can occur with SSRIs, medication should be slowly tapered at 25 per cent per week after chronic use. The usual treatment period is at least four to six months, and often extends throughout a school year.

The anxiolytic benzodiazepines have hypnotic effects and suppress night terrors in both adults and young people. Alprazolam has some effectiveness in overanxious and avoidant children. In adolescent panic disorder, clonazepam was superior to placebo, but side-effects of disinhibition and irritability were noted (Kutcher *et al.* 1995). While benzodiazepines are efficacious in adult generalized anxiety and panic disorders, limitations include psychomotor impairment, dependence potential, and disrupted sleep architecture with REM rebound on discontinuation. However, benzodiazepines like clonazepam may be appropriate in treating resistant parasomnias. The primary current use in anxiety disorders is for acute symptom management while titrating the slower-acting serotonergic medications. For panic disorder, clonazepam is initiated at 0.25–0.5 mg b.i.d. and titrated to 1–2 mg b.i.d. in adolescents. Alprazolam is started at 0.125–0.25 mg in the morning for school avoidance. Ideally, benzodiazepines are tapered within a few weeks as symptoms are controlled.

Summary

In children and adolescents with insomnia, the contribution of anxiety should be evaluated. Children with anxious temperament manifest chronic sleep disturbances from early life, resulting in poor sleep habits. When children develop anxiety disorders, heightened arousal is associated with difficulty initiating sleep, poor sleep quality, and sleep panic attacks. Because anxiety disorders are recurrent, therapeutic strategies not only address the acute disorder, but also prevent future sleep behavioural problems. The comprehensive approach to these vulnerable children focuses on education of the parents, behaviour management, sleep hygiene, and empowering the child with self-soothing and anxiety management strategies. SSRIs are preferred for ongoing pharmacotherapy, but antihistamines, trazodone or benzodiazepines may be used for acute management of insomnia.

REFERENCES

American Psychiatric Association (1994) *Diagnostic and Statistical Manual of Mental Disorders, 4th Edn.* Washington, DC: American Psychiatric Association.

Dantendorfer, K., Frey, R., Maierhofer, D., Saletu, B. (1996) 'Sudden arousals from slow wave sleep and

panic disorder: Successful treatment with anticonvulsants – a case report.' *Sleep*, **19**, 744–746.

Francis, G., Beidel, D. (1995) 'Cognitive–behavioral psychotherapy.' *In:* March, J.S. (Ed.) *Anxiety Disorders in Children and Adolescents*. New York: Guilford Press, pp. 321–340.

Garland, E.J. (1995) 'The relationship of sleep disturbances to childhood panic disorder.' *In:* Schaefer, C.E. (Ed.) *Clinical Handbook of Sleep Disorders in Children*. Northvale, NJ: Jason Aaronson, pp. 285–310.

Kutcher, S., Reiter, S., Gardner, D. (1995) 'Pharmacotherapy: Approaches and applications.' *In:* March, J.S. (Ed.) *Anxiety Disorders in Children and Adolescents*. New York: Guilford Press, pp. 341–385.

Mellman, T.A., Uhde, T.W. (1990) 'Sleep in panic and generalized anxiety disorders.' *In:* Ballenger, J.C. (Ed.) *Neurobiology of Panic Disorder. Frontiers of Clinical Neuroscience 8*. New York: Wiley-Liss, pp. 365–376.

Nowell, P.D., Reynolds, C.F., Buysse, D.J., Dew, M.A., Kupfer, D.J. (1999) 'Paroxetine in the treatment of primary insomnia: Preliminary clinical and electroencephalogram sleep data.' *Journal of Clinical Psychiatry*, **60**, 89–95.

Ollendick, T.H., Haggopian, L.P., Huntzinger, R.M. (1991) 'Cognitive–behavior therapy with nighttime fearful children.' *Journal of Behavior Therapy and Experimental Psychiatry*, **22**, 113–121.

Scharf, M.B., Sachais, B.A. (1990) 'Sleep laboratory evaluation of the effects and efficacy of trazodone in depressed insomniac patients.' *Journal of Clinical Psychiatry*, **51** (Suppl.), 13–17.

Simonds, J.F., Parraga, H. (1984) 'Sleep behaviors and disorders in children and adolescents evaluated at psychiatric clinics.' *Developmental and Behavioral Pediatrics*, **5**, 6–10.

24
SLEEP AND DEPRESSION

Ronald E. Dahl and Daniel S. Lewin

There are important links between sleep and mood regulation in children and adolescents, but the interactions are complex, and the details and directionality of the effects are not well understood at this time. There is evidence that emotional distress can interfere with sleep, and that sleep deprivation can produce alterations in mood and motivation. There are also substantial amounts of data indicating that children and adolescents with emotional disorders such as major depression report high rates of sleep complaints. In addition, there is preliminary evidence that sleep problems during the first two decades can predict future mood disturbances and disorders in early adulthood (Rao *et al.* 1996, Johnson *et al.* 2000).

Despite the compelling evidence of strong links between sleep and mood problems, it is also necessary to acknowledge important caveats and limitations to our understanding. For example, EEG sleep studies in depressed children and adolescents have revealed relatively limited evidence for objective sleep changes associated with depression in children (Dahl *et al.* 1996b). More importantly, these findings do not provide assistance in making clinical diagnoses or directing treatment decisions at the present time (Dahl 1996).

One of the critical issues for the field is to elucidate the developmental pathophysiology of mood disorders and examine specific links to sleep/arousal regulation. For example, it has been hypothesized that sleep disruption and deprivation may sometimes contribute to affect dysregulation and clinically significant impairments in mood and motivation. This is an important hypothesis because of the implication that intervening early to address the sleep problem might alter the course of depression in at least some children. Another set of hypotheses suggest that sleep changes may reflect genetic vulnerability toward affective disorders, and thus may help to target individuals for early intervention or prevention.

Initially in this chapter a background description of several features of mood disorders in children and adolescents is provided. This is followed by a discussion of links between sleep and depression.

Depression in children and adolescents
DEFINITIONS AND EPIDEMIOLOGY
While sadness or depressed mood arises in the course of most children's lives there has been increasing recognition of serious and pervasive disorders of mood regulation in young people that are associated with significant morbidity (*i.e.* impairment in psychosocial function) and mortality (*i.e.* suicide) (Sells and Blum 1996, Wichstrom 2000). Currently, depressive illnesses are classified into three broad categories (American Psychiatric Association 1994).

(1) *Major Depressive Disorder:* requires at least two weeks of sad or irritable mood, or decreased interest in most activities, at least one-half the time as well as an additional four depressive symptoms (including sleep disturbance). This contrasts with adjustment disorder in which depressed mood is milder and relatively brief following a serious life stressor.

(2) *Dysthymic Disorder:* involves chronic depressed and irritable mood without evidence of major depressive episodes.

(3) *Bipolar Affective Illness or Cyclothymic Disorder:* involves periods of depressed mood with alternating periods of mania or hypomania.

Estimates of the prevalence of major depression disorder (MDD) are approximately 1.5–2.5 per cent in prepubertal children, increasing to 4–5 per cent during adolescence. The prevalence of bipolar illness is estimated to be between 0.2 and 0.4 per cent among pre-pubertal children and 1 per cent among adolescents. Sex differences in depressive illness emerge at puberty with a female-to-male ratio of 2:1 that endures throughout adulthood. Bipolar disorders are equally common in males and females.

AETIOLOGY AND PATHOGENESIS

Many types of emotional trauma have been associated with the early (and also later) onset of depressive disorders (*e.g.* physical and sexual abuse, loss of a parent, loss of a sibling or close friend), but the single most important risk factor of an early depressive illness is having at least one depressed parent. To date, the best evidence suggests that there are both genetic and shared environmental sources of transmission. Important environmental variables include disruption of the parental role, decreased family support, and increased parent–child discord. Several physiological changes may be due to both genetics and environment; for example, abnormalities of growth hormone regulation and CNS serotonin and norepi-nephrine function are seen in early onset depression. Additional abnormalities directly related to sleep will be discussed later in this chapter.

CLINICAL MANIFESTATIONS

Typically, depressed children have periods of *disturbed mood* that are often accompanied by somatic complaints, decreased school performance, apathy, loss of interest, social withdrawal, irritability, and sleep and appetite changes. Depressed children of all ages are also likely to have somatic complaints, oppositional behaviour, cognitive changes (*i.e.* feelings of worthlessness and guilt), and occasional psychotic features related to mood disorder (*i.e.* auditory hallucinations and paranoid ideation). *Anxiety* symptoms are common among children with major depression and they may *antedate* depressive symptomatology.

Suicidal ideation and gestures are particularly common among adolescents, and risk must be assessed whenever depression is suspected. Among adolescents, depressive illnesses are also frequently associated with tobacco, alcohol or substance use, promiscuous sexual behaviour, and risk-taking behaviour.

An episode of *mania* indicates a bipolar affective disorder. Most typically during manic episodes children have periods of prolonged excitation, euphoria, rapid speech, grandiosity, and also sensation-seeking, promiscuous and sexualized behaviour. The need for sleep is

decreased. Delusions of invulnerability may lead to dangerous behaviour such as running in front of cars and jumping off buildings. When children and adolescents with bipolar disorder are depressed, they often present as anergic (*i.e.* low energy and slow) and hypersomnic, and manifest symptoms of psychosis.

ASSESSMENT AND DIAGNOSIS

Any persistent disturbance of mood (*e.g.* withdrawal, irritability and aggression) that is associated with functional impairment (*i.e.* deterioration of school or social function) should raise the suspicion of an affective disorder. The primary goals of clinical assessment are to assess: (a) mood symptoms; (b) the extent to which symptoms interfere with usual daily activities; and (c) suicidal risk. It is particularly important to identify patients at risk for suicide (Shaffer 1988) and to take immediate preventative action. Both the child and parents contribute important information to be used in the diagnosis of depression. Definitive diagnoses are best achieved by structured or semi-structured diagnostic interviews.

MANAGEMENT AND TREATMENT

Most common mood problems among children will respond to a few sessions of supportive counselling concerning such causes of the problem as family discord, school failure, difficulty with peers or other specific stressors. If family discord appears to be prominent, problem-solving interventions should involve the entire family.

The management of children and adolescents with severe mood disorders usually requires combinations of (a) psychotherapy including cognitive–behaviour therapy or interpersonal therapy, (b) pharmacotherapy especially with selective serotonin reuptake inhibitors (SSRIs) or tricyclic antidepressants, and (c) improvement in the child and family's understanding and ability to cope with affective disturbances ('psychoeducation'). Bipolar disorder requires prophylaxis with a mood-stabilizing agent—either lithium or an anticonvulsant such as valproic acid or carbamazepine.

Sleep and depression

Sleep disturbance is one of nine diagnostic criteria for affective disorders (American Psychiatric Association 1994). Considerable overlap exists in the neurobehavioural systems underlying the regulation of sleep, emotion and attention (Dahl 1996). There are three lines of evidence regarding the association between sleep and depression: (1) depressed patients' high rates of sleep complaints (difficulty initiating and maintaining sleep); (2) evidence that insufficient sleep causes decrements in mood regulation; and (3) objective evidence of sleep changes among depressed youths. Each of these will be discussed in detail.

SUBJECTIVE SLEEP DISTURBANCES IN MDD

As many as 90 per cent of depressed children and adolescents report significant changes in sleep duration and poor sleep quality (Morielli *et al.* 1996), with 75 per cent meeting criteria for insomnia (Ryan *et al.* 1987). There are several plausible explanations for increased subjective complaints and sleep problems among depressed children and adolescents. With few exceptions, a physically and mentally relaxed state is necessary for sleep onset

to occur. In depressed patients, rumination, negative thoughts and worry are associated with heightened physical and mental arousal that is not compatible with sleep onset. Being alone in a dark room trying to fall asleep can be a difficult time for a child to inhibit negative thoughts—these distressing thoughts and images may in turn result in increased arousal and interfere with sleep. Insufficient sleep and the resulting daytime somnolence can contribute to daytime tiredness, decreased motivation, and impaired functioning in school and social domains. Interventions focused on improving sleep habits and sleep quality may play an important role in breaking the vicious cycle of insomnia, hypersomnolence and mood disturbance.

This cycle of mood and sleep disturbance may be due to neurobiological changes associated with the depressive disorders (*e.g.* decreased serotonin) or fundamental changes in sleep/arousal regulation that contribute to poor sleep. A third possibility is that mood regulation and sleep regulation share some level of vulnerability.

In addition to insomnia and poor sleep quality, hypersomnia is sometimes associated with depression; this manifestation of sleep changes is more common in adolescent than in childhood depression (Ryan *et al.* 1987). In these cases it is important to consider the possible overlap with sleep–wake schedule problems. Late and erratic bedtimes are quite frequent in adolescents and can lead to a variety of sleep problems including insomnia and daytime sleepiness. Late and erratic bedtimes and difficulty getting to sleep are even more troublesome in depressed adolescents. These problems may be independent or overlapping, and in some cases sleep phase delay may be an important risk factor for adolescents who have a history of depression or who have high environmental or family loadings for affective disorders.

Bipolar disorder is associated with another pattern of sleep disturbance that is characterized by a drastically reduced need for sleep during manic phases during which there is a general increase in energy and heightened mood (American Psychiatric Association 1994). During the depressive phases of their illness, bipolar patients' sleep is comparable to that of patients with unipolar depression.

Depressed patients also tend to perceive the quality of their sleep as being poor and non-restorative. Laboratory-based studies of children and adolescents do not consistently confirm these reported decrements in sleep quality. It is possible that the biochemical and cognitive changes of depression cause a change in the perception of sleep quality. Alternative explanations are that sleep disruption, particularly in younger children, is masked by a more powerful sleep drive, and that children do not consistently report sleep disturbance.

CAN INSUFFICIENT SLEEP CAUSE PROBLEMS IN MOOD REGULATION?
Despite an absence of well-controlled research studies to directly answer this question, there is convergence of evidence that some *changes in mood and motivation are among the most important effects of sleep loss* (Chapter 1). Irritability, 'moodiness', and low frustration-tolerance are the most frequently described symptoms in sleep-deprived children and adolescents. However, this is not a simple issue of less sleep leading to depressed mood, since in some situations sleepy children exhibit disinhibited behaviour such as silliness, impulsivity and anger.

Common evidence suggests that sleep deprivation leads to *mood lability*. Not only does there appear to be greater variability in emotional states following sleep loss, but also *less control over emotional responses* in many adolescents. For example, if faced with a frustrating task a sleep-deprived teenager may be more likely to become angry or aggressive. Yet, in response to something humorous, the same subject might act more silly or inane. Unpublished laboratory observations (by the present authors) include several adolescents reporting increased crying reactions during sad scenes in videotaped movies when sleep-deprived, and many subjects reporting increased irritability and impatience, and low frustration-tolerance when asked to perform tedious computer tasks. Such findings suggest a decrease in inhibition or conscious control over emotions following sleep loss. It is also important to point out that some subjects seemed to show no measurable changes in any emotion when sleep-deprived.

These preliminary observations involve a high degree of variability across subjects and require replication with larger samples to better characterize individual differences. However, the findings fit within a general pattern of similar observations regarding *effortful control*. That is, the primary emotional changes following sleep loss suggest a decrease in the ability to control, inhibit or modify emotional responses according to long-term goals, social rules, or other learned principles. Executive function and effort to control emotion involve regions of the prefrontal cortex (PFC) of the brain and fit with evidence that these neurobehavioural systems in PFC may be particularly affected by sleep deprivation (Horne 1993, Drummond *et al.* 2000).

An important clinical issue is raised by this pattern. Specifically, a decrease in PFC control over feelings following sleep loss could have serious consequences regarding many high-risk behaviours among adolescents. Disinhibition of emotional responses could influence aggression, sexual behaviour, the use of alcohol and drugs, and risky driving. Further, there is some indication that the disinhibitory effects of sleep deprivation can increase the risk of impulsive suicidal gestures and suicidal ideation; this obviously has quite significant implications for clinical and social policy issues with depressed adolescents.

OBJECTIVE SLEEP CHANGES IN DEPRESSION

Studies of depressed adults have yielded extensive objective evidence of abnormalities in EEG sleep (Reynolds and Kupfer 1987). In depressed children and adolescents, however, EEG sleep studies have not revealed the same magnitude of changes (Lahmeyer *et al.* 1983; Puig-Antich *et al.* 1983, 1984, 1989; Emslie *et al.* 1987, 1994; Appelboom-Fondu *et al.* 1988; Dahl *et al.* 1990, 1991, 1995, 1996b; Kahn *et al.* 1989, Kutcher *et al.* 1992). The strongest evidence for changes in sleep is seen in the interval surrounding sleep onset. Not only do many depressed children and adolescents take rather longer to fall asleep, but they also show changes in neuroendocrine secretory patterns in this interval of time (Dahl *et al.* 1996a).

Some REM changes have been observed in association with early onset depression, including some evidence for increased REM density and reduced REM latency; however, the effect sizes appear to be smaller in younger samples than those found in samples of depressed adults (Emslie *et al.* 1990). The importance of methodological issues regarding

standardizing sleep–wake schedules in the interval preceding the sleep study, as well as careful attention to adaptation and inpatient/outpatient differences, should be emphasized.

Finally, when challenged with a cholinergic agent (arecoline), depressed children who had shown no baseline differences in REM latency did demonstrate significantly shorter REM latency than normal control children (Dahl *et al.* 1994). Similar cholinergic sensitivity to REM sleep regulation was reported in depressed adolescents by McCracken *et al.* (1997). Together these preliminary findings suggest that underlying differences in sleep dysregulation in depressed children might be 'unmasked' in a study using an arecoline challenge.

A second important issue to consider regarding objective changes in sleep physiology and mood disorders is that of long-term clinical course. Work by the Pittsburgh research group found that prolonged sleep latency and increased serum cortisol in the interval surrounding sleep onset (as measured during adolescence) predicted more frequent onsets of depressive episodes into early adulthood (Rao *et al.* 1996).

PRAGMATIC CLINICAL ISSUES AT THE INTERFACE OF SLEEP AND DEPRESSION

One additional dimension of consideration, particularly among adolescents, is the possible *contribution of secondary factors* such as the use of caffeine, nicotine, alcohol or other drugs and erratic sleep–wake schedules (or sleep phase delay) that increase during adolescence. Not only may these influences have negative effects on sleep, but they can also be important causes of mood problems in adolescents. However, the causal direction of these effects is not clearly delineated. For example, the links between depression and nicotine dependence have been hypothesized in each direction, with some evidence that some youths may use substances to try to regulate affect because of the mood problems, and other evidence clearly suggesting that smoking may increase the risk for developing depression (Patten *et al.* 2000).

At the most pragmatic level, one of the greatest concerns is the reciprocal effects or the potential for negative spirals of *interacting effects between sleep and mood problems*. That is, depression may contribute to sleep difficulties and disruptions, as well as to behaviours and habits tending toward late-night schedules and the use of substances that further interfere with sleep. These disruptions in sleep may in turn contribute to greater difficulties with mood regulation and may increase the use of stimulants and other substances. Therefore it is easy to see how these interactions could lead to a negative spiral with increasing sleep and circadian problems and further deterioration of mood and motivation.

Regarding *treatment implications*, there are a few principles to emphasize. Because of the interacting domains it is often important for treatment to focus on *each* component as an independent entity. Specifically the objectives should be to (a) optimize sleep (including the identification and treatment of sleep-related problems such as late erratic bedtimes and poor sleep habits, with use of behavioural interventions to target sleep onset insomnia), (b) assess and treat the mood disorder with a combination of psychotherapy and pharmacotherapy, and (c) assess the use and abuse of stimulants, caffeine and other substances, and plan treatments accordingly.

There are cases where the treatment efforts for depression and sleep disturbance may overlap. For example, a primary goal of cognitive behavioural therapy involves reducing

rumination on distressing anxiety-provoking thoughts. This intervention, if successful, improves both day- and night-time symptoms. In a similar way, helping the adolescent and family develop better sleep habits or hygiene, and follow a more stable sleep–wake schedule, can involve tasks and goals that are part of treatment plans for the depression and also family therapy.

Clearly, there remain more questions than answers in our current understanding of sleep and mood interactions in children and adolescents. There is evidence that psychotherapeutic and pharmacological approaches to improving sleep and mood disturbance appear to be efficacious. Long-term clinical progress and prevention programmes will require additional research. These efforts must involve a more advanced understanding of the common neurobehavioural systems and mechanisms.

REFERENCES

American Psychiatric Association (1994) *Diagnostic and Statistical Manual of Mental Disorders, 4th Edn.* Washington DC: APA.

Appelboom-Fondu, J., Kerkhofs, M., Mendlewicz, J. (1988) 'Depression in adolescents and young adults – polysomnographic and neuroendocrine aspects.' *Journal of Affective Disorders*, **14**, 35–40.

Dahl, R. (1996) 'The regulation of sleep and arousal: development and psychopathology.' *Development and Psychopathology*, **8**, 3–27.

—— Puig-Antich, J., Ryan, N.D., Nelson, B., Dachille, S., Cunningham, S.L., Trubnick, L., Klepper, T.P. (1990) 'EEG sleep in adolescents with major depression: The role of suicidality and inpatient status.' *Journal of Affective Disorders*, **19**, 63–75.

—— Ryan, N.D., Birmaher, B., Al-Shabbout, M., Williamson, D.E., Neidig, M., Nelson, B., Puig-Antich, J. (1991) 'Electroencephalographic sleep measures in prepubertal depression.' *Psychiatry Research*, **38**, 201–214.

—— —— Perel, J., Birmaher, B., Al-Shabbout, M., Nelson, B., Puig-Antich, J. (1994) 'Cholinergic REM induction test with arecoline in depressed children.' *Psychiatry Research*, **51**, 269–282.

—— —— Birmaher, B., Al-Shabbout, M., Nelson, B. (1995) 'EEG sleep measures in child depression.' *Sleep Research*, **24**, 157. *(Abstract.)*

—— Birmaher, B., Al-Shabbout, M., Nelson, B. (1996a) 'Altered sleep/growth hormone in childhood depression.' *Sleep Research*, **25**, 158. *(Abstract.)*

—— Ryan, N.D., Matty, M.K., Birmaher, B., Al-Shabbout, M., Williamson, D.E., Kupfer, D.J. (1996b) 'Sleep onset abnormalities in depressed adolescents.' *Biological Psychiatry*, **39**, 400–410.

Drummond, S.A., Brown, G.G., Gillin, J.C., Stricker, J.L., Wong, E.C., Buxton, R.B. (2000) 'Altered brain response to verbal learning following sleep deprivation.' *Nature*, **403**, 655–657.

Emslie, G.J., Roffwarg, H.P., Rush, A.J., Weinberg, W.A., Parkin-Feigenbaum, L. (1987) 'Sleep EEG findings in depressed children and adolescents.' *American Journal of Psychiatry*, **144**, 668–670.

—— Rush, A.J., Weinberg, W.A., Rintelmann, J.W., Roffwarg, H.P. (1990) 'Children with major depression show reduced rapid eye movement latencies.' *Archives of General Psychiatry*, **47**, 119–124.

—— —— —— —— —— (1994) 'Sleep EEG features of adolescents with major depression.' *Biological Psychiatry*, **36**, 573–581.

Horne, J.A. (1993) 'Human sleep, sleep loss and behaviour: implications for the prefrontal cortex and psychiatric disorder.' *British Journal of Psychiatry*, **162**, 413–419.

Johnson, E.O., Chilcoat H.D., Breslau, N. (2000) 'Trouble sleeping and anxiety/depression in childhood.' *Psychiatry Research*, **94**, 93–102.

Kahn, A., Van de Merckt, C., Rebuffat, E., Mozin, M.J., Sottiaux, M., Blum, D., Hennart, P. (1989) 'Sleep problems in healthy preadolescents.' *Pediatrics*, **84**, 542–546.

Kutcher, S.P., Williamson, P., Marton, P., Szalai, J. (1992) 'REM latency in endogenously depressed adolescents.' *British Journal of Psychiatry*, **161**, 399–402.

Lahmeyer, H.W., Poznanski, E.O., Bellur, S.N. (1983) 'EEG sleep in depressed adolescents.' *American Journal of Psychiatry*, **140**, 1150–1153.

McCracken, J.T., Poland, R.E., Lutchmansingh, P., Edwards, C. (1997) 'Sleep electroencephalographic abnormalities in adolescent depressives: effects of scopolamine.' *Biological Psychiatry*, **42**, 577–584.

Morielli, A., Ladan, S. Ducharme, F.M., Brouillette, R.T. (1996) 'Can sleep and wakefulness be distinguished in children by cardiorespiratory and videotape recordings?' *Chest*, **109**, 680–687.

Patten, C.A., Choi, W.S., Gillin, J.C., Pierce, J.P. (2000) 'Depressive symptoms and cigarette smoking predict development and persistence of sleep problems in US adolescents.' *Pediatrics*, **106**, e23.

Puig-Antich, J., Goetz, R., Hanlon, C., Tabrizi, M.A., Davies, M., Weitzman, E.D. (1983) 'Sleep architecture and REM sleep measures in prepubertal major depressives. Studies during recovery from the depressive episode in a drug-free state.' *Archives of General Psychiatry*, **40**, 187–192.

—— Novacenko, H., Davies, M., Chambers, W.J., Tabrizi, M.A., Krawiec, V., Ambrosini, P.J., Sachar, E.J. (1984) 'Growth hormone secretion in prepubertal children with major depression. I. Final report on response to insulin-induced hypoglycemia during a depressive episode.' *Archives of General Psychiatry*, **41**, 455–460.

—— Goetz, R., Davies, M., Kaplan, T., Davies, S., Ostrow, L., Asnis, L., Twomey, J., Iyengar, S., Ryan, N.D. (1989) 'A controlled family history study of prepubertal major depressive disorder.' *Archives of General Psychiatry*, **46**, 406–418.

Rao, U., Dahl, R.E., Ryan, N.D., Birmaher, B., Williamson, D.E., Giles, D.E., Rao, R., Kaufman, J., Nelson, B. (1996) 'The relationship between longitudinal clinical course and sleep and cortisol changes in adolescent depression.' *Biological Psychiatry*, **40**, 474–484.

Reynolds, C.F., Kupfer D.J. (1987) 'Sleep research in affective illness: state of the art circa 1987.' *Sleep*, **10**, 199–215.

Ryan, N.D., Puig-Antich, J. Ambrosini, P., Rabinovich, H., Robinson, D., Nelson, B., Iyengar, S., Twomey, J. (1987) 'The clinical picture of major depression in children and adolescents.' *Archives of General Psychiatry*, **44**, 854–861.

Sells, C.W., Blum, R.W. (1996) 'Morbidity and mortality among US adolescents: An overview of data and trends.' *American Journal of Public Health*, **86**, 513–519.

Shaffer, D. (1988) 'The epidemiology of teen suicide: An examination of risk factors.' *Journal of Clinical Psychiatry*, **49** (Suppl.), 36–41.

Wichstrom, L. (2000) 'Predictors of adolescent suicide attempts: A nationally representative longitudinal study of Norwegian adolescents.' *Journal of the American Academy of Child and Adolescent Psychiatry*, **39**, 603–610.

25
SLEEP AND TRAUMA IN CHILDREN

Avi Sadeh

The relationships between stress, trauma and sleep are complex and intriguing. The questions of whether to 'sleep tight' or 'sleep light' or 'to sleep or not to sleep' appear to be existential under real or imagined threat. The literature on sleep and dreaming suggests that these phenomena are very sensitive to physiological and psychological stress. Similarly, it has been documented that sleep-related issues such as darkness, separation and being alone may arouse significant fears and anxieties in many children and thus represent a significant stressor in their lives. Furthermore, sleep problems, insufficient sleep and chronic sleep deprivation can become a significant source of stress to the sleepless youngster and his family. This short review focuses on the relationships between stress, trauma and sleep in children. The research findings from studies in this field have often been incongruent and unpredictable. A theoretical model is developed to explain these findings and to create a more coherent picture.

Defining stress and trauma

Stress and trauma are concepts with complex medical and psychosocial connotations. They usually refer to unusual events, significant change or threat, demanding special biobehavioural or psychological adaptive responses by the individual in order to maintain psychophysiological equilibrium and well-being. The psychological impact of stress is mediated by many factors including the specific characteristics of the event (*e.g.* intensity, duration, predictability), the child's subjective interpretation of the event, his resiliency and coping skills, and his support systems. The term 'trauma' is usually reserved for events that are exceedingly challenging to adaptation and may potentially lead to significant negative outcomes. When we assess stress and trauma in children it is particularly important to pay special attention to the child's subjective interpretation, while considering his developmental phase and cognitive development as key factors.

Regardless of the specific stressful event and its unique characteristics, stress researchers have generated some common principles. Selye (1983) defined a general adaptive pattern that characterizes responses to diverse nonspecific stressors. The general adaptive syndrome (GAS) is characterized by: (1) the alarm phase, in which the activity of the adrenocortical system increases dramatically and facilitates hypervigilance, increased activity and readiness for action; (2) the stage of resistance which represents the organism's attempt to regain and maintain homeostasis; and (3) the stage of exhaustion, which results from a depletion of the adaptive energies and may cause irreversible damage to cardiovascular, digestive, immune and circulatory systems. Within Selye's framework, atypical alternations in rest–

activity cycles, hypervigilance, fatigue and sleep–wake disorders represent nonspecific components of the GAS.

Selye's model emphasizes the role of hypervigilance, which is incompatible with sleep, and the stage of exhaustion that may be compatible with excessive sleep. Other models underline a different pattern of response to extreme and uncontrollable stress that is characterized by withdrawal and energy conservation that is compatible with increased sleep (Engel and Schmale 1972). Specific models addressing traumas in children differentiated between the effects of acute stress and those of chronic, ongoing or repeated stress (Terr 1991). Acute stress or trauma may lead to hypervigilance and nightmares, which represent active coping efforts, whereas chronic unavoidable or repeated traumatization may lead to detachment, dissociation and apathy that is compatible with Engel and Schmale's conservation–withdrawal theory.

Methodologically, there are two basic ways to address the topic of trauma. One way is to study groups of children who were exposed to a similar traumatic event (*e.g.* sexual abuse, violence, natural catastrophe). The second approach is to study children who have a clinical diagnosis related to stress or trauma. The chronic impact of traumatic events is diagnostically labelled post-traumatic stress disorder (PTSD). Sleep- and dreaming-related disturbances play a central role in PTSD (Ross *et al.* 1989, Pillar *et al.* 2000). The diagnostic criteria for PTSD in DSM-IV (APA 1994) include recurrent distressing dreams (nightmares), difficulty falling and staying asleep, and hypervigilance. However, the research on sleep and PTSD yields contradictory results that are not easy to reconcile into a coherent picture (Pillar *et al.* 2000).

Characteristic sleep problems or sleep variations and their aetiology

The literature on stress, trauma and sleep suggests that there are two seemingly contradictory response modes that have empirical validity (Sadeh 1996). A new model for understanding the relationships between stress and sleep could resolve the apparent contradictions between these response modes. This model could be described as the 'turn on'/'shut off' stress–vigilance regulation. The main assumption of the model is that the adaptive response to stress could be classified as either a 'turn on' response characterized by a state of alarm, hypervigilance, active coping attempts and sleep avoidance or disrupted sleep, or a 'shut off' response characterized by exhaustion, withdrawal, passivity, dissociation and escape into sleep. In the following section the relationship between trauma and sleep is reviewed and assessed according to this organizing theme.

THE 'TURN ON' RESPONSE—SLEEP AVOIDANCE OR DISRUPTED SLEEP

A real or perceived threat triggers the well-established alarm (fight–flight) response. This response is mediated by the adrenocortical system and facilitates hypervigilance (Selye 1983, Field and Reite 1984). The alarm response requires heightened preparedness to perceive and to behaviourally cope with the immediate threat. Under such circumstances sleep is the least protected state of the organism and therefore should be avoided or maintained at a level that would be most responsive to the environment.

The 'turn on' mode is well supported by the literature, which indicates that under stress, sleep is avoided as evidenced by shorter sleep, difficulties in falling or staying asleep, and

sleep fragmentation. For instance, following a short separation from their mothers, both young monkeys and human infants exhibit a stage of agitation, increased activity level, and sleep fragmentation (Field and Reite 1984, Field 1991). Sleep difficulties have been reported following the loss of a parent (Hancock 1978, Harris 1991). Child abuse and particularly sexual abuse has also been associated with sleep problems including sleep fragmentation and nightmares (Mead and Mead 1986, Rimsza *et al.* 1988, Moore 1989, Sadeh *et al.* 1995, Choquet *et al.* 1997, Glod *et al.* 1997, Calam *et al.* 1998). Stress related to war and disasters appears to lead to similar sleep disruptions and nightmares (Dollinger *et al.* 1984, Pynoos *et al.* 1987, Vogel and Vernberg 1993, Ellis *et al.* 1998). In a normative sample of school-age children, stressful life events have been associated with more fragmented sleep (Sadeh *et al.* 2000).

THE 'SHUT OFF' RESPONSE —ESCAPE INTO SLEEP
Under certain circumstances, particularly when stress is perceived as unavoidable or chronic, the best way for the organism to cope is to retreat, preserve energy, and dissociate if possible from experiencing the impact of the stress (Engel and Schmale 1972, Terr 1991). Sleep could be considered as a good shelter for dissociating from extraneous stress, particularly if there is no way to influence the situation. Indeed, some studies on stress and sleep have provided evidence that supports this notion, often in contrast to the anticipated results.

Infant studies have documented an increase in sleep time or an increase in the proportion of quiet sleep in response to stress (see Sadeh 1996). Researchers suggested that this increase in sleep time or in quiet sleep proportion raises the stimulus barrier and protects the infant from additional external stimulation. This protective mode is also seen in children living under conditions of a chronic threat of terror. Under such circumstances, children slept longer and had fewer bad dreams in comparison to children who lived in secure areas (Rofe and Lewin 1982). Additional support for the idea that sleep sometimes protects from stress could be derived from the data on children's sleep in Israel under the threat and the actual attacks of ballistic missiles during the Gulf war (Lavie *et al.* 1993). Contrary to what was expected, when their sleep was monitored using actigraphy, children revealed high resiliency to the stressful circumstances, only waking up briefly during a missile attack and resuming their sleep with no significant difficulties as soon as the event was terminated. It is important to note, however, that children's responses to war-related stress are mediated by their limited cognitive skills, their flexible adaptive resources, and the reality-interpretation provided by their parents. Thus, these responses often diverge from the anticipated negative course. This phenomenon is artistically explored to its extreme in the Oscar-winning movie *Life is Beautiful*.

The most striking support for the 'shut off' response comes from the literature on PTSD in adults. Despite many descriptions of sleep disruptions in PTSD patients, research based on objective measures often fails to validate these complaints (Pillar *et al.* 2000). The differences between subjective complaints and objective findings are striking. Furthermore, studies have documented elevated awakening thresholds in PTSD patients, suggesting that sleep is more protected in these patients (Dagan *et al.* 1991).

One major factor that regulates which mode of response ('turn on' or 'shut off') predom-

inates is the type of trauma or stress. Short and acute stress turns on the hypervigilance mode, whereas chronic or repeated uncontrollable stress shuts off the system. Psychological characteristics such as individual coping style may also play a significant role in determining the predominance of the 'turn on'/'shut off' responses. The 'turn on' mode appears to be more compatible with an active, task-oriented coping style, whereas the 'shut off' mode is more likely to serve the repressive, dissociative coping style. This hypothesis is yet to be scientifically examined, but from a methodological standpoint it is possible that these two coping styles mask each other, thus leading to some of the confusing findings in the literature on relationships between stress, trauma and sleep.

Special consideration of management

When traumatized children are admitted to psychiatric inpatient units it is often surprising how well they adapt in terms of their sleep on the unit, considering the earlier complaints of their caregivers prior to admission (Sadeh *et al.* 1995). It appears that providing these children with a secure setting that includes a stable and strict sleep regime is perhaps the most crucial element in coping with trauma- and stress-related sleep difficulties. If sexual abuse within the family is suspected, it is important to bear in mind that sexual abuse often occurs at night or is associated with the child's bedroom, and sleep avoidance or sleep disruptions may reflect the disturbing fact that it is unsafe to sleep at home.

In the home setting, when a child's sleep is acutely disrupted by anxieties, fears and memories about a traumatic event, the immediate response of parents and other caregivers is to strengthen the child's sense of security. The most common way to achieve this is by co-sleeping with the child. Co-sleeping often occurs by letting the child sleep with the parents in their bed or by a parent sleeping next to the child in the child's bedroom. Co-sleeping next to the child in his bedroom for a limited period is a preferred strategy, as it conveys a message of stability with regard to sleeping habits while reducing excessive anxieties and fears by parental presence and reassurance.

If sleep problems persist after a traumatic event and beyond the acute response phase, then psychosocial intervention should be introduced as early as possible. The intervention could be in the form of a specific technique designed to help the child cope with anxieties, tension and hypervigilance (*e.g.* relaxation techniques), or in the form of broader psychotherapeutic interventions directed at helping the family and the child in particular cope and adjust to the aftermath of the trauma.

Finally, the possibility of post-traumatic 'shut off' response in terms of overextended sleep and sleepiness, which is hardly addressed in the clinical PTSD literature, should be considered as well, particularly in cases of chronic or repeated ongoing stress. In such cases, restricting sleep may lead to positive clinical response, as demonstrated in studies on sleep restriction for clinical depression (King *et al.* 1987, Wirz-Justice and Van den Hoofdakker).

REFERENCES

APA (1994) *Diagnostic and Statistical Manual of Mental Disorders, 4th Edn.* Washington DC: American Psychiatric Association.
Calam, R., Horne, L., Glasgow, D., Cox, A. (1998) 'Psychological disturbance and child sexual abuse: a

follow-up study.' *Child Abuse and Neglect*, **22**, 901–913.

Choquet, M., Darves-Bornoz, J.M., Ledoux, S., Manfredi, R., Hassler, C. (1997) 'Self-reported health and behavioral problems among adolescent victims of rape in France: results of a cross-sectional survey.' *Child Abuse and Neglect*, **21**, 823–832.

Egan, Y., Lavie, P., Bleich, A. (1991) 'Elevated awakening thresholds in sleep stage 3–4 in war-related post-traumatic stress disorder.' *Biological Psychiatry*, **30**, 618–622.

Dollinger, S.J., O'Donnell, J. P., Staley, A.A. (1984) 'Lightning-strike disaster: Effects on children's fears and worries.' *Journal of Consulting and Clinical Psychology*, **52**, 1028–1038.

Ellis, A., Stores, G., Mayou, R. (1998) 'Psychological consequences of road traffic accidents in children.' *European Child and Adolescent Psychiatry*, **7**, 61–68.

Engel, G.L., Schmale, A.H. (1972) 'Conservation–withdrawal: a primary regulatory process for organismic homeostasis.' *Ciba Foundation Symposium*, **8**, 57–75.

Field, T.M. (1991) 'Young children's adaptations to repeated separations from their mothers.' *Child Development*, **62**, 539–547.

—— Reite, M. (1984) 'Children's responses to separation from mother during the birth of another child.' *Child Development*, **55**, 1308–1316.

Glod, C.A., Teicher, M.H., Hartman, C.R., Harakal, T. (1997) 'Increased nocturnal activity and impaired sleep maintenance in abused children.' *Journal of the American Academy of Child and Adolescent Psychiatry*, **36**, 1236–1243.

Hancock, E. (1978) 'The case of Ann: a sleep disturbance in a 3-year-old child.' *Social Work in Health Care*, **3**, 243–255.

Harris, E.S. (1991) 'Adolescent bereavement following the death of a parent: an exploratory study.' *Child Psychiatry and Human Development*, **21**, 267–281.

King, B.H., Baxter, L.R., Stuber, M., Fish, B. (1987) 'Therapeutic sleep deprivation for depression in children.' *Journal of the American Academy of Child and Adolescent Psychiatry*, **26**, 928–931.

Lavie, P., Amit, Y., Epstein, R., Tzischinsky, O. (1993) 'Children's sleep under the threat of attack by ballistic missiles.' *Journal of Sleep Research*, **2**, 34–37.

Mead, J.M., Mead, N.E. (1986) 'Postmolestation regression in children.' *American Journal of Psychiatry*, **143**, 559. *(Letter.)*

Moore, M.S. (1989) 'Disturbed attachment in children: A factor in sleep disturbance, altered dream production and immune dysfunction. I. Not safe to sleep: Chronic sleep disturbance in anxious attachment.' *Journal of Child Psychotherapy*, **15**, 99–111.

Pillar, G., Malhotra, A., Lavie, P. (2000) 'Post-traumatic stress disorder and sleep – what a nightmare!' *Sleep Medicine Reviews*, **4**, 183–200.

Pynoos, R.S., Frederick, C., Nader, K., Arroyo, W., Steinberg, A., Eth, S., Nunez, F., Fairbanks, L. (1987) 'Life threat and posttraumatic stress in school-age children.' *Archives of General Psychiatry*, **44**, 1057–1063.

Rimsza, M.E., Burke, R.A., Locke, C. (1988) 'Sexual abuse: somatic and emotional reactions.' *Child Abuse and Neglect*, **12**, 201–208.

Rofe, Y., Lewin, I. (1982) 'The effect of war environment on dreams and sleep habits.' *Series in Clinical and Community Psychology: Stress and Anxiety*, **8**, 67–79.

Ross, R.J., Ball, W.A., Sullivan, K.A., Caroff, S.N. (1989) 'Sleep disturbance as the hallmark of posttraumatic stress disorder.' *American Journal of Psychiatry*, **146**, 697–707.

Sadeh, A. (1996) 'Stress, trauma, and sleep in children.' *Child and Adolescent Psychiatric Clinics of North America*, **5**, 685–700.

—— McGuire, J.P., Sachs, H., Seifer, R., Tremblay, A., Civita, R., Hayden, R.M. (1995) 'Sleep and psychological characteristics of children on a psychiatric inpatient unit.' *Journal of the American Academy of Child and Adolescent Psychiatry*, **34**, 813–819.

—— Raviv, A., Gruber, R. (2000) 'Sleep patterns and sleep disruptions in school-age children.' *Developmental Psychology*, **36**, 291–301.

Selye, H. (1983) 'The stress concept: Past, present and future.' *In:* Cooper, C.L. (Ed.) *Stress Research.* Chichester: John Wiley, pp. 1–20.

Terr, L.C. (1991) 'Childhood traumas: an outline and overview.' *American Journal of Psychiatry*, **148**, 10–20.

Vogel, J.M., Vernberg, E.M. (1993) 'Psychological responses of children to natural and human-made disasters: I. Children's psychological responses to disasters.' *Journal of Clinical Child Psychology*, **22**, 464–484.

Wirz-Justice, A., Van den Hoofdakker, R.H. (1999) 'Sleep deprivation in depression: what do we know, where do we go?' *Biological Psychiatry*, **46**, 445–453.

26
SLEEP PROBLEMS IN ATTENTION DEFICIT HYPERACTIVITY DISORDER

Penny Corkum

Attention deficit hyperactivity disorder (ADHD) comprises three core symptoms—inattention, impulsivity and hyperactivity—and is the most common problem presented to children's mental health services (Barkley 1998). The current diagnostic classification, the DSM-IV (Barkley 1994), identifies three subtypes of ADHD: predominantly inattentive, predominantly hyperactive–impulsive, and combined subtypes. The prevalence of the disorder is conservatively estimated at 3–6 per cent of school-age children, with boys being diagnosed at least three times more frequently than girls. Although once thought of as a childhood disorder, it is now believed that the symptoms of ADHD can persist across the life-span, with age- and sex-specific changes in its manifestation. The disorder has been found to have a negative impact on an individual's functioning within the family, school and community.

In addition to the core symptomatology, ADHD is associated with other problems (*e.g.* academic underachievement, poor social relations) and shows a high rate of comorbidity with other clinical disorders (Barkley 1998). The rates of comorbidity in latency-aged (6- to 12-year-old) children with ADHD vary depending on the sample and methodology. However, the majority of children with ADHD meet diagnostic criteria for at least one other psychiatric disorder (Tannock 1998). Other externalizing disorders such as oppositional defiant disorder and conduct disorder are the most common comorbid diagnosis with ADHD, with an estimated rate between 40 and 90 per cent. Internalizing disorders, such as anxiety and mood disorders, and intellectual impairments are also frequently comorbid with ADHD, with an estimated frequency of approximately 25 per cent. It is believed that many of the problems thought to be associated with ADHD may in fact be attributable to the comorbid disorder (Jensen *et al.* 1997).

In addition to comorbid disorders associated with ADHD, it is also believed that these children suffer from a variety of sleep difficulties. One particular sleep problem, 'restless sleep', was included in DSM-III (American Psychiatric Association 1980), although it has not been included in subsequent revisions. Also, items assessing sleep problems have been included in a number of popular child rating scales (*e.g.* Conners' Parent Rating Scale—Goyette *et al.* 1978). These rating scales, including the sleep items, continue to be used for diagnostic purposes in both clinical and research settings. It appears that the inclusion of sleep problems has been based primarily on clinical observations that identified an association between ADHD and sleep problems, rather than a theory that implicated sleep disturbances in ADHD.

The study of sleep problems in children with ADHD is also critical given that the most common treatment for this disorder, stimulant medication, is associated with sleep difficulties. It is estimated that 75 per cent of children diagnosed with ADHD are treated with stimulant medication (Barkley 1998). Of the children prescribed methylphenidate, 70–80 per cent show a marked reduction in core and associated symptoms (Spencer *et al.* 1996). However, an increase in the rate of sleep problems has been one of the most consistent side-effects found in acute trials (Barkley 1998), long-term studies (Schachar *et al.* 1997) and cross-sectional studies (Stein 1999).

Characteristic sleep problems

In order to delineate the type, frequency and significance of sleep problems in children with ADHD, we conducted a systematic review of the literature (Corkum *et al.* 1998). Based on this literature search, 16 studies were found that directly addressed sleep in children with ADHD in comparison with normally developing children (Small *et al.* 1971, Feinberg *et al.* 1974, Haig *et al.* 1974, Nahas and Krynicki 1977, Khan and Rechtschaffen 1978, Stahl *et al.* 1979, Busby *et al.* 1981, Poitras *et al.* 1981, Greenhill *et al.* 1983, Porrino *et al.* 1983, Busby and Pivik 1985, Kaplan *et al.* 1987, Trommer *et al.* 1988, Ramos Platon *et al.* 1990, Palm *et al.* 1992, Tirosh *et al.* 1993). These studies were divided into two categories: those that employed subjective measures (*e.g.* questionnaires), and those that used objective ones (*e.g.* polysomnographs, actigraphy).

Based on the two studies employing subjective measures, the prevalence of sleep problems was estimated to be between 25 and 50 per cent, compared with 7 per cent among normal controls (Kaplan *et al.* 1987, Trommer *et al.* 1988). At the time of the review, no study had examined sleep disturbances in children with ADHD compared to other clinical groups, therefore making it impossible to determine if increased parental reports of sleep problems (*e.g.* difficulty falling asleep, restless sleep, night wakings, early morning awakening) were unique to a diagnosis of ADHD, reflected general psychological disturbances, and/or were attributable to comorbid disorders. Since the review was published, Marcotte *et al.* (1998) compared children diagnosed with ADHD and those diagnosed with a specific learning disability (LD). It was found that the clinical groups (ADHD, LD, ADHD+LD) differed from a community-based control group, but did not differ from each other in their sleep-related problems. This finding calls into question the specificity of sleep problems to a diagnosis of ADHD.

The results of the studies that employed objective measures of sleep were analysed using a 'box-score' approach that allowed for comparison across studies that differed on a number of methodological issues (*e.g.* definition of ADHD, inclusion and exclusion criterion, type of recording). The findings were inconsistent across these studies (Table 26.1). The inconsistencies were attributed to small sample sizes that could result in type II errors, and/or inadequate and inconsistently applied diagnostic criteria for ADHD. Only three relatively consistent findings across the studies were found. First, nine out of 10 studies reviewed found that the ADHD group did not differ from the normal control group on total sleep time. Second, four out of six studies reviewed found that children with ADHD were more restless during sleep. Third, the majority of studies examining the impact of stimulant

TABLE 26.1
Results of studies employing objective measures*

Sleep variable (number of studies)	ADHD groups more/longer/better	ADHD and control groups similar	ADHD groups less/shorter/worse
Sleep onset latency (n=9)	3/9	4/9	2/9
Total sleep time (n=10)	1/10	9/10	0/10
Sleep efficiency (n=8)	0/8	5/8	3/8
Movements (n=6)	4/6	2/6	0/6
REM sleep (n=9)	N/A**	4/9	N/A**
NREM sleep (n=10)	N/A**	5/10	N/A**

*See text for references.
**Not applicable (results not easily compiled into these categories).

medication on sleep found that there were changes in the sleep parameters (*e.g.* prolonged sleep latency, increased length of onset to first REM cycle), but these changes were considered to be non-pathological. The lack of consistent findings of sleep problems in ADHD children using objective methodology is in stark contrast to high rates of sleep problems reported by parents.

A recent study using objective measures further suggests that it may be the instability of the sleep–wake patterns (*i.e.* increased variability from night to night) of children with ADHD that distinguishes their sleep patterns from those of control children, rather than quantitative differences in any particular sleep-related variable (Gruber *et al.* 2000).

Aetiological factors

Given the fivefold increase in parent-reported sleep problems in children with ADHD, it is unlikely that the relationship between ADHD and sleep problems is a spurious finding. However, the exact aetiology of sleep difficulties in this population remains unknown.

The most common explanation for sleep problems in children with ADHD is that these problems are intrinsic to ADHD (*i.e.* internally generated and specific to an ADHD diagnosis). It has been proposed that children with ADHD may suffer from a primary sleep disorder (Guilleminault *et al.* 1982, Weinberg and Brumback 1990, Dahl *et al.* 1991, Sheldon *et al.* 1991, Picchietti *et al.* 1994), with the strongest interpretation of this postulate indicating that ADHD symptoms may be secondary to the sleep disorder or at least that the sleep disorder exacerbates the ADHD symptoms. Another explanation is that sleep problems in children with ADHD may be due to dysregulation of arousal (Greenhill *et al.* 1983, Busby and Pivik 1985, Tirosh *et al.* 1993, Lecendreux *et al.* 2000). Since dysregulation of arousal has been viewed as a core component of ADHD, sleep difficulties could result in sleep deprivation that might exacerbate problems with attention, impulsivity and hyperactivity.

An alternative explanation is that sleep problems in children with ADHD may be extrinsic (*i.e.* behavioural) in nature. It may be that the sleep problems most commonly associated with ADHD are a manifestation of challenging behaviour, rather than internally generated. We conducted two empirical studies to test the relative contribution of intrinsic and extrinsic factors to sleep problems in children with ADHD. The first tested the specificity of sleep problems to ADHD, while the second attempted to verify parental reports of sleep problems using objective measures.

The results of the first study (Corkum *et al.* 1999) highlight the potential contribution of comorbid disorders and stimulant medication treatment to the existence of sleep problems in this population. In this study, children aged 6 to 12 years were assigned to four groups based on clinical diagnostic interviews: unmedicated ADHD (n=79); medicated ADHD (n=22); clinical comparison (n=35); and healthy non-clinical comparison (n=36). These groups were compared on two sleep questionnaires completed by the parents that assessed current sleep problems and factors associated with sleep difficulties (*i.e.* sleep routines, sleep practices, child and family sleep history). The major findings were that: (1) dyssomnias (*i.e.* bedtime resistance, sleep onset problems, difficulty arising) were related to confounding factors (*i.e.* comorbid opposition defiant disorder and stimulant medication) rather than ADHD; (2) parasomnias (*i.e.* sleepwalking, night awakenings, night terrors) were similar between the clinical and non-clinical groups; and (3) the DSM-IV combined subtype of ADHD was associated with sleep-related involuntary movements (*e.g.* sleep talking, teeth grinding, restless sleep, jerky movements during sleep). However, sleep-related involuntary movements were more highly associated with separation anxiety.

The second study (Corkum *et al.* 2001) underscores the discrepancy between parent reports of sleep problems and verification of these sleep problems using objective measures. The study used multiple sleep measures and evaluated six sleep parameters (*viz.* bedtime resistance, sleep duration, sleep onset, night awakenings, motor activity and morning arising) for two groups of children—ADHD and normal comparison—who ranged from 7 to 11 years of age. The ADHD group members were selected only if they displayed pervasiveness in their symptomatology and were medication naive. Parents completed a retrospective questionnaire that evaluated sleep problems over a six-month period. Additionally, each child was required to wear an actigraph for seven consecutive nights, and the child's parents completed a sleep diary during this time period. As expected, parents of children with ADHD reported significantly more sleep problems than parents of normally developing children. However, the majority of these differences were not verified through the actigraphy or sleep diary data, with the exception of longer sleep duration for children with ADHD and parent reports that described increased bedtime resistance. It was also found that parent–child interactions during bedtime routines were more challenging in the ADHD group.

The results of the above two studies highlight the possibility that many of the reported sleep problems in children with ADHD may not be specific to a diagnosis of ADHD, but rather may be related to comorbid disorders and/or treatment with stimulant medication. Also, sleep problems in this population may be related to difficult parent–child interactions associated with bedtime routines, which may contribute to more negative parental perception

of the child's sleep. However, the relative contribution of intrinsic and extrinsic factors to sleep problems in children with ADHD requires further investigation. Current treatment of sleep problems in this population should take into consideration both intrinsic and extrinsic factors.

Special considerations of management
From a clinical perspective, it is prudent to carefully assess for sleep problems in children with ADHD, including both medication-naive children and children receiving pharmacological treatment. This is particularly important as sleep problems in children have been reported as a significant stressor for parents, and treatment of sleep problems has resulted in improvements in daytime functioning. The assessment of sleep needs to cover a wide range of sleep problem areas, as well as to consider information concerning the child's primary and comorbid diagnoses and medication use. Given the current research, treatment should address both extrinsic (behavioural) and intrinsic (physiological) components of sleep problems.

Treatment of disordered sleep in children with ADHD has received only limited formal investigation, with the vast majority of studies concentrating on pharmacological interventions. Clonidine has been the most widely studied pharmacological treatment, and results have indicated significant improvements in sleep quality in the majority of subjects, but also increased daytime sedation, hypotension and rebound hypertension (Prince *et al.* 1996). Individual case studies examining the use of imipramine (Hilton *et al.* 1991) and bupropion (Malek-Ahmadi 1999) have also demonstrated improved sleep.

The impact of various stimulant medication schedules has also been investigated. Two studies compared the impact of stimulant medication delivered b.i.d. (two doses a day) and t.i.d. (three doses a day), and both found that a third dose failed to demonstrate a substantial effect on sleep (Kent *et al.* 1995, Stein *et al.* 1996). However, Chatoor *et al.* (1983) examined the effect of a nocturnally administered dose of stimulant medication and found significant changes in sleep architecture (*e.g.* delay in first REM period, and decreased percentage of REM sleep). It was noted that some children might benefit from a dose later in the day because of the improved bedtime behaviour that results.

Only two reported case studies employing behavioural interventions have been published. A combination of behavioural modification and chronotherapy was successfully used to treat a 10-year-old girl with ADHD and delayed sleep phase insomnia (Dahl *et al.* 1991). In the second study, Bergman (1976) reported a successful behavioural intervention targeted at insomnia in a 7-year-old boy diagnosed with ADHD.

Given the limited research on appropriate interventions for sleep problems in children with ADHD, the clinician would be well advised to focus on both intrinsic and extrinsic factors associated with sleep problems in children with ADHD, including the possibility of a primary sleep disorder existing. Particular attention should be paid to sleep hygiene issues, such as a regular sleep schedule and consistency of parental limit-setting at bedtime. Further intervention studies are needed to clarify the most appropriate approach and to delineate the relative contributions of intrinsic and extrinsic influences on sleep problems in children with ADHD.

REFERENCES

American Psychiatric Association (1980) *Diagnostic and Statistical Manual of Mental Disorders, 3rd Edn.* Washington DC: APA.

Barkley, R.A. (1994) *Diagnostic and Statistical Manual of Mental Disorders, 4th Edn.* Washington DC: APA.

—— (1998) *Attention Deficit Hyperactivity Disorder. A Handbook for Diagnosis and Treatment. 2nd Edn.* New York: Guilford Press.

Bergman, R.L. (1976) 'Treatment of childhood insomnia diagnosed as "hyperactivity".' *Journal of Behavior Therapy and Experimental Psychiatry*, **7**, 199. *(Abstract.)*

Busby, K., Pivik, R.T. (1985) 'Auditory arousal thresholds during sleep in hyperkinetic children.' *Sleep*, **8**, 332–341.

—— Firestone, P., Pivik, R.T. (1981) 'Sleep patterns in hyperkinetic and normal children.' *Sleep*, **4**, 366–381.

Chatoor, I., Wells, K.C., Conners, C.K., Seidel, W.T., Shaw, D. (1983) 'The effects of nocturnally administered stimulant medication on EEG sleep and behaviour in hyperactive children.' *Journal of the American Academy of Child and Adolescent Psychiatry*, **22**, 337–342.

Corkum, P., Tannock, R., Moldofsky, H. (1998) 'Sleep disturbances in children with attention-deficit/hyperactivity disorder.' *Journal of the American Academy of Child and Adolescent Psychiatry*, **37**, 637–646.

—— Moldofsky, H., Hogg-Johnson, S., Humphries, T., Tannock, R. (1999) 'Sleep problems in children with attention-deficit/hyperactivity disorder: Impact of subtype, comorbidity and stimulant medication.' *Journal of the American Academy of Child and Adolescent Psychiatry*, **38**, 1285–1293.

—— Tannock, R., Moldofsky, H., Hogg-Johnson, S., Humphries, T. (2001) 'Actigraphy and parental ratings of sleep in children with attention-deficit/hyperactivity disorder.' *Sleep*, **24**, 303–312.

Dahl, R.E., Pelham, W.E., Worsen, M. (1991) 'The role of sleep disturbances in attention deficit disorder symptoms: A case study.' *Journal of Pediatric Psychology*, **16**, 229–239.

Feinberg, I., Hibi, S., Braun, M., Cavness, C., Westerman, G., Small, A. (1974) 'Sleep amphetamine effects in MBDS and normal subjects.' *Archives of General Psychiatry*, **31**, 723–731.

Goyette, C., Conners, C.K., Ulrich, R. (1978) 'Normative data on the Revised Conners' Parent and Teacher Rating Scales.' *Journal of Child Psychology*, **6**, 221–236.

Greenhill, L., Puig-Antich, J., Goetz, R., Hanlon, C., Davies, M. (1983) 'Sleep architecture and REM sleep measures in prepubertal children with attention deficit disorder with hyperactivity.' *Sleep*, **6**, 91–101.

Gruber, R., Sadeh, A., Raviv, A. (2000) 'Instability of sleep patterns in children with attention-deficit/hyperactivity disorder.' *Journal of the America Academy of Child and Adolescent Psychiatry*, **39**, 495–501.

Guilleminault, C., Winkle, R., Korobkin, R., Simmons, B. (1982) 'Children and nocturnal snoring: evaluation of the effects of sleep related respiratory resistive load and daytime functioning.' *European Journal of Pediatrics*, **139**, 165–171.

Haig, J.R., Schroeder, C.S., Schroeder, S.R. (1974) 'Effects of methylphenidate on hyperactive children's sleep.' *Psychopharmacologia*, **37**, 185–188.

Hilton, D.K., Martin, C.A., Heffron, W.M., Hall, B.D., Johnson, G.L. (1991) 'Imipramine treatment of ADHD in a fragile X child.' *Journal of the American Academy of Child and Adolescent Psychiatry*, **30**, 831–834.

Jensen, P.S., Martin, B.A., Cantwell, D.P. (1997) 'Comorbidity in ADHD: Implications for research, practice, and DSM IV.' *Journal of the American Academy of Child and Adolescent Psychiatry*, **36**, 1065–1079.

Kaplan, B.J., McNicol, J., Conte, R.A., Moghandam, H.K. (1987) 'Sleep disturbance in preschool-aged hyperactive and nonhyperactive children.' *Pediatrics*, **80**, 839–844.

Kent, J.D., Blader, J.C., Koplewicz, H.S., Abikoff, H., Foley, C.A. (1995) 'Effects of a late-afternoon methylphenidate administration on behaviour and sleep in attention-deficit hyperactivity disorder.' *Pediatrics*, **96**, 320–325.

Khan, A., Rechtschaffen, A. (1978) 'Sleep patterns and sleep spindles in hyperkinetic children.' *Sleep Research*, **7**, 137. *(Abstract.)*

Lecendreux, M., Knofal, E., Bouvard, M., Falissard, B., Mouren-Siméoni, M-C. (2000) 'Sleep and alertness in children with ADHD.' *Journal of Child Psychology and Psychiatry*, **41**, 803–812.

Malek-Ahmadi, P. (1999) 'Bupropion, periodic limb movement disorder, and ADHD.' *Journal of the American Academy of Child and Adolescent Psychiatry*, **38**, 637–638.

Marcotte, A.C., Thacher, P.V., Butters, M., Bortz, J., Acebo, C., Carskadon, M.A. (1998) 'Parental report of sleep problems in children with attentional and learning disorders.' *Developmental and Behavioral Pediatrics*, **19**, 178–186.

179

Nahas, A.D., Krynicki, V. (1977) 'Effects of methylphenidate on sleep stages and ultradian rhythms in hyperactive children.' *Journal of Nervous and Mental Disease*, **164**, 66–69.

Palm, L., Persson, E., Bjerre, I., Elmqvist, D., Blennow, G. (1992) 'Sleep and wakefulness in preadolescent children with deficits in attention, motor control and perception.' *Acta Paediatrica*, **81**, 618–624.

Picchietti, D.L., England, S.J., Walters, A.S., Willis, K., Verrico, T. (1994) 'Periodic limb movement disorder and restless legs syndrome in children with attention-deficit hyperactivity disorder.' *Journal of Child Neurology*, **13**, 588–594.

Poitras, L., Bylsma, F.W., Simeon, J., Pivik, R.T. (1981) 'Cortical sleep spindle activity in hyperkinetic children.' *Sleep Research*, **10**, 117. *(Abstract.)*

Porrino, L.J., Rapoport, J.L., Behar, D., Sceery, W., Ismond, D., Bunney, W.E. (1983) 'A naturalistic assessment of the motor activity of hyperactive boys.' *Archives of General Psychiatry*, **40**, 681–687.

Prince, J.B., Wilens, T.E., Biederman, J., Spencer, T.J., Wozniak, J.R. (1996) 'Clonidine for sleep disturbances associated with attention-deficit hyperactivity disorder: A systematic chart review of 62 cases.' *Journal of the American Academy of Child and Adolescent Psychiatry*, **35**, 599–605.

Ramos Platon, M.J., Vela Bueno, A., Espinar Sierra, J., Kales, S. (1990) 'Hypnopolygraphic alterations in attention deficit disorder (ADD) children.' *International Journal of Neuroscience*, **53**, 87–101.

Schachar, R.J., Tannock, R., Cunningham, C., Corkum, P.V. (1997) 'Behavioral, situational, and temporal effects of treatment of ADHD with methylphenidate.' *Journal of the American Academy of Child and Adolescent Psychiatry*, **36**, 754–763.

Sheldon, S.H., Irby, S., Applebaum, J., Golbin, A., Levy, H.B., Spire, J.B. (1991) 'Sleep pressure in children with attentional deficits.' *Sleep Research*, **20**, 448. *(Abstract.)*

Small, A., Hibi, S., Feinberg, I. (1971) 'Effects of dextroamphetamine sulfate on EEG sleep patterns of hyperactive children.' *Archives of General Psychiatry*, **25**, 369–380.

Spencer, T., Biederman, J., Wilens, T., Harding, M., O'Dovvell, D., Griffin, S. (1996) 'Pharmacotherapy of attention-deficit hyperactivity disorder across the life cycle.' *Journal of the American Academy of Child and Adolescent Psychiatry*, **35**, 409–432.

Stahl, M.L., Orr, W.C., Griffiths, W.J. (1979) 'Nocturnal levels of growth hormone in hyperactive children of small stature.' *Journal of Clinical Psychiatry*, **40**, 225–227.

Stein, M.A., Blondis, T.A., Schnitzler, E.R., O'Brien, T., Fishkin, J., Blackwell, B., Szumowski, E., Roizen, N.J. (1996) 'Methylphenidate dosing: twice daily versus three times daily.' *Pediatrics*, **98**, 748–756.

—— (1999) 'Unravelling sleep problems in treated and untreated children with ADHD.' *Journal of Child and Adolescent Psychopharmacology*, **9**, 157–168.

Tannock, R. (1998) 'Attention deficit hyperactivity disorder: Advances in cognitive, neurobiological, and genetic research.' *Journal of Child Psychology and Psychiatry*, **39**, 65–99.

Tirosh, E., Sadeh, A., Munvez, R., Lavie, P. (1993) 'Effects of methylphenidate on sleep in children with attention-deficit hyperactivity disorder.' *American Journal of Diseases of Children*, **147**, 1313–1315.

Trommer, B.L., Hoeppner, J.B., Rosenberg, R.S., Armstrong, K.J., Rothstein, J.A. (1988) 'Sleep disturbance in children with attention deficit disorder.' *Annals of Neurology*, **24**, 322. *(Abstract.)*

Weinberg, W.A., Brumback, R.A. (1990) 'Primary disorder of vigilance: A novel explanation of inattentiveness, daydreaming, boredom, restlessness and sleepiness.' *Journal of Pediatrics*, **116**, 720–725.

27
SLEEP IN CHILDREN WITH AUTISM AND ASPERGER SYNDROME

Amanda Richdale

Autism

Autism is a pervasive developmental disorder. Children with autism exhibit both deviance and delay in social development, communication and behaviour, and over 70 per cent have a concurrent intellectual impairment (American Psychiatric Association [APA] 1994). The disorder is biologically based, with a strong genetic component, and may also co-occur with a number of other medical or neurological conditions. About one in 1000 children are affected and there is a male predominance (Peeters and Gillberg 1999). Apart from the primary characteristics of autism, a number of secondary features may occur including hyperactivity, inattention, impulsiveness, eating problems, sound sensitivity, exaggerated or odd responses to sensory stimuli, self-injurious behaviour, aggression, tantrums and sleep difficulties, and epilepsy is common (APA 1994).

SLEEP PROBLEMS

Sleep problems in autism have been recognized for several decades and have been recently reviewed (Stores and Wiggs 1998, Richdale 1999). Sleep problems are common in autism. Around two-thirds of children with autism exhibit sleep problems at any one time (Table 27.1), and the majority are likely to have a problem during childhood (DeMeyer 1979, Richdale and Prior 1995). This is at least twice the rate found in typically developing children (Clarkson *et al.* 1986, Armstrong *et al.* 1994). In children with an intellectual impairment the frequency of sleeping difficulties is variable. In her review, Johnson (1996) found that 34 to 80 per cent of these children had sleep problems. While these rates appear similar to those for autism, they generally refer to groups with a range of disabilities. Wiggs and Stores (1996a) noted that sleep problems were particularly prevalent in children with autism as compared with other disability groups. Sleep problems are often long-term in children with an intellectual impairment (Bramble 1997, Quine 1991) or autism (Richdale and Prior 1995). In autism, sleep problems can occur at all levels of intellectual ability (Richdale and Prior 1995, Patzold *et al.* 1998).

Sleep problems in children with autism appear to be more prevalent in younger children (DeMeyer 1979, Richdale and Prior 1995), and are generally related to sleep onset and maintenance. Sleep problems reported by various authors (DeMeyer 1979, Hoshino *et al.* 1984, Clements *et al.* 1986, Richdale and Prior 1995, Patzold *et al.* 1998, Taira *et al.* 1998, Hering *et al.* 1999, Schreck and Mulick 2000) include: irregular sleep–wake patterns;

TABLE 27.1
Prevalence of sleep problems in children with autism

Study	Autism				Comparison groups			
	Subjects N	Age range	Level of disability*	Sleep problems (%)	Subjects N	Age range	Level of disability*	Sleep problems (%)
De Meyer (1979)	32	Early childhood		100[a]	—	—	—	Not reported
Hoshino et al. (1984)	75	3–15 years	IQ: <50–71+	65[a]	75	3–15 years	Normal range	—
Clements et al. (1986)	16	<15 years	Severe II	56.3[c]	139	<15 years	Severe II	31.7[c]
Richdale and Prior (1995)	39[d]	2.7–19 years	IQ: <20–119	75.4[b]	61	2.9–14.9 years	IQ: 45 to normal range	57.4[b]
	27	4.3–14.3 years	IQ: 57–119	44.4[c]	26	4.1–14.3 years	IQ: 45–154	26.9[c]
Wiggs and Stores (1996)	25	10±3.7[e] years	Severe II	68[c]	183	10±3.7[e] years	Severe II	40.4
Patzold et al. (1998)[f]	38	7.8±2.6 years	Severe II to normal range	76.3[b] / 63.2[c]	36	8.4±2.6 years	Severe II to normal range	37.1[b] / 22.9[c]
Taira et al. (1998)	88	Preschool to high school		65.1[a]	—	—	—	—
Herring et al. (1999)	22	3–12 years		54.4[c]	—	—	—	—

*II = intellectual impairment.
[a]Percentage of children who had or currently have sleep problems.
[b]Past sleep problems.
[c]Current sleep problems.
[d]Combination of data for low- and high-functioning groups.
[e]Average of all subjects in study.
[f]This study included seven children with Asperger syndrome.

problems with sleep onset, including long sleep latencies and problematic sleep routines; early morning waking; generally poor sleep; shortened night sleep; variable or late sleep onset and wake times; night waking; excessive co-sleeping; and an increased frequency of dyssomnias. Not all these studies included comparison groups, and group size and the age of the children was variable. Night waking problems do not appear to be due to an increased frequency of waking, rather the issues are the length of time spent awake and/or the behaviours engaged in while awake (DeMeyer 1979, Patzold et al. 1998). Early morning waking (waking before 6.00 a.m. and as early as 2.00 a.m.) appears to be more prevalent in younger children. It has been suggested that sleep problems may be of aetiological significance for autism (Richdale and Prior 1995, Stores and Wiggs 1998).

There is little research regarding the parasomnias in autism. Richdale and Prior (1995) and Patzold et al. (1998) found that bad dreams, nightmares or sleep talking did not occur more frequently than in typical children. However, DeMeyer (1979) noted that night terrors were more common in autism. Recently, Schreck and Mulick (2000) reported that parasomnias were more frequent in autism than in other groups of children. In particular, parents reported nightmares, environmental disturbances, disoriented awakening, bruxism and apnoea to be problematic. The significance of the parasomnias in autism awaits further investigation.

As well as parent report, Hering et al. (1999) used actigraphy to investigate sleep in autism, confirming the presence of early waking in those children identified with a sleep problem, compared to an age- and sex-matched control group. No other differences were found, and the authors suggested that parents of children with autism were less tolerant of disturbances and may be biased in their reporting of sleep difficulties. Several factors may account for their conclusions, including small group size, age, and failure to report: (a) sleep latency; (b) length of night-waking episodes; (c) behavioural disturbances surrounding sleep onset, and night and early waking; and (d) bedtime routines. Further studies using objective measures of sleep are required. Recent research using actigraphy demonstrated moderate to strong correlations between sleep measures from diaries and those obtained via actigraphy, but night waking was particularly susceptible to underestimation (Sadeh 1996). However, actigraphy does not give an indication of extrinsic issues surrounding sleep, such as routines and behaviour. Sadeh has suggested that the two methods are complimentary in the determination of sleep problems in children.

BEHAVIOUR PROBLEMS AND FAMILY STRESS
Levels of psychopathology in autism are generally high (Patzold et al. 1998); difficult and challenging behaviours are common, and social and communication problems are a hallmark of the disorder (APA 1994). Difficult and challenging daytime behaviour is associated with sleep problems in children with an intellectual impairment (Quine 1991, Wiggs and Stores 1996a, Richdale et al. 2000). Quine also reported a link between communication difficulties and the presence of sleep problems in children with an intellectual impairment. Hoshino et al. (1984) noted that sleep difficulties were associated with more challenging behaviours, while Patzold et al. (1998) found that increased psychopathology was associated with sleep problems in autism. Similarly, Schreck (1997) found a link between abnormalities in social interaction and communication, and sleep problems in autism. Thus, children with autism

and sleep problems are likely to exhibit more severe levels of the problematic behaviours generally associated with the disorder.

Autism is associated with significantly higher levels of family stress compared with other disorders such as Down syndrome (Fisman and Wolf 1991), and it is likely that the presence of sleep problems will exacerbate the stress burden of families. The impact of sleep difficulties on parents and families has not been specifically addressed in autism. DeMeyer (1979) reported that mothers in particular were significantly affected and experienced extreme tiredness and irritability, and in families of children with an intellectual impairment (including autism) sleep problems are associated with increased parental stress (Richdale et al. 2000).

Thus, more severe psychopathology, social and communication problems, and parent stress appear to be linked to concurrent sleep problems in autism. This is of particular concern given the high levels of psychopathology and family stress generally reported for these children. Any sleep problems therefore become additional burdens for parents and have a negative impact on the children's behaviour.

AETIOLOGICAL FACTORS

Sleep problems in autism may: (1) occur as part of the challenging and difficult behaviours present in the majority of these children, (2) be a manifestation of some factor(s) intrinsic to the disorder, or (3) be a combination of both (Richdale 1999). However, the aetiology of sleep problems is currently unknown. Nevertheless a number of potential factors may be involved.

There is evidence that improved sleep and improved *daytime behaviour* in children with an intellectual impairment are linked (Bramble 1997). Risperidone [a serotonin (5HT2) and dopamine (D2) antagonist] treatment of aggression in a group of males with autism led to improvement in co-occurring sleep onset and maintenance problems (Horrigan and Barnhill 1997a). Others have demonstrated that lack of adequate sleep results in an increase in challenging behaviours in children with an intellectual impairment (Kennedy and Meyer 1996). Additionally, the failure of Hering et al. (1999) to find objective evidence for sleep problems such as settling, night waking and shortened night sleep may also indicate that the major sleep issues in autism are extrinsic and are manifestations of difficult and challenging behaviours, rather than an intrinsic abnormality in the control of the sleep–wake cycle.

Children with autism can exhibit high levels of *anxiety* (Patzold et al. 1998), variability in level of arousal (Hutt et al. 1964), stereotypical behaviour that is believed to serve an arousal function (Johnson 1996), and adherence to routines and rituals (APA 1994). Anxiety is associated with sleep problems in typically developing children (Clarkson et al. 1986) and may be an important factor in autism, particularly in higher-functioning children whose cognitive abilities may allow magnification of any fears. The association between sleep problems and more active daytime behaviour (Richdale and Prior 1995) and reports that young, higher-functioning children with autism are more likely to wake spontaneously than other children (Patzold et al. 1998) also suggest an association between arousal factors and sleep difficulties.

The routines and rituals that form part of the behavioural criteria for a diagnosis of autism may manifest as inappropriate *bedtime routines and rituals*. Adherence to inappropriate bedtime routines can be an exacerbating factor, as sleep problems are likely to emerge when the conditions of the routine are not fulfilled. Parents of children with autism have reported that sleep problems were likely to occur if bedtime routines, many of which were inappropriate, were not followed (Patzold *et al.* 1998).

Social and communication difficulties are primary characteristics of autism and may play a prominent role in sleep disorders, particularly in children who are more severely impaired. The sleep–wake cycle is a circadian rhythm and is primarily entrained by the light–dark cycle. However, to some extent sleep and wake times can be chosen and this is generally guided by social cues. Social cues can play a role in entraining the sleep–wake rhythm (Aschoff *et al.* 1971) and are important in entraining the sleep–wake patterns of infants (Ma *et al.* 1993). In autism, failure to perceive these cues or their importance may therefore result in sleep difficulties.

Melatonin is produced by the pineal gland and is important for sleep regulation. Its main physiological role appears to be rhythm synchronization to photoperiodic cues, and it appears to assist in phase-setting the circadian pacemaker (Arendt 1997). Melatonin synthesis occurs via the essential amino acid tryptophan and the neurotransmitter serotonin. Blood serotonin is elevated in up to a third of children with autism. Blood tryptophan has been reported to be both elevated and reduced. However, the relationship between blood and brain levels of tryptophan and serotonin, and any impact on melatonin synthesis, has not been established. Some studies have reported an abnormal melatonin rhythm in autism, and children in one study also had sleep problems (for a review, see Richdale 1999). Alterations to the melatonin rhythm may affect the timing and maintenance of sleep in autism. A late-peaking melatonin rhythm may be related to sleep-onset problems, while reduced rhythm amplitude may be related to both night waking and early morning waking (Richdale 1999). It has been suggested that abnormalities in the melatonin rhythm may be related to sleep difficulties in autism (Patzold *et al.* 1998), but this issue remains to be investigated. Sadeh (1997) reported that in normal infants, development of the melatonin rhythm was associated with the establishment of a mature sleep–wake rhythm.

Polysomnographic abnormalities may also be related to sleep difficulties, and several studies have been conducted (*e.g.* Ornitz 1972, Tanguay *et al.* 1976). Children with autism and controls were in early to middle childhood, and no major differences in sleep parameters, including the amount of time spent in REM sleep, were reported. NREM sleep was not analysed. Maturational delay in the development of REM was suggested, particularly in relation to vestibular control. Two recent reports (Elia *et al.* 1991, Diomedi *et al.* 1999) on adolescents and young adults with autism have examined the overnight sleep EEG. In general, NREM sleep was not different in autism. Some significant differences were reported for REM sleep measures but these were not consistent between the studies. Polysomnography is clearly an area for further exploration. In particular it would be of interest to compare children with autism and sleep problems to those without. *Epilepsy* may also need to be considered as a contributing factor in some cases. Any relationship between sleep problems in autism and putative sites for brain pathology remain to be explored.

Thus, there are likely to be a number of extrinsic and intrinsic factors contributing to the development and maintenance of sleep problems in autism, which may vary with individual cases. A systematic investigation of behavioural, physiological and biochemical factors associated with autism and believed to affect the development and maintenance of an appropriate sleep–wake cycle is needed.

Asperger syndrome (AS)

AS is a pervasive developmental disorder (DSM-IV) (APA 1994) first described by Hans Asperger (1944/1991). Children with the disorder have significant impairments in social interaction and behaviour, including routines and rituals, but no clinically significant cognitive or language delay. Nevertheless, there are generally significant communication difficulties, particularly with pragmatics (Kugler 1998). There is debate regarding the differentiation of AS and high-functioning autism and the adequacy of DSM-IV diagnostic criteria (*e.g.* Kugler 1998, Manjiviona and Prior 1999). Boys predominate, and while the prevalence rate is uncertain, AS may be more common than autism. A biological cause with a genetic component is postulated (Gillberg 1993).

SLEEP PROBLEMS

Little is known about sleep problems in children with AS, but sleep issues similar to those in autism may be expected (Richdale 1999). Patzold *et al.* (1998) included seven boys with AS in their sleep study, reporting that there were no qualitative differences from the children with autism. A 7-year-old boy with AS and bedtime settling problems participated in Weiskop *et al.*'s (1999) study but the family withdrew prior to completion. Descriptive data for 10 children with AS (including the seven from Patzold *et al.*'s study) show some similarities between autism and AS, particularly for the severity of past sleep problems (S. Cotton and A. Richdale, unpublished data). Nevertheless, there are also some notable differences, particularly shorter sleep latency and longer night sleep at the time of study in AS compared to autism. In other respects the sleep parameters in the AS group appear to be intermediate between autism and typically developing children. However, this is only indicative of possible sleep issues in this group.

Descriptions of sleep in two 17-year-old males (Berthier *et al.* 1992), a group of eight "patients" with AS (Bergeron *et al.* 1997), and one 25-year-old man (Godbout *et al.* 1998) with AS and Fahr's disease (idiopathic encephalic calcification) are reported. Berthier *et al.*'s subjects both suffered recurrent hypersomnia during the preceding year. One showed reduced sleep efficiency due to increased night waking, decreased REM time with increased REM density, and periodic limb movements, and the second had sleep-onset REM, but otherwise normal sleep stages. The authors concluded that the adolescents' symptoms were consistent with the Kleine–Levin syndrome. Bergeron *et al.* reported long sleep latency, increased stage 1 sleep, frequent waking, REM sleep abnormalities and periodic leg movements in their group. Severely reduced slow wave sleep, an increase in stage 1 sleep and awakenings, and a reduction in sleep spindles, but no EEG abnormalities, were characteristic of Godbout *et al.*'s subject. The young man also reported no dreams or sense of dreaming. It was postulated that brain changes associated with Fahr's disease might be related to the

sleep abnormalities. Additionally, Simblett and Wilson (1993) described a young woman with AS whose presenting problems included sleep difficulties with early morning waking, and Horrigan and Barnhill (1997b) referred to a 17-year-old male with AS who had insomnia and whose sleep had been "problematic since childhood".

Most recently, Godbout *et al.* (2000) reported an EEG study of seven males and one female with AS aged 7 to 53 years, compared with an age- and gender-matched control group. Compared with controls, the AS group showed decreased sleep during the first two-thirds of the night indicating sleep onset and maintenance difficulties, and decreased sleep spindles. Seven AS subjects had some signs of REM disruption and three subjects suffered from periodic limb movements. These findings are consistent with some of those previously reported and are further indication that sleep is likely to be disrupted in this population.

While little can be generalized about sleep in AS, data suggest that young children are likely to go through a period of significant sleep difficulties, possibly related to settling and night waking. There is also some evidence for structural sleep abnormalities, periodic limb movements during sleep, and sleep onset and maintenance problems, though much of this evidence is from older individuals. Further comment is speculative and there is an urgent need for large-scale studies.

AETIOLOGICAL FACTORS

It is likely that some of the causes underlying sleep problems in autism are also causative in AS. High rates of psychopathology and anxiety are found (Tonge *et al.* 1999), and these are associated with sleep problems in other groups of children and adolescents (Stores 1996). When anxiety levels are high in AS children, autistic behaviours such as rigidity and adherence to routines are exacerbated (Attwood 1998). At such times sleep problems may develop or become pronounced. These behaviours may, in particular, predispose children with AS to significant bedtime settling problems, and suggest that sleep may often be problematic in this population. Children with AS, especially in adolescence, are also susceptible to depression (Attwood 1998), which is usually associated with sleeping problems (Stores 1996).

The role of social cues in assisting in the development and maintenance of the sleep–wake rhythm (Aschoff *et al.* 1971, Ma *et al.* 1993) may also be important. Considerable social difficulties are a defining criterion of the disorder. Like children with autism, those with AS may have trouble using such cues to synchronize their sleep–wake cycles when they are younger. The similar severity of past sleep problems in autism and AS noted above supports this notion. As AS is often diagnosed at a later age, it is possible that these children will present with sleep problems before their primary diagnosis is made. Further speculation awaits future research findings.

Management of sleep problems in autism and Asperger syndrome

Frequent and often severe sleep problems that may be associated with increased problematic behaviour and family stress indicate that intervention for sleep problems is essential. However, intervention is rarely addressed in the literature. Sleep assessment should form part of any clinical evaluation and include a thorough history, parent description and a

sleep diary, which should be kept for at least one week, and preferably two or more weeks. Objective measures such as actigraphy, home polysomnography or video-recording may provide valuable additional information. Our studies suggest that there is considerable inter- and intra-individual variability in sleep patterns, and some parents report what appear to be cyclical changes in sleep. These factors also need to be kept in mind. Baseline data and subsequent identification of antecedent and consequent events should form the basis of any intervention. Pertinent child (*e.g.* age, IQ, behaviours) and family factors (*e.g.* beliefs, sleeping arrangements, work commitments) that may affect the suitability of any intervention must also be considered. It is my experience that epilepsy is rarely reported as diagnosed in children with autism and sleep problems. Thus, undiagnosed epilepsy may be a factor in some cases, and its successful treatment (Chapter 15) might well contribute to improvements in sleep.

While sedative *medication* appears to be the most frequently prescribed intervention strategy for children with an intellectual impairment and sleep problems, there is little evidence that it is very effective (Wiggs and Stores 1996b, Bramble 1997). Many parents do not like medication being prescribed for their child, and medication is often ineffective in resolving sleep problems in young children with autism (DeMeyer 1979). Children with autism can also exhibit paradoxical and unexpected responses to medications (Peeters and Gillberg 1999) and, since AS is also an autistic spectrum disorder, similar paradoxical responses may occur in this group too. Clearly, medication for any coexisting psychiatric diagnosis might be helpful (Stores 1996).

Where the sleep onset and night-waking problems predominate, an intervention based on *behavioural principles*, together with *good sleep hygiene*, is most likely to be effective. There are several case reports of successful behavioural interventions for these problems in children with autism (Wolf *et al.* 1964, Howlin 1984, Durand *et al.* 1996, Piazza *et al.* 1997, Weiskop *et al.* 2001). A number of approaches can be taken including extinction, graduated extinction, faded bedtime, fading with parental presence, and bedtime scheduling. Lancioni *et al.* (1999) believe that extinction is a potentially stressful approach to intervention. However, others have found that extinction is successful for treating sleep problems in children with an intellectual impairment (Bramble 1997, Didden *et al.* 1998), including autism (Weiskop *et al.* 1999, 2001). Behavioural and other approaches to intervention are reviewed by France *et al.* (1996), Durand (1998) and Lancioni *et al.* (1999). Care is needed in the design and implementation of any intervention, and parents require considerable ongoing support to achieve and maintain success (Weiskop *et al.* 2001). Reasons for the failure of behavioural approaches to sleep intervention include inadequate therapist knowledge and family support, and parental resistance to behavioural approaches (Wiggs and Stores 1996b).

It is likely that various forms of behavioural interventions will be effective in treating sleep problems in children with AS. Psychological approaches can be effective in treating other problems in AS (Szatmari 1991), and stress management, relaxation and cognitive behaviour therapy (CBT) are used to treat issues such as anxiety (Attwood 1998). Thus, while traditional behavioural approaches such as extinction or graduated extinction may be preferable for younger children with AS, techniques such as relaxation, stress management and CBT may be helpful for older children.

Circadian sleep–wake disorders, such as delayed sleep phase syndrome and fragmented or irregular sleep patterns, are likely to respond to interventions that alter the phase of the sleep–wake rhythm such as *chronotherapy*, which involves altering sleep timing by a variety of means (see Chapter 5). This has been used successfully to treat a fragmented and irregular sleep–wake pattern in a severely intellectually impaired 8-year-old girl with autism (Piazza *et al.* 1998). Bright light (*phototherapy*) can also be used to treat sleep rhythm disorders. As a general guide, bright light in the morning phase advances the sleep–wake rhythm, while bright light in the evening delays it. Guilleminault *et al.* (1993) successfully used phototherapy to treat intractable sleep problems in five of 14 youngsters with severe levels of intellectual impairment, with success being maintained over several years.

Jan and O'Donnell (1996) have reported that *melatonin* is useful in the treatment of intractable sleep problems in children with severe disabilities, including autism. Melatonin has been used successfully to treat adult sleep problems (Arendt 1997), including those in an adult with AS whose insomnia had not responded to the use of hypnotic medication (Horrigan and Barnhill 1997b). While there are no adverse reports of long-term melatonin administration, caution is warranted in prescribing it for children and young adults with autism (Lord 1998); there is some suggestion of an impact on the timing of puberty and on fertility. Arendt (1997) provides a comprehensive review of melatonin's safety.

Conclusion

Sleep problems (particularly problems with sleep onset and maintenance) are common and often severe in autism. Little is known about sleep problems in children with AS. However, given that this is an autistic spectrum disorder, that children with AS exhibit high rates of psychopathology, that anxiety is common, and that depression may also occur, sleep problems are likely to be prevalent.

Systematic research regarding their nature, precipitating and maintaining factors, and aetiological significance is lacking. In general, treatment should be individualized and psychological approaches are likely to be most helpful, with behavioural interventions being preferable approaches to treatment of the most common sleeplessness problems. In other cases, different approaches including medication may be warranted, particularly in intractable cases.

REFERENCES

American Psychiatric Association (1994) *Diagnostic and Statistical Manual of Mental Disorders, 4th Edn.* Washington DC: APA.

Arendt, J. (1997) 'Safety of melatonin in long-term use.' *Journal of Biological Rhythms*, **6**, 673–681.

Armstrong, K.L., Quinn, R.A., Dadds, M.R. (1994) 'The sleep patterns of normal children.' *Medical Journal of Australia*, **161**, 202–205.

Aschoff, J., Fatranská, M., Giedke, H., Doerr, P., Stamm, D., Wisser, H. (1971) 'Human circadian rhythms in continuous darkness: Entrainment by social cues.' *Science*, **171**, 213–215.

Asperger, H. (1944/1991) 'Autistic psychopathy in childhood.' *In:* Frith, U. (Ed.) *Autism and Asperger Syndrome.* Cambridge: Cambridge University Press, pp. 37–92. (Translated by U. Frith.)

Attwood, T. (1998) *Asperger's Syndrome.* London: Jessica Kingsley.

Bergeron, C., Godbout, R., Mottron, L., Stop, E. (1997) 'Sleep and dreaming in Asperger's syndrome.' *Sleep Research*, **26**, 541. *(Abstract.)*

Berthier, M.L., Santamaria, J., Encabo, H., Tolosa, E.S. (1992) 'Recurrent hypersomnia in two adolescent males with Asperger's syndrome.' *Journal of the American Academy of Child and Adolescent Psychiatry*, **31**, 735–738.

Bramble, D. (1997) 'Rapid-acting treatment for a common sleep problem.' *Developmental Medicine and Child Neurology*, **39**, 543–547.

Clarkson, S., Williams, S., Silva, P.A. (1986) 'Sleep problems in middle childhood – a longitudinal study of sleep problems in a large sample of Dunedin children aged 5–9 years.' *Australian Paediatrics Journal*, **22**, 31–35.

Clements, J., Wing, L., Dunn, G. (1986) 'Sleep problems in handicapped children: A preliminary study.' *Journal of Child Psychology and Psychiatry*, **27**, 399–407.

DeMeyer, M.K. (1979) 'Sleeping problems.' *In: Parents and Children in Autism.* New York: John Wiley, pp. 89–100.

Didden, R., Curfs, L.M.G., Sikkema S.P.E., de Moor, J. (1998) 'Functional assessment and treatment of sleeping problems with developmentally disabled children: six case studies.' *Journal of Behavior Therapy*, **29**, 85–97.

Diomedi, M., Curatolo, P., Scalise, A., Placidi, F., Gigli, G.L. (1999) 'Sleep abnormalities in mentally retarded autistic subjects: Down's syndrome with mental retardation and normal subjects.' *Brain and Development*, **21**, 548–553.

Durand, M.V. (1998) *Sleep Better! A Guide to Improving Sleep for Children with Special Needs.* Baltimore: Paul H. Brookes.

—— Gernert-Dott, P., Mapstone, E. (1996) 'Treatment of sleep disorders in children with developmental disabilities.' *Journal of the Association for Persons with Severe Handicaps*, **21**, 114–122.

Elia, M., Ferri, R., Musumeci, S.A., Bergonzi, P. (1991) 'Rapid eye movement modulation during night sleep in autistic subjects.' *Brain Dysfunction*, **4**, 348–354.

Fisman, S., Wolf, L. (1991) 'The handicapped child: Psychological effects of parental, marital, and sibling relationships.' *Psychiatric Clinics of North America*, **14**, 199–217.

France, K.G., Henderson, J.M.T., Hudson, S.M. (1996) 'Fact, act, and tact. A three stage approach to treating the sleep problems of infants and young children.' *Child and Adolescent Psychiatric Clinics of North America*, **5**, 581–599.

Gillberg, C. (1993) 'Autism and related behaviours.' *Journal of Intellectual Disability Research*, **37**, 343–372.

Godbout, R., Bergeron, C., Stip, E., Mottron, L. (1998) 'A laboratory study of sleep and dreaming in a case of Asperger's syndrome.' *Dreaming*, **8**, 75–88.

—— —— Limoges, E., Stip, E., Mottron L. (2000) 'A laboratory study of sleep in Asperger's syndrome.' *Neuroreport*, **11**, 127–130.

Guilleminault, C., Crowe McCann, C., Quera-Salva, M., Cetel, M. (1993) Light therapy as treatment of dyschronosis in brain impaired children.' *European Journal of Pediatrics*, **152**, 754–759.

Hering, E., Epstein, R., Elroy, S., Iancu, D.R., Zelnik, N. (1999) 'Sleep patterns in autistic children.' *Journal of Autism and Developmental Disorders*, **29**, 143–147.

Horrigan J.P., Barnhill L.J. (1997a) 'Risperidone and explosive aggressive autism.' *Journal of Autism and Developmental Disorders*, **27**, 313–323.

—— —— (1997b) 'More on melatonin.' *Journal of the American Academy of Child and Adolescent Psychiatry*, **36**, 1014. *(Letter.)*

Hoshino, Y., Watanabe, H., Yashima, Y., Kaneko, M., Kumashiro, H. (1984) 'An investigation on the sleep disturbance of autistic children.' *Folia Psychiatrica et Neurologica Japonica*, **38**, 45–51.

Howlin, P. (1984) 'A brief report on the elimination of long term sleeping problems in a 6-year-old autistic boy.' *Behavioural Psychotherapy*, **12**, 257–260.

Hutt, C., Hutt, S.J., Lee, D., Ounsted, C. (1964) 'Arousal and childhood autism.' *Nature*, **204**, 908–909.

Jan, J.E., O'Donnell, M.E. (1996) 'Use of melatonin in the treatment of paediatric sleep disorders.' *Journal of Pineal Research*, **21**, 193–199.

Johnson, C.R. (1996) 'Sleep problems in children with mental retardation and autism.' *Child and Adolescent Psychiatric Clinics of North America*, **5**, 673–683.

Kennedy C.H., Meyer K.A. (1996) 'Sleep deprivation, allergy symptoms, and negatively reinforced problem behavior.' *Journal of Applied Behavior Analysis*, **29**, 133–135.

Kugler, B. (1998) 'The differentiation between autism and Asperger syndrome.' *Autism*, **2**, 11–32.

Lancioni, G.E., O'Reilly, M.F., Basili, G. (1999) 'Review of strategies for treating sleep problems in persons with severe and profound intellectual or multiple disabilities.' *American Journal on Mental Retardation*, **104**, 170–186.

Lord, C. (1998) 'What is melatonin? Is it a useful treatment for sleep problems in autism?' *Journal of Autism*

and Developmental Disorders, **28**, 345–346.

Ma, G., Segawa, M., Nomura, Y., Kondo, Y., Yanagitani, M., Higurashi, M. (1993) 'The development of sleep–wakefulness rhythms in normal infants and young children.' *Tohoku Journal of Experimental Medicine*, **171**, 29–41.

Manjiviona, J., Prior, M. (1999) 'Neuropsychological profiles of children with Asperger syndrome and autism.' *Autism*, **3**, 327–356.

Ornitz, E.M. (1972) 'Development of sleep patterns in autistic children.' *In:* Clemente, C.D., Pupura, D.P., Mayer, E.F. (Eds.) *Sleep and the Maturing Nervous System.* New York: Academic Press, pp. 363–381.

Patzold, L.M., Richdale, A.L., Tonge, B.J. (1998) 'An investigation into the sleep characteristics of children with autism and Asperger's disorder.' *Journal of Paediatrics and Child Health*, **34**, 528–533.

Peeters, T., Gillberg, C. (1999) *Autism: Medical and Educational Aspects. 2nd Edn.* London: Whurr.

Piazza, C.C., Fisher, W.W., Sherer, M. (1997) 'Treatment of multiple sleep problems in children with developmental disabilities: faded bedtime with response cost versus bedtime scheduling.' *Developmental Medicine and Child Neurology*, **39**, 414–418.

—— Hagopian, L.P., Hughes, C.R., Fisher, W.W. (1998) 'Using chronotherapy to treat severe sleep problems: A case study.' *American Journal on Mental Retardation*, **102**, 358–366.

Quine, L. (1991) 'Sleep problems in children with a mental handicap.' *Journal of Mental Deficiency Research*, **35**, 269–290.

Richdale, A.L. (1999) 'Sleep problems in autism: prevalence, cause and intervention.' *Developmental Medicine and Child Neurology*, **41**, 60–66.

—— Prior, M.R. (1995) 'The sleep/wake rhythm in children with autism.' *European Child and Adolescent Psychiatry*, **4**, 175–186.

—— Gavidia-Payne, S., Francis, A., Cotton, S. (2000) 'Stress, behaviour and sleep problems in children with an intellectual disability.' *Journal of Intellectual and Developmental Disability*, **25**, 147–161.

Sadeh, A. (1996) 'Evaluating night wakings in sleep-disturbed infants: A methodological study of parental reports and actigraphy.' *Sleep*, **19**, 657–762.

—— (1997) 'Sleep and melatonin in infants: A preliminary study.' *Sleep*, **20**, 185–191.

Schreck, K.A. (1997) 'Preliminary analysis of sleep disorders in children with developmental disabilities.' Doctoral dissertation, Ohio State University, Ohio, USA.

—— Mulick, J.A. (2000) 'Parental report of sleep problems in children with autism.' *Journal of Autism and Developmental Disorders*, **30**, 127–135.

Simblett, G.J., Wilson, D.N. (1993) 'Asperger's syndrome: three cases and a discussion.' *Journal of Intellectual Disability Research*, **37**, 85–94.

Stores, G. (1996) 'Practitioner review: Assessment and treatment of sleep disorders in children and adolescents.' *Journal of Child Psychology and Psychiatry*, **37**, 907–925.

—— Wiggs, L. (1998) 'Abnormal sleep patterns associated with autism: A brief review of research findings, assessment methods and treatment strategies.' *Autism*, **2**, 157–170.

Szatmari, P. (1991) 'Asperger's syndrome: Diagnosis, treatment, and outcome.' *Psychiatric Clinics of North America*, **14**, 81–93.

Taira, M., Takase, M., Sasaki, H. (1998) 'Sleep disorder in children with autism.' *Psychiatric and Clinical Neurosciences*, **52**, 182–183.

Tanguay, P.E., Ornitz, E.M., Forsythe, A.B., Ritvo, E.R. (1976) 'Rapid eye movement (REM) activity in normal and autistic children during REM sleep.' *Journal of Autism and Childhood Schizophrenia*, **6**, 275–288.

Tonge, B.J., Brereton, A.V., Gray, K.M., Einfeld, S.L. (1999) 'Behavioural and emotional disturbance in high-functioning autism and Asperger syndrome.' *Autism*, **3**, 117–130.

Weiskop, S., Matthews, J., Richdale, A. (1999) 'A parent training program for parents of young children with autism and sleep problems.' *In: Conference Papers and Proceedings, 1999 National Autism Conference, Hobart, Australia*, pp. 227–235.

—— —— (2001) 'Treatment of sleep problems in a 5-year-old boy with autism using behavioural principles.' *Autism. (In press.)*

Wiggs, L., Stores, G. (1996a) 'Severe sleep disturbances and daytime challenging behaviour in children with severe learning disabilities.' *Journal of Intellectual Disability Research*, **40**, 518–528.

—— —— (1996b) 'Sleep problems in children with severe intellectual disabilities: What help is being provided?' *Journal of Applied Research in Intellectual Disabilities*, **9**, 160–165.

Wolf, M., Risley, T., Mees, H. (1964) 'Application of operant conditioning procedures to the behaviour problems of an autistic child.' *Behaviour Research and Therapy*, **1**, 305–312.

191

28
DISTURBANCES OF SLEEP IN THE CHRONIC FATIGUE SYNDROME

Gregory Stores

The chronic fatigue syndrome (CFS) is a contentious topic. The continuing debate (sometimes acrimonious) about its aetiology is reflected in the other terms used to describe the syndrome: postviral fatigue syndrome, myalgic encephalomyelitis (ME) and neurasthenia. The term CFS is preferable because of its essentially descriptive nature.

Discussion of the condition has been helped in recent years by the development of definitions of CFS for purposes of diagnosis in the individual case and for research (Sharpe *et al.* 1991, Fukada *et al.* 1994). The main defining characteristics can be stated as:
- severe disabling mental and physical fatigue made worse by minor exertion
- at least six months in duration (three months in children)
- absence of physical and major psychiatric causes of chronic fatigue.

Other symptoms such as muscle pain, sleep disorder and mood disturbance are common. Wessely *et al.* (1998) have provided a comprehensive account of chronic fatigue and its management; the UK Royal Colleges have issued a guidance report (1997); and the Association for Child Psychology and Psychiatry (1999) has published an account of CFS in children including recommendations for clinical practice.

This last account is welcome because the vast majority of the literature on CFS concerns adults despite evidence that the condition may not be uncommon in children, although its prevalence is not really known (Marcovitch 1997). However often it occurs, CFS is usually a challenge to general practitioners, paediatricians, child psychiatrists and others to whom children with the condition are referred. The Royal Colleges report encourages further research on CFS including its management in children.

Sleep studies in patients with CFS
Most reported studies of sleep have involved adult subjects but the findings are potentially instructive about younger patients. It is clear that sleep complaints of various types appear to be common in adults and also in children with CFS (Marcovitch 1991). The findings are of three main types, according to which aspect of sleep has been investigated.

SLEEP COMPLAINTS
A number of sleep complaints have been reported, not obviously all originating in any one way. In the studies by Whelton *et al.* (1992), Morriss *et al.* (1993) and Schaefer (1995), difficulty getting to sleep, waking at night, unrefreshing sleep and daytime napping were often reported. This remained so when psychiatric and specific sleep disorders had been

excluded and comparisons made with suitable controls (Sharpley *et al.* 1997), and where the possible contribution to sleep disturbance of psychiatric disorder had been controlled (Morriss *et al.* 1997). Usually, possible sleep disorders underlying the sleep complaints (Chapter 3) have not been considered.

SLEEP DISORDERS

In a number of studies, detailed assessments including PSG have revealed specific sleep disorders in a (small) proportion of CFS patients, emphasizing the need to exclude such conditions as obstructive sleep apnoea, periodic limb movements in sleep (sometimes in combination with the restless legs syndrome), and narcolepsy or related disorder (Whelton *et al.* 1988, Krupp *et al.* 1993, Morehouse *et al.* 1994, Ambrogetti and Olson 1994, Buchwald *et al.* 1994, Morehouse and Braha 1995, Le Bon *et al.* 2000). Terman *et al.* (1998) reported that a proportion of adults with CFS have features similar to those of seasonal affective disorder (SAD) including hypersomnia, although others have failed to detect any seasonal fluctuation in CFS symptoms (Garcia-Borreguero *et al.* 1998).

PSG ABNORMALITIES

A variety of nonspecific PSG abnormalities (often not accompanied by clinical symptoms) have been described in CFS patients with or without psychiatric disorder (Morriss *et al.* 1993, Fischler *et al.* 1997, Sharpley *et al.* 1997, Morehouse *et al.* 1998). These are: delayed onset of sleep; poorly sustained sleep with reduced time asleep while in bed (poor 'sleep efficiency'); and, in some patients, a reduced interval between sleep onset and the first period of REM sleep ('short REM latency'). The significance of these findings is unclear, but, collectively, they suggest poor-quality sleep.

The same is true of the findings in a home PSG study of teenagers (age 11–18 years) with CFS diagnosed according to accepted criteria (Stores *et al.* 1998). None of the patients had any formal psychiatric disorder. Compared with controls matched for age and sex, they showed significantly higher levels of sleep disruption by both brief and longer awakenings without any change in other conventional sleep variables. These arousals were often of the type that would be unaccompanied by clinically detectable awakening. The overall fragmentation of sleep seems likely to have impaired the patients' sleep quality (see Chapter 2).

A number of sleep complaints and PSG abnormalities have (inconsistently) been reported in patients, including children and adolescents, with fibromyalgia, which has a debatable relationship to CFS (Wessely *et al.* 1998).

Caution is needed in interpreting these reports of various sleep abnormalities in people with CFS. Because the studies have varied in regard to diagnostic criteria, sleep assessments, comorbidity, ascertainment bias, use and type of controls, and numbers and age of subjects, permissible generalizations are limited and much further effort is required to clarify the many issues involved.

Relationship between sleep disturbance and chronic fatigue syndrome
Sleep and CFS might be linked in a number of ways.

- It is important to consider both daytime activity patterns and nocturnal aspects. For example, difficulty getting off to sleep can be caused by daytime inactivity, especially if naps are taken during the day. Long periods awake in bed can lead to conditioned insomnia (Chapter 4). Alternatively, persistently going to bed late may cause the delayed sleep phase syndrome (Chapter 5) with a physiological inability to go to sleep, considerable difficulty getting up in the morning and excessive sleepiness during the day.
- Psychological or psychiatric aspects are further possible factors. For example, if there is an aversion to school, this abnormal sleep pattern may be a preferred way of avoiding going there. Waking at night or feeling unrefreshed after sleeping (other sleep complaints reported in patients with CFS) are not obviously the result of daytime inactivity and may be due to coexisting anxiety or depression, or sleep disturbance for some other reason.
- It is conceivable that physical pathology underlying CFS in some patients could play a causal role in the development of certain sleep abnormalities.
- Rather than the sleep complaint being the result of the chronic fatigue condition, it is possible (as indicated above) that in some cases a sleep disorder is the primary *cause* of CFS symptoms. This possibility arises because of the overlap between CFS symptoms and the complaints of people whose sleep has been reduced or disturbed, *i.e.* fatigue, low mood, physical symptoms, and poor memory and concentration. Even where sleep disturbance is not the primary cause of the CFS symptoms, it is possible for these symptoms to be made worse by persistent sleep disturbance.

Clinical implications

Irrespective of differing views about the aetiology of CFS, as part of the overall comprehensive assessment of people with CFS, including young patients (Association of Child Psychology and Psychiatry 1999), it is appropriate to enquire explicitly about sleep problems and to describe them in detail. In this way, it should be possible to identify ways in which the young person's sleep can be improved, in the expectation that this will be beneficial, including helping the child to cope with other problems. As discussed in Chapter 5, a distinction needs to be made between sleepiness and fatigue. The two may coexist but the causes of each tend to be different. Sleep hygiene principles (Chapter 3) are likely to be an important part of treatment for any child. If enquiries suggest that there is a specific sleep disorder such as a sleep-related breathing problem, special investigations will be required for diagnosis and also appropriate treatment as discussed in earlier chapters.

REFERENCES

Ambrogetti, A., Olson, L.G. (1994) 'Consideration of narcolepsy in the differential diagnosis of chronic fatigue syndrome.' *Medical Journal of Australia*, **160**, 426–429.
Association for Child Psychology and Psychiatry (1999) *Chronic Fatigue Syndrome: Helping Children and Adolescents.* London: Association for Child Psychology and Psychiatry.
Buchwald, D., Pascualy, R., Bombardier, C., Kith, P. (1994) 'Sleep disorders in patients with chronic fatigue.' *Clinical Infectious Diseases*, **18**, Suppl. 1, S68–S72.
Fischler, B., Le Bon, O., Hoffman, G., Cluydts, R., Kaufman, L., De Meirleir, K. (1997) 'Sleep anomalies in the chronic fatigue syndrome. A comorbidity study.' *Neuropsychobiology*, **35**, 115–122.
Fukada, K., Straus, S., Hickie, I., Sharpe, M.C., Dobbins, J.G., Komaroff, A. (1994) 'The chronic fatigue

syndrome: a comprehensive approach to its definition and study.' *Annals of Internal Medicine*, **121**, 953–959.

Garcia-Borreguero, D., Dale, J.K., Rosenthal, N.E., Chiara, A., O'Fallon, A., Bartko, J.J., Straus, S.E. (1998) 'Lack of seasonal variation of symptoms in patients with chronic fatigue syndrome.' *Psychiatry Research*, **77**, 71–77.

Krupp, L.B., Jandorf, L., Coyle, P.K., Mendelson, W.B. (1993) 'Sleep disturbance in chronic fatigue syndrome.' *Journal of Psychosomatic Research*, **37**, 325–331.

Le Bon, O., Fischler, B., Hoffman, G., Murphy J.R., De Meirleir, K., Cluydts, R., Pelc, I. (2000) 'How significant are primary sleep disorders and sleepiness in the chronic fatigue syndrome?' *Sleep Research Online*, **3**(2), 43–48. (http://www.sro.org/2000/LeBon/43/)

Marcovitch, H. (1991) 'Chronic fatigue states in children.' *In:* Jenkins, R., Mowbray, J. (Eds.) *Post-viral Fatigue Syndrome.* Chichester: Wiley, pp. 335–344.

—— (1997) 'Managing chronic fatigue syndrome in children.' *British Medical Journal*, **314**, 1635–1636.

Morehouse, R., Braha, D. (1995) 'Sleep characteristics in patients with chronic fatigue syndrome.' *Sleep Research*, **24**, 409. *(Abstract.)*

—— MacDonald, D., Hause, D., Marrie, T., Braha, D. (1994) 'Leg movements in sleep and complaints of restless legs in patients with chronic fatigue syndrome.' *Sleep Research*, **23**, 373. *(Abstract.)*

—— Flanigan, M., MacDonald, D.D., Braha, D., Shapiro, C. (1998) 'Depression and short REM latency in subjects with chronic fatigue syndrome.' *Psychosomatic Medicine*, **60**, 347–351.

Morriss, R., Sharpe, M., Sharpley, A.L., Cowen, P.J, Hawton, K., Morris, J. (1993) 'Abnormalities of sleep in patients with the chronic fatigue syndrome.' *British Medical Journal*, **306**, 1161–1163.

—— Wearden, A.J., Battersby, L. (1997) 'The relation of sleep difficulties to fatigue, mood and disability in chronic fatigue syndrome.' *Journal of Psychosomatic Research*, **42**, 597–605.

Royal College of Physicians, Royal College of Psychiatrists, Royal College of General Practitioners (1997) *Chronic Fatigue Syndrome. 2nd printing with amendments.* London: Royal College of Physicians.

Schaefer, K.M. (1995) 'Sleep disturbance and fatigue in women with fibromyalgia and chronic fatigue syndrome.' *Journal of Obstetric, Gynecological and Neonatal Nursing*, **24**, 229–233.

Sharpe, M.C., Archard, L.C., Banatvala, J.E., Borysiewicz, L.K., Clare, A.W., David, A., Edwards, R.H., Hawton, K.E., Lambert, H.P., *et al.* (1991) 'A report—chronic fatigue syndrome: guidelines for research.' *Journal of the Royal Society of Medicine*, **84**, 118–121.

Sharpley, A., Clements, A., Hawton, K., Sharpe M. (1997) 'Do patients with "pure" chronic fatigue syndrome (neurasthenia) have abnormal sleep?' *Psychosomatic Medicine*, **59**, 592–596.

Stores, G., Fry, A., Crawford, C., Wiggs, L. (1998) 'Sleep abnormalities demonstrated by home polysomnography in teenagers with chronic fatigue syndrome.' *Journal of Psychosomatic Research*, **45**, 85–92.

Terman, M., Levine, S.M., Terman, J.S., Doherty, S. (1998) 'Chronic fatigue syndrome and seasonal affective disorder: Comorbidity, diagnostic overlap, and implications for treatment.' *American Journal of Medicine*, **105** (Suppl.), 115S–124S.

Wessely, S., Hotopf, M., Sharpe, M. (1998) *Chronic Fatigue and its Syndromes.* Oxford: Oxford University Press.

Whelton, C., Saskin, P., Salit, I. (1988) 'Post-viral fatigue syndrome and sleep.' *Sleep Research*, **17**, 307. *(Abstract.)*

—— Salit, I., Moldofsky, H. (1992) 'Sleep, Epstein–Barr virus infection, musculoskeletal pain, and depressive symptoms in chronic fatigue syndrome.' *Journal of Rheumatology*, **19**, 939–943.

29
SLEEP IN OTHER PSYCHIATRIC DISORDERS OF CHILDHOOD AND ADOLESCENCE

Gregory Stores

High rates of sleep disorder of the various types have been reported consistently in child psychiatric groups (Salzarulo and Chevalier 1983, Simonds and Parraga 1984, Sadeh *et al.* 1995), but research on the details of these disorders has been relatively sparse and mainly confined to the psychiatric conditions reviewed in the last few chapters. However, there are some reports on other child and adolescent psychiatric conditions, general accounts of which are available in Graham *et al.* (1999) and/or the additional references provided.

Conduct disorder

Conduct disorder (persistent failure to control behaviour appropriately within socially defined rules) and oppositional–defiant behaviour in younger children (with the accent on aggression and defiance) have been the subject of virtually no sleep research directed specifically to them, despite the commonness with which these difficult behavioural problems occur. Coble *et al.* (1984) reported that, compared with age-matched controls, the polysomnography of prepubertal boys with a diagnosis of conduct disorder showed less sleep and more arousals during sleep, but more slow wave sleep. These findings can be interpreted as preliminary evidence of a reduction in the duration and (to some extent) the quality of overnight sleep. Compatible findings are those reported by Lavigne *et al.* (1999) that within a large group of 2- to 5-year-olds, parental reports of shorter sleep were associated with various problems including difficult behaviour, and the evidence outlined in Chapter 1 that sleep disturbance predisposes children to socially undesirable behaviour including that of an ADHD type. From general principles, it might be expected that children with antisocial behaviour will have less than satisfactory sleep patterns, including irregular sleep habits, because of such associated factors as poor parenting, generally disordered families and unregulated way of life. *Substance abuse* (Gillin and Drummond 2000) could be an additional factor, but this is another area of neglect in sleep research considering the large number of children and adolescents affected in this way.

Eating disorders

Sleep disturbance associated with eating disorders has attracted somewhat more attention by researchers (Benca and Casper 2000). Adolescents and others with *anorexia nervosa* do not usually complain about their sleep, although polysomnographic studies have shown

that sleep is often curtailed with various abnormalities of sleep architecture. Patients with *bulimia nervosa* may describe binge eating at night after initially falling asleep, with only partial recollection of eating. The various unresolved issues concerning sleep abnormalities and eating disorders include the contribution made by associated psychiatric illness, especially depression, as distinct from some intrinsic aspect of the eating disorder itself or, in the case of anorexia nervosa, the effects of starvation and weight loss on sleep.

Sleep-related eating disorder, characterized by often bizarre eating practices at night (Schenck *et al.* 1993), may begin in childhood. The behaviour is mainly linked to sleep-walking but may also occur in people with other sleep disorders or psychiatric disturbance including mood disorders, anxiety or substance abuse. The relationship of the condition to daytime eating disorder is debatable (Winkelman *et al.* 1999).

Tourette syndrome

There are various intriguing sleep aspects of the neuropsychiatric condition Tourette syndrome. Consistently high rates of clinical sleep disturbance have been reported (including sleeplessness and parasomnias), and polygraphic studies have demonstrated a variety of abnormalities associated with impaired sleep efficiency and quality (Glaze *et al.* 1983). Possible explanations include seemingly integral aspects of the disorder; others implicate comorbid conditions.

Sleep disturbances have been reported as more frequent than expected in family members of patients with the condition (Nee *et al.* 1980). More directly relevant to broken sleep is the fact that, unlike in many other movement disorders, the characteristic tics are present during sleep in all stages and are likely to disrupt sleep continuity. A different type of sleep instability has been suggested in the form of an increased tendency to sudden partial arousals from slow wave sleep. This is thought to account for the reported high frequency of sleep-walking and night terrors in patients with Tourette syndrome (Barabas *et al.* 1984a) and possibly other abnormal behaviours including coprolalia during sleep (Burd and Kerbeshian 1988). In early studies, nocturnal enuresis (thought at the time to be an arousal disorder) was also reported to be associated with Tourette syndrome. These arousal disorders were taken to suggest basic neurotransmitter abnormalities especially involving serotonin (Barabas *et al.* 1984b). Sleep has been said to improve with successful treatment of the syndrome (Jankovic *et al.* 1984).

An alternative to sleep disturbances being an intrinsic part of Tourette syndrome is the possibility that they are caused by commonly associated psychiatric disorders, notably attention deficit hyperactivity disorder (ADHD) (Allen *et al.* 1992) and obsessive–compulsive disorder (OCD). Drake *et al.* (1992) suggested that patients with Tourette syndrome associated with one or other of these disorders might show sleep abnormalities associated with slow wave sleep or REM sleep respectively, reflecting different biochemical abnormalities. However, it has been argued that rather than being discrete disorders, Tourette syndrome, ADHD and OCD are part of a behavioural spectrum (Comings 1995). The more recent preliminary report by Vorderholzer *et al.* (1997) of frequent periodic limb movements during sleep in young unmedicated adults with Tourette syndrome adds to the speculation about possible underlying neurotransmitter abnormalities.

Schizophrenia

Long-standing attempts to identify diagnostically useful characteristics in the polysomnograms of adults with schizophrenia have been unsuccessful (Benson and Zarcone 2000). Comparable studies in young patients are very limited and equally unhelpful diagnostically, despite the suggestion that sleep is more disrupted in adolescent schizophrenic patients than in those with major depressive disorder (Riemann *et al.* 1995). However, clinical experience indicates that sleep complaints are very common and can be very striking, taking the form of difficulty getting to sleep, disrupted overnight sleep (including frightening parasomnias) and even a reversal of normal sleep–wake patterns. It remains an open question how far these sleep abnormalities are attributable to the schizophrenic illness itself or to such comorbid conditions as depression, substance abuse, or sleep disruption including circadian sleep–wake cycle disorders due to a disorganized way of life. Excessive daytime sleepiness may be the result of such factors as these or over-sedation from medication. Douglass *et al.* (1991) have reported that some patients diagnosed as schizophrenic actually have narcolepsy with prominent hallucinatory phenomena intruding into the awake state.

In general, antipsychotic drugs improve both polysomnographic and clinical aspects of sleep, partly through their sedative action, but side-effects (notably akathisia) can disrupt sleep. Sleep hygiene should be strongly encouraged as part of overall management. Just as sleep complaints can be a first sign of the onset of serious psychiatric disorder (Ford and Kamerow 1989), a recurrence of sleep complaints can be an early feature of relapse (Van Kammen *et al.* 1986).

Additional psychiatric conditions

Prominent sleep disturbance is a well-recognized clinical feature of *manic and hypomanic states*. The manic patient usually feels a reduced need to sleep, although a loss of sleep immediately preceding a manic episode might contribute to the mania (Wehr 1991). By the same token, promotion of adequate sleep is an important part of treating mania. Mood stabilizing drugs (lithium, carbamazepine and sodium valproate) generally have a sedating effect, especially lithium, the use of which, however, has been linked to the development of sleepwalking (Landry *et al.* 1999) and restless legs syndrome (Terao *et al.* 1991).

Little research attention has been paid to sleep aspects of *obsessive–compulsive disorder* (OCD). The sleep-disrupting effects of anxiety (Chapter 23) are likely to apply in many patients, and prolonged checking behaviours at bedtime will delay sleep onset. The limited polysomnographic data suggest that sleep quality (including that of adolescents with OCD) is poor, but for reasons that need to be clarified (Rapoport *et al.* 1981, Insel *et al.* 1982).

In addition to the main depressive disorders reviewed in Chapter 24, *seasonal affective disorder* (SAD), which can occur in children and adolescents (Glod and Baisden 1999), is characterized by excessive sleepiness or other sleep disturbances.

Psychiatric states of *organic origin* will usually have prominent sleep disturbance of an acute or chronic type depending on the underlying process. In the more insidious forms of brain disease, behavioural change (including sleep disturbance) can be misinterpreted as psychological in origin as in the child with subacute sclerosing panencephalitis reported by Forrest and Stores (1996).

Sleep-related violence (Broughton and Shimizu 1997) is occasionally described in children and adolescents and may be attributable to sleepwalking (Oswald and Evans 1985), REM sleep behaviour disorder (Sheldon and Jacobsen 1998), or (very rarely and in an essentially non-directed way) nocturnal seizures. In their description of the use of sleep studies in the assessment of night-time violence, Mahowald *et al.* (1992) refer to *psychogenic dissociative states* as part of the differential diagnosis.

'*Pseudoparasomnias*' can also occur, even in young people (Molaie and Deutsch 1997), in which polysomnography demonstrates that at the time the patient appears to be asleep he is actually awake. It is also of importance to both child psychiatrists and paediatricians that in *Munchausen syndrome by proxy* complaints about the child's sleep can be a presenting feature (Griffith and Slovick 1989).

REFERENCES

Allen, R.P., Singer, H.S., Brown, J.E., Salam, M.M. (1992) 'Sleep disorders in Tourette syndrome: A primary or unrelated problem?' *Pediatric Neurology*, **8**, 275–280.

Barabas, G., Matthews, W.S., Ferrari, M. (1984a) 'Disorders of arousal in Gilles de la Tourette's syndrome.' *Neurology*, **34**, 815–817.

—— —— —— (1984b) 'Somnambulism in children with Tourette syndrome.' *Developmental Medicine and Child Neurology*, **26**, 457–460.

Benca, R.M., Casper, R.C. (2000) 'Eating disorders.' *In:* Kryger, M., Roth, T., Dement, W.C. (Eds.) *Principles and Practice of Sleep Medicine, 3rd Edn.* Philadelphia: W.B. Saunders, pp. 1169–1175.

Benson, K.L., Zarcone, V.P. (2000) 'Schizophrenia.' *In:* Kryger, M., Roth, T., Dement, W.C. (Eds.) *Principles and Practice of Sleep Medicine, 3rd Edn.* Philadelphia: W.B. Saunders, pp. 1159–1167.

Broughton, R.J., Shimizu, T. (1997) 'Dangerous behaviors by night.' *In:* Shapiro, C., McCall Smith, A. (Eds.) *Forensic Aspects of Sleep.* Chichester: Wiley, pp. 65–83.

Burd, L., Kerbeshian, J. (1988) 'Nocturnal coprolalia and phonic tics.' *American Journal of Psychiatry*, **145**, 132. *(Letter.)*

Coble, P.A., Taska, L.S., Kupfer, D.J., Kasdin, A.E., Unis, A., French, N. (1984) 'EEG sleep 'abnormalities' in preadolescent boys with a diagnosis of conduct disorder.' *Journal of the American Academy of Child Psychiatry*, **23**, 438–447.

Comings, D.E. (1995) 'Tourette's syndrome: a behavioral spectrum disorder.' *Behavioral Neurology of Movement Disorders*, **65**, 293–303.

Douglass, A.B., Hays, P., Pazderka, F., Russell, J.M. (1991) 'Florid refractory schizophrenias that turned out to be treatable variants of HLA-associated narcolepsy.' *Journal of Nervous and Mental Disease*, **179**, 12–17.

Drake, M.E., Hietter, S.A., Bogner, J.E., Andrews, J.M. (1992) 'Cassette EEG sleep recordings in Gilles de la Tourette syndrome.' *Clinical Electroencephalography*, **23**, 142–146.

Ford, D.E., Kamerow, D.B. (1989) 'Epidemiological study of sleep disturbances and psychiatric disorders: An opportunity for prevention?' *Journal of the American Medical Association*, **262**, 1479–1484.

Forrest, G., Stores, G. (1996) 'Subacute sclerosing panencephalitis presenting with psychosis and possible sexual abuse.' *European Child and Adolescent Psychiatry*, **5**, 110–113.

Gillin, J.C., Drummond, S.P.A. (2000) 'Medication and substance abuse.' *In:* Kryger, M., Roth, T., Dement, W.C. (Eds.) *Principles and Practice of Sleep Medicine, 3rd Edn.* Philadelphia: W.B. Saunders, pp. 1176–1195.

Glaze, D.G., Frost, J.D., Jancovic, J. (1983) 'Sleep in Gilles de la Tourette's syndrome: disorder of arousal.' *Neurology*, **33**, 586–592.

Glod, C.A., Baisden, N. (1999) 'Seasonal affective disorder in children and adolescents.' *Journal of the American Psychiatric Nurses Association*, **5**, 29–33.

Graham, P., Turk, J., Verhulst, F. (1999) *Child Psychiatry: A Developmental Approach. 3rd Edn.* Oxford: Oxford University Press.

Griffith, J.L., Slovick, L.S. (1989) 'Munchausen syndrome by proxy and sleep disorders medicine.' *Sleep*, **12**, 178–183.

Insel, T.R., Gillin, J.C., Moore, A., Mendelson, W.B., Lowenstein, R.J., Murphy, D.L. (1982) 'The sleep of patients with obsessive–compulsive disorder.' *Archives of General Psychiatry*, **39**, 1372–1377.

Jancovic, J., Glaze, D.G., Frost, J.D. (1984) 'Effects of tetrabenazine on tics and sleep of Gilles de la Tourette syndrome.' *Neurology*, **34**, 688–692.

Landry, P., Warnes, H., Nielson, T., Montplaisir, J. (1999) 'Somnambulistic-like behaviour in patients attending a lithium clinic.' *International Clinical Psychopharmacology*, **14**, 173–175.

Lavigne, J.V., Arend, R., Rosenbaum, D., Smith, A., Weissbluth, M., Binns, H.J., Christoffel, K.K. (1999) 'Sleep and behavior problems among preschoolers.' *Journal of Developmental and Behaviroal Pediatrics*, **20**, 164–169.

Mahowald, M.W., Schenck, C.H., Rosen, G.M., Hurwitz, T.D. (1992) 'The role of a sleep disorder center in evaluating sleep violence.' *Archives of Neurology*, **49**, 604–607.

Molaie, M., Deutsch, G.K. (1997) 'Psychogenic events presenting as parasomnia.' *Sleep*, **20**, 402–405.

Nee, L.E., Caine, E.D., Polinsky, R.J., Eldridge, R., Ebert, M.H. (1980) 'Gilles de la Tourette's syndrome. Clinical and family study of 50 cases.' *Annals of Neurology*, **7**, 41–49.

Oswald, I., Evans, J. (1985) 'On serious violence during sleepwalking.' *British Medical Journal*, **149**, 120–121.

Rapoport, J., Elkins, R., Langer, D.H., Sceery, W., Buchsbaum, M.S., Gillin, C., Murphy, D.L., Zahn, T.P., Lake, R., *et al.* (1981) 'Childhood obsessive–compulsive disorder.' *American Journal of Psychiatry*, **138**, 1545–1554.

Riemann, D., Kammerer, J., Low, H., Schmidt, M.H. (1995) 'Sleep in adolescents with primary major depression and schizophrenia: a pilot study.' *Journal of Child Psychology and Psychiatry*, **36**, 313–326.

Sadeh, A., McGuire, J.P.D., Saches, H., Seifer, R., Tremblay, A., Civita, R., Hayden, R.M. (1995) 'Sleep and psychological characteristics of children on a psychiatric inpatient unit.' *Journal of the American Academy of Child and Adolescent Psychiatry*, **74**, 813–819.

Salzarulo, P., Chevalier, A. (1983) 'Sleep problems in children and their relationships with early disturbances of waking–sleeping rhythms.' *Sleep*, **6**, 47–51.

Schenck, C.H., Hurwitz, T.D., O'Connor, K.A., Mahowald, M.W. (1993) 'Additional categories of sleep-related eating disorders and the current status of treatment.' *Sleep*, **16**, 457–466.

Sheldon, S.H., Jacobsen, J. (1998) 'REM-sleep motor disorder in children.' *Journal of Child Neurology*, **13**, 257–260.

Simonds, J.F., Parraga, H. (1984) 'Sleep behaviors and disorders in children and adolescents evaluated at psychiatric clinics.' *Developmental and Behavioral Pediatrics*, **5**, 6–10.

Terao, T., Terao, M., Yoshimura, R., Abe, K. (1991) 'Restless legs syndrome induced by lithium.' *Biological Psychiatry*, **30**, 1167–1170.

Van Kammen, D.P., Van Kammen, W.B., Peters, J.L., Rosen, J., Slauski, R.C., Neylan, T., Linnoila, M. (1986) 'CSF, MHPG, sleep and psychosis in schizophrenia.' *Clinical Neuropharmacology*, **9**, 575–577.

Vorderholzer, U., Müller, N., Haag, C., Riemann, D., Straube, A. (1997) 'Periodic limb movements during sleep are a frequent finding in patients with Gilles de la Tourette's syndrome.' *Journal of Neurology*, **244**, 521–526.

Wehr, T.A. (1991) 'Sleep loss as a possible mediator of diverse causes of mania.' *British Journal of Psychiatry*, **159**, 576–578.

Winkelman, J.W., Herzog, D.B., Fava, M. (1999) 'The prevalence of sleep-related eating disorder in psychiatric and non-psychiatric populations.' *Psychological Medicine*, **29**, 1461–1466.

SECTION SIX

ENVOI

30
FUTURE DEVELOPMENTS

Gregory Stores and Luci Wiggs

Hopefully, the preceding chapters will have amply demonstrated that sleep disturbance occupies a particularly important position in very many disorders of development of a primarily physical or psychological origin. The case for much more attention being paid to sleep disturbance in children with such disorders may be summarized as follows.

- It is common, indeed likely to be affecting most children with such disorders.
- Especially if persistent and severe (as is likely to be the case), sleep disturbance causes significant additional difficulties for the child and the family, impairing their ability to cope with other problems.
- The child's developmental difficulties (of both cognitive and behavioural types) may well be exacerbated by persistent sleep disruption.
- Although not generally appreciated, sufficient is already known about children's sleep and its many types of disorder to allow an accurate diagnosis in most individual cases.
- Given diagnostic accuracy (in terms of the child's underlying sleep disorder rather than simply the symptom of sleep disturbance), an appropriate choice can be made from the range of treatments that are available.
- Committed use of treatment, selected in this way, is likely to at least lessen the child's sleep problem (even if it is severe and of long standing), to the benefit of the child himself and other family members.

Public education

Unfortunately, this happy state of affairs, although achievable in principle, often seems not to be attained in practice. This view is supported partly by empirical evidence (Wiggs and Stores 1996) but also by inference from the fact that, as discussed in the opening chapter, sleep and its disorders feature so little (if at all) in the training of professionals contributing to the care of children with disorders of development. Inevitably, comprehensive services for children with sleep problems are very few and far between. In the absence of more widespread interest and experience in each child's own locality, the effectiveness of national centres providing advice is necessarily limited despite the assessment and advice being valued by many parents (Stores and Wiggs 1998).

The future, therefore, should not be seen to lie entirely in the provision of centres with a specialized interest in sleep disorders. Improvement is required at all levels, both lay and professional.

Basic health education should include information about the central role of adequate sleep in the maintenance of health and well-being. In the case of parents, there would be a

distinct advantage if planning for parenthood included ways of promoting sleep habits from an early age (often antenatal classes are organized with the moment of delivery as the end-point rather than quite possibly the start of the most challenging phase of parenting practice and responsibility).

There have been few attempts to instruct parents of very young children in the hope of preventing the development of sleep problems. Of course, parental instruction is unlikely to be effective in preventing some sleep disorders (*e.g.* sleep-related breathing problems). However, it is worth considering the possibility that even those sleep disorders that may not be responsive to preventive techniques and parental instruction might be identified more rapidly if parents were made aware of the basic features of common sleep disorders and their daytime consequences. On the other hand, for sleep disorders in which parenting practices are likely to be implicated, instruction and advice is likely to be of help. Encouragingly, recent research suggests that administering advice to parents even in sim-plified form (such as a booklet and limited personal contact with a therapist) is almost as effective as conventionally administered, therapist-led behavioural programmes for the treatment of sleeplessness problems in children with severe intellectual impairments (Mont-gomery and Stores 2000). The possibility that similar methods might be equally useful as a preventive measure needs investigation.

It is essential that parents of developmentally delayed children (and their professional advisors) should know that sleep disturbance is not an inevitable accompaniment of their child's basic condition and that treatment can be very effective.

Service provision and professional training

Needless to say, it is no use raising parental expectations without an informed professional service providing accurate diagnosis and effective treatment. Such a service for all children can be envisaged as operating at three levels (Stores 2001):

- *primary care*, for the relatively straightforward sleep problems such as settling and night-waking problems or nocturnal enuresis, which are already treated effectively by some health visitors or general-practice-based psychologists
- community or hospital *paediatric services* for more difficult diagnostic or treatment problems, preferably working in close association with colleagues in child psychiatry where psychological complications are prominent (although *child psychiatrists* themselves should be well versed in children's sleep disorders in general, including physical aspects)
- *specialized sleep disorder services*, perhaps on a regional basis, for diagnostic or treatment purposes where attempts at the primary and secondary levels have not been adequate.

For such a system to operate effectively, teaching and training of all personnel involved at these three levels need to improve dramatically. Because of the educational shortcomings to which reference was made in Chapter 1, no professional group is exempt. That is, adequate instruction and experience needs to be provided routinely in the training of general prac-titioners, health visitors, health psychologists, clinical and educational psychologists, community and hospital paediatricians, paediatric neurologists, child and adolescent psychiatrists, specialists in children with intellectual impairments, and any other group contributing to child healthcare services in the broadest sense.

Each of these groups will need a special emphasis and varying degrees of detail in their training, but for all of them certain aspects of sleep and its disorders could form a basic core curriculum, the substance of which is readily available in the sources of further information recommended in the opening chapter. Ways of promoting effective improvements in professional teaching and training in sleep-disorder medicine have been discussed by Sateia *et al.* (2000). Table 30.1 contains a suggested framework for basic training in children's sleep disorders that would be suitable for all those involved in child healthcare. The introduction of such content into teaching and training courses would represent a much needed advance in awareness of these important aspects of child development and pathology, and an understanding of how help can be provided.

Other requirements

There are countless other research possibilities and clinical issues arising from the accounts provided in earlier chapters. Some that are relevant to children's sleep disorders in general (such as the need to study further the effects of persistent sleep disturbance on learning and behaviour and to devise appropriate measures for this purpose) are discussed elsewhere (Stores 2001). However, there are some special considerations regarding children with disorders of development.

Incorporation into clinical practice of the information already available about the diagnosis and management of children's sleep disorders would improve standards of care to a very large extent. It is obvious from the preceding chapters, however, that much more remains to be described about sleep disturbance in children with developmental problems, who, in many ways, are a particularly neglected group in this respect. Four aspects can be summarized.

(1) Aspects in need of systematic research include some very basic *epidemiological issues and clinical descriptions*. These include the occurrence of the various types of sleep disorder in children with disorders of development. As mentioned previously, it is not unreasonable to assume that any child with such a disorder is likely to have significant sleep disturbance. Screening questions as suggested in Chapter 3 should be asked routinely, and positive responses followed up by detailed enquiries about the nature of the underlying sleep disorder. This alone would help ensure a more balanced view of the pattern of sleep disorders compared with the patchy account available at present caused by the omission of even basic enquiries.

For the purposes of clinical practice as well as research, more sophisticated enquiries will be required for a definitive diagnosis where this depends partly on physiological findings. A case in point is sleep-disordered breathing (widely distributed in neurodevelopmentally disordered children in particular), for which a different approach is needed in children compared with adults to avoid cases being missed or the degree of severity being misjudged (Marcus 2000). Similarly, accounts based on children in general may need to be modified when applied to those with developmental disorders. Possible differences include the clinical manifestations of some of the parasomnias, the official classification of which is based on the stage of sleep with which they are usually associated (Chapter 6). This classification presupposes normal overnight sleep architecture, which cannot be assumed, especially in

TABLE 30.1
Suggested framework for training in children's sleep disorders for paediatricians, primary care doctors and other child healthcare personnel

Subject matter

1. *General issues*
   - Children's sleep disorders in the general population and high-risk groups (paediatric, psychiatric, intellectually impaired)
   - Developmental effects: psychological, physical, family

2. *Basic aspects of sleep and its disorders*
   - Normal sleep including developmental changes in sleep physiology of clinical significance
   - Types of sleep disturbance: sleep loss, poor quality sleep, mistiming of sleep phase
   - Aetiological factors: physical, psychological
   - Classification of children's sleep disorders
   - Assessment: clinical, special investigations

3. *Sleeplessness and its treatment*
   - Definition and prevalence
   - Infants: Excessive crying, colic, night-time feeds
   - Toddlers: Napping
     - Settling problems
     - Recommendations for bedtime
     - Behavioural treatments
     - Medication issues
   - Middle childhood: Night-time fears
     - Night waking including early morning waking
   - Adolescence: Circadian sleep–wake cycle disorders

4. *Excessive sleepiness and its treatment*
   - Definition and persistence
   - Insufficient sleep and circadian rhythm disorders
   - Poor quality sleep, *e.g.* obstructive sleep apnoea
   - Conditions with increased sleep requirements, *e.g.* narcolepsy

5. *Parasomnias and their management*
   - Primary sleep parasomnias related to different sleep stages, *e.g.* head-banging, sleepwalking, sleep terrors, nightmares
   - Parasomnias secondary to physical disorder (*e.g.* nocturnal epilepsies) or psychological disorder (*e.g.* panic attacks)
   - Differential diagnosis

Competencies
- Taking a sleep history and performing the relevant clinical assessments
- Use of and interpretation of sleep diaries
- Knowing indications for special investigations including polysomnography
- Basics of interpreting results of special investigations
- Knowing uses and limitations of drug treatments
- Organizing basic behavioural treatments
- Recognizing indications for referral to specialized services

children (or adults for that matter) with central nervous system pathology. While the need for a whole new system for classifying the parasomnias in such patients is debatable, the possibility should be considered that not all the usually described manifestations (including timing) of the various parasomnias may apply.

This issue will only be resolved by detailed investigation of night-time episodes of behavioural disturbance in developmentally disordered children. This is a particularly neglected

area compared with investigations of sleeplessness problems. It is also a difficult subject, not least because communication about subjective features may be a problem. However, the effort to achieve a precise diagnosis is worthwhile in order to avoid uncertainty and potentially inappropriate treatment. This point was made in the study by Hunt and Stores (1994) of children with tuberous sclerosis. It was found that in a high proportion of cases the nature of night-time events was unclear from the description available. In these circumstances there is a risk that the episodes would be assumed to be epileptic in nature and in some instances erroneously treated as a consequence.

(2) One of the difficulties in interpreting many of the earlier studies of sleep abnormalities in children with an intellectual impairment was the inclusion of aetiologically very mixed groups. To understand the pathogenesis of the sleep disturbance there is much in favour of identifying the profile of sleep disorders in relatively homogenous categories regarding the nature of the underlying condition, and ideally severity, age, comorbidity and other factors of likely causal significance.

Subgrouping according to specific syndrome raises the possibility that *behavioural phenotypes* may include characteristic types of sleep disturbance. The difficulties of identifying behavioural features ascribable to the biological origins of particular developmental disorders have been discussed by Flint (1996). The care required in convincingly demonstrating this attribution applies equally to disordered sleep.

At present there is little evidence of sleep disturbances "consistently associated with, and specific to a syndrome with a chromosomal or genetic aetiology" (Flint 1996). As demonstrated in earlier chapters, the requirement of consistency is commonly met, but specificity is not. In Smith–Magenis syndrome (Chapter 14) there is a suggestion of a specific pattern of disrupted overnight sleep, persisting from an early age, comprising short bursts of sleep and prolonged awakenings terminating in very early waking with extremely disturbed behaviour. The inappropriate laughing or singing, and other disruptive and destructive behaviour during the night reported in some children with Sanfilippo syndrome (Chapter 11) also seems to be an unusual combination, although a similar type of disturbance (including laughing episodes during night-time awakenings) has been reported to occur in a high proportion of girls with Rett syndrome (Chapter 13) and also in a significant proportion of children with autistic spectrum disorders (Wiggs and Stores 2000). These possibilities of specific types of sleep disturbance can be considered adequately only by means of detailed reporting in the syndromes in question and also in children with other disorders for comparison.

(3) It should be axiomatic that all children with sleep disturbance, including those with severe disorders of physical or psychological development, receive the same high standard of *investigation and care*. As discussed in Chapter 3, polysomnography is indicated in only the minority of cases of sleep disturbance. Where hospital recordings are necessary (*e.g.* to include detailed respiratory monitoring), a setting and procedure specially devised for children, such as the service described by Brouillette *et al.* (2000), are the ideal but are rarely available, and there is a need for much more provision of this type for selected cases.

However, as cooperation for special investigations such as sleep recordings may be difficult to obtain in children with serious behavioural or emotional problems, there is a

need for minimally intrusive recording systems where their use is really required. As also described in Chapter 3, home polysomnography can be useful where less detailed sleep studies are sufficient for addressing the particular issue in question, but further developments in the standardization of this procedure when used for children with developmental disorders would be useful. One potentially valuable method, capable of providing quite detailed information about sleep physiology in a minimally intrusive way, involves recording by means of a single EEG channel with analysis based on neural network theory (Tarrasenko *et al.* 2001). Actometry (also described in Chapter 3) is an exciting area for the future, offering a practical and useful way of assessing basic sleep–wake patterns, although validation of the scoring procedure with developmentally disordered populations would be helpful. Personal experience, and reports in the literature, suggest that recording failures are few (even in very disturbed children) when the procedure is followed in a careful and sensitive way.

(4) A recurrent theme throughout this book has been the need for accurate diagnosis of each child's sleep disorder in order to choose and employ the form of *treatment* appropriate for that sleep disorder. This principle applies to children with developmental disorders with no less force than to other children with disturbed sleep. There is, however, a need for more careful research on the effectiveness of the various types of treatment specifically in children with a developmental disorder.

As described earlier (Chapters 4 and 7), it has been demonstrated that behavioural methods of treatment for even severe and long-standing sleeplessness problems can be very effective in children with difficult behaviour, and possibly other complications. However, success is not invariable and there is much to be discovered about the causes of treatment failures. Possibilities for investigation include mistaken diagnosis, wrong choice of treatment, inadequate implementation of the treatment programme (*e.g.* from lack of parental conviction or consistency, or from inadequate therapist guidance), or non-acceptance of the procedure by the child. A possible example of this last point, requiring reinforcement or modification of the approach, is the intolerance of the changes of routine required by the treatment programme in children with autism.

The many other aspects of treatment that call for informed research include the place of various measures used for the relief of sleep-related breathing problems and their consequences in the many conditions of which they are a part, and the contentious issue of the role of melatonin in the management of sleep–wake cycle disorders in particular. Systematic investigation of the efficacy of *preventive measures* should also be emphasized. Overall, the field is replete with research possibilities of both practical importance and theoretical interest.

REFERENCES

Brouillette, R.T., Waters, K.A., Morielli, A. (2000) 'Establishing and running a pediatric sleep laboratory.' *In:* Loughlin, G.M., Carroll, J.L., Marcus, C.L. (Eds.) *Sleep and Breathing in Children: A Developmental Approach.* New York: Marcel Dekker, pp. 767–781.

Flint, J. (1996) 'Behavioural phenotypes: Window onto the biology of behaviour.' *Journal of Child Psychology and Psychiatry,* **37**, 355–367. *(Annotation.)*

Hunt, A., Stores, G. (1994) 'Sleep disorder and epilepsy in children with tuberous sclerosis: a questionnaire-based study.' *Developmental Medicine and Child Neurology,* **36**, 108–115.

Marcus, C.L. (2000) 'Obstructive sleep apnea: Differences between children and adults.' *Sleep*, **23**, S140–S141.

Montgomery, P., Stores, G. (2000) 'Behavioural treatment of severe sleep disorders in children with learning disability (mental retardation): a randomised controlled trial of treatment delivery methods.' *Journal of Sleep Research*, **9**, Suppl. 1, S135. *(Abstract.)*

Sateia, M.D., Owens, J., Dube, C., Goldberg, G. (2000) 'Advancement in sleep medicine education.' *Sleep*, **23**, 1021–1023.

Stores, G. (2001) *A Clinical Guide to Sleep Disorders in Children and Adolescents.* Cambridge: Cambridge University Press.

—— Wiggs, L. (1998) 'Clinical services for sleep disorders.' *Archives of Disease in Childhood*, **79**, 495–497.

Tarrasenko, L., Zamora, M., Pardey, J. (2001) 'Neural network analysis of sleep disorders.' *In:* Dybowski, R., Gant, V. (Eds.) *Clinical Applications of Artificial Neural Networks.* Cambridge: Cambridge University Press. *(In press)*

Wiggs, L., Stores, G. (1996) 'Sleep problems in children with severe intellectual disabilities: What help is being provided?' *Journal of Applied Research in Intellectual Disabilities*, **9**, 160–165.

—— —— (2000) 'Sleep disorders in children and adolescents with autistic spectrum disorders.' *Journal of Sleep Research*, **9**, Suppl. 1, S209. *(Abstract.)*

INDEX

Suicidal ideation, 162
Suprachiasmatic nucleus (SCN), 12, 107–108
    in Prader–Willi syndrome, 62
Surgical management
    in cerebral palsy, 110, 113
    in Down syndrome, 57, 70
    in mucopolysaccharidoses, 77
    see also Adenotonsillectomy
Syringobulbia, 126
Syringomyelia, 126

T
Teachers, 51
Teeth grinding, 39
Teething, 26
Theophylline, 70, 143, 144, 149
Tics, in Tourette syndrome, 197
Tidal volume, 140
Tinnitus, 129–130
Tiredness
    physical, 30
    sleepy, 30
Tobacco (nicotine) consumption, 28, 32, 166
Tonsillectomy, *see* Adenotonsillectomy
Tonsils, enlarged, 33, 34, 148–149
Topiramate, 109
Tourette syndrome, 90, 197
Toxic states, 36
Tracheomalacia, 67
Tracheostomy
    in cerebral palsy, 110, 113
    in craniofacial anomalies, 66, 70
    in mucopolysaccharidoses, 77
    in neuromuscular diseases, 118
    in Prader–Willi syndrome, 62
Training, professional, 3, 203, 204–205, *206*
Transitional sleep, 11
Trauma, 169–173
    defining, 169–170
    see also Stress
Trazodone, 158
Treacher–Collins syndrome (TCS), 64, *65*, 67–68, *69*
Treatment of sleep disorders, 22–23, 208
    see also Behavioural treatments; Medication;
        Surgical management; *other specific treat-
        ments*
Tricyclic antidepressants, 42, 116–117, 158

Trisomy 21, *see* Down syndrome
Tryptophan, 185
TSC genes, 79
Tuberous sclerosis complex (TSC), 79–82, 103, 207
    management aspects, 80–81
    sleep problems and aetiological factors, 79–80

U
Uncomfortable conditions, 147–148
Upper airway hypotonia, 111–112
Upper airway obstruction (UAO), 4, 33–35
    in craniofacial anomalies, 64–66, 67–69
    in Down syndrome, 55, 66–67
    medical conditions causing, 149
    in mucopolysaccharidoses, 75
    see also Obstructive sleep apnoea; Sleep-dis-
        ordered breathing
Upper airways resistance syndrome (UARS), 33–34
Uvulopalatopharyngoplasty, 70

V
Valproate, sodium, 101
Ventilatory control dysfunction, 65–66, 112, *115*
Ventilatory support, mechanical, 117–118
Video recordings, 21
Violence, sleep-related, 199
Visual impairment, 32, 120–125
    aetiological factors, 123
    management issues, 123–124
    research needs, 124
    sleep problems, 120–122
    see also Blindness
Vitamin B_{12}, 124

W
Wakefulness, 10
Waking problems, *see* Early morning waking;
        Night-waking problems
War-related stress, 171
Werdnig–Hoffmann disease (SMA type I), 113, *117*
Wheezing, 137, 138
Williams syndrome, 32, 89–90
Wind-down period, 26
Worry, 28

Z
Zeitgeber, 12

PROPERTY OF

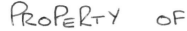
MANSFIELD DISTRICT **PCT NHS**
CHILD HEALTH DEPT.
COMMUNITY HOSPITAL
STOCKWELL GATE
MANSFIELD
NOTTS. NG18 5QJ